Lecture Notes in Computer Science 8462

Commenced Publication in 197
Founding and Former Series E
Gerhard Goos, Juris Hartmanis,

T0183212

Anna Spagnolli   Luca Chittaro
Luciano Gamberini (Eds.)

Persuasive Technology

9th International Conference, PERSUASIVE 2014
Padua, Italy, May 21-23, 2014
Proceedings

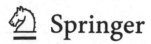 Springer

Volume Editors

Anna Spagnolli
Luciano Gamberini
Università degli Studi di Padova
Dipartimento di Psicologia Generale
via Venezia, 8, 35131 Padova, Italy
E-mail: {anna.spagnolli, luciano.gamberini}@unipd.it

Luca Chittaro
Università di Udine
Dipartimento di Matematica ed Informatica
via delle Scienze, 206, 33100 Udine, Italy
E-mail: luca.chittaro@uniud.it

ISSN 0302-9743   e-ISSN 1611-3349
ISBN 978-3-319-07126-8 e-ISBN 978-3-319-07127-5
DOI 10.1007/978-3-319-07127-5
Springer Cham Heidelberg New York Dordrecht London

Library of Congress Control Number: 2014938108

LNCS Sublibrary: SL 3 – Information Systems and Application, incl. Internet/Web and HCI

Typesetting: Camera-ready by author, data conversion by Scientific Publishing Services, Chennai, India

Printed on acid-free paper

Springer is part of Springer Science+Business Media (www.springer.com)

Preface

Persuasive Technology is an interdisciplinary research field that focuses on the design and development of technologies aimed at changing users' attitudes or behaviors through persuasion and social influence, but not through coercion or deception. PERSUASIVE, the International Conference on Persuasive Technology, is the leading venue to meet and discuss the latest theories and applications of persuasive technology in a growing number of domains, ranging from personal health and safety to corporate and governmental campaigns. Previous PERSUASIVE conferences were held at Eindhoven, Stanford, Oulu, Copenhagen, Claremont, Columbus, Linkoping, and Sydney.

This volume collects the papers presented at the ninth edition of the conference (PERSUASIVE 2014) that took place in Padua, Italy, during May 21-23, 2014. PERSUASIVE 2014 was chaired by Luciano Gamberini and Anna Spagnolli (HTLab and Human Inspired Technologies Research Centre – HIT, University of Padova, Italy), and by Luca Chittaro (Human-Computer Interaction Lab, University of Udine, Italy) and benefited from the collaboration of 40 scholars composing the scientific committee. In addition to the themes of persuasive technology dealt with in the previous editions of the conference, this edtion highlighted a special theme, i.e., persuasive, motivating, empowering videogames. Adding game elements has become one of the most challenging and acclaimed strategies to turn applications of information and communication technology into systems that persuade, motivate, and empower users to take action. The program succeeded in building bridges between the persuasion and the videogames, serious games, and game-based learning communities by including nine papers on this topic.

The papers comprising this volume result from a thorough selection process. The 58 papers submitted to the conference were examined by at least three experts on the topics of the paper in a double-blind review process. Based on these evaluations, 36% of the submissions (21 papers) were accepted as long and 10% (6 papers) as short presentations in the conference program. All 27 accepted papers underwent a second round of revisions before being included in this volume. We would like to thank all the experts who carefully read the submissions and generously gave of their time to provide advice to the authors. We would also like to thank the authors, for the effort they made in this iterative revision process, which is more typical of journals rather than conferences.

In addition to the oral presentations included in this volume, the conference also featured a poster session, a demo session, and a doctoral consortium. This resulted in more than 50 further contributions, available in the adjunct proceedings published by University of Padua Press. PERSUASIVE 2014 also offered two international workshops, the Second International Workshop on Behavior Change Support Systems (BCSS) and the Workshop on

Persuasive Technologies in Challenging Contexts. All together, the conference brought together contributions from 19 countries in Asia, Europe, and North America.

The conference organization benefited from advice from prior organizers of Persuasive conferences, in particular Harri Oinas-Kukkonen, Magnus Bang, and Shlomo Berkovsky. It also benefited from the support of five sponsors, Dipartimento di Psicologia Generale, Università degli Studi di Padova, Air France Global Meetings, Noldus, and DataBiz and from the collaboration with Comune di Padova.

It is our hope that this volume will contribute to increasing awareness of the many ways in which persuasive technology can help change our behavior to better address societal challenges, and illustrate how the field is expanding in breadth as well as depth to meet such challenges.

May 2014   Anna Spagnolli
                                                                  Luca Chittaro
                                                              Luciano Gamberini

Organization

Scientific Committee

Alexander Felfernig	Graz University of Technology, Austria
Alessio Malizia	Brunel University, UK
Anna Spagnolli	University of Padua, Italy
Anthony Jameson	German Research Center for Artificial Intelligence, Germany
B.J. Fogg	Stanford University, California, USA
Carlo Galimberti	Catholic University of Milan, Italy
Cees Midden	Eindhoven University of Technology, The Netherlands
Cheryl Campanella Bracken	Cleveland State University, Ohio, USA
Curtis P. Haugtvedt	Ohio State University, Ohio, USA
Fahri Yetim	University of Oulu, Finland
Floriana Grasso	University of Liverpool, UK
Giulio Jacucci	Helsinki Institute for Information Technology, Finland
Harri Oinas-Kukkonen	Oulu University, Finland
Hanna Schraffenberger	LIACS, Leiden University, The Netherlands
Ian Bogost	Georgia Institute of Technology, Georgia, USA
Jaap Ham	Eindhoven University of Technology, The Netherlands
Jang-Han Lee	Chung-Ang University, Korea
Jill Freyne	CSIRO, Australia
Jilles Smids	Eindhoven University of Technology, The Netherlands
Johan Åberg	Linköping University, Sweden
Judith Masthoff	University of Aberdeen, UK
Julita Vassileva	University of Saskatchewan, Canada
Kyung-Hyan Angie Yoo	William Paterson University, New Jersey, USA
Luca Chittaro	University of Udine, Italy
Luciano Gamberini	University of Padua, Italy
Magnus Bang	Linkoping University, Sweden
Maurity Kaptein	Eindhoven University of Technology, The Netherlands
Manfred Tscheligi	ICT&S Center, University of Salzburg, Austria
Mark Gilzenrat	CNN Digital, Georgia, USA
Nadja Decarolis	Università degli Studi di Bari, Italy
Oliviero Stock	FBK-IRST, Italy

Peter de Vries	University of Twente, The Netherlands
Rilla Khaled	IT University of Copenhagen, Denmark
Robert Biddle	Carleton University, Canada
Samir Chatterjee	Claremont Graduate University, California, USA
Sarvnaz Karimi	CSIRO, Australia
Sebastian Deterding	Rochester Institute of Technology, NY, USA
Shlomo Berkovsky	National ICT, Australia
Sriram Iyengar	The University of Texas, Texas, USA
Stephen Intille	MIT, Massachusetts, USA
Timothy Bickmore	Northeastern University, Massachusetts, USA
Tom MacTavish	Illinois Institute of Technology, Illinois, USA
Ulrike Gretzel	University of Wollongong, Australia

Additional Reviewers

Pippin Barr	University of Malta, Malta
Jiri Baum	Sabik Software Solutions, Australia
Brock R. Dubbels	McMaster University, Hamilton, Canada
Marco Guerini	Trento RISE, Trento, Italy
Antti Jylhä	University of Helsinki, Finland
Sitwat Langrial	University of Oulu, Finland
Sanjoy Moulik	University of California, Irvine
Rita Orji	University of Saskatchewan, Canada
Andreas Riener	Johannes Kepler University, Linz, Austria
Peter Ruijten	Eindhoven University of Technology, The Netherlands
Agnis Stibe	University of Oulu, Finland
Frank Verberne	Eindhoven University of Technology, The Netherlands

Organizing Committee

Luciano Gamberini	HTLab, University of Padua (General Chair)
Anna Spagnolli	University of Padua (Organizing Chair)
Luca Chittaro	University of Udine (Program Chair)

Sponsorships and Collaborations

Dipartimento di Psicologia Generale 'Vittorio Benussi'

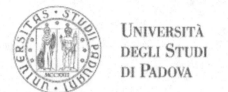

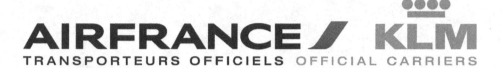

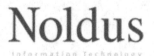

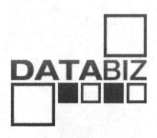

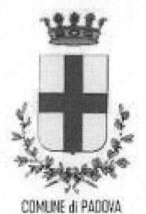

Table of Contents

Covert Persuasive Technologies: Bringing Subliminal Cues to Human-Computer Interaction

Oswald Barral[1], Gabor Aranyi[2], Sid Kouider[3], Alan Lindsay[2], Hielke Prins[3], Imtiaj Ahmed[1], Giulio Jacucci[1], Paolo Negri[4], Luciano Gamberini[4], David Pizzi[2], and Marc Cavazza[2]

[1] Helsinki Institute for Information Technology (HIIT), Department of Computer Science, University of Helsinki, Finland
{barralme,imtiaj.ahmed,giulio.jacucci}@helsinki.fi
[2] School of Computing, Teesside University, UK
{g.aranyi,a.lindsay,d.pizzi,m.o.cavazza}@tees.ac.uk
[3] Laboratoire de Sciences Cognitives et Psycholinguistique (LSCP), École Normale Supérieure, France
{sid.kouider,hielke.prins}@ens.fr
[4] Department of General Psychology, University of Padova, Italy
{paolo.negri,luciano.gamberini}@unipd.it

Abstract. The capability of machines to covertly persuade humans is both exciting and ethically concerning. In the present study we aim to bring subliminal masked stimulus paradigms to realistic environments, through Virtual Environments. The goal is to test if such paradigms are applicable to realistic setups while identifying the major challenges when doing so. We designed a study in which the user performed a realistic selection task in a virtual kitchen. For trials below one-second reaction time, we report significant effect of subliminal cues on the selection behavior. We conclude the study with a discussion of the challenges of bringing subliminal cueing paradigms to realistic HCI setups. Ethical concerns when designing covertly persuasive systems are discussed as well.

Keywords: Covert persuasion·subliminal cueing·masked cues.

1 Introduction

Psychologists and neuroscientists have been studying for long the possibility to impact users' behavior in an unobservable manner, by means of subliminal cues. Nevertheless, studies on the field have historically been done in an extremely controlled manner, using non-realistic interfaces. In the present study we aim to bring such subliminal cueing paradigms into more realistic human-computer interaction setups using naturalistic interfaces, while identifying the major challenges of doing so. We will first quickly review the background on subliminal cueing, followed by the definition of covert persuasive technologies, closely related to this work. At the end of this introduction we will give an overview of the system and study designed.

A. Spagnolli et al. (Eds.): PERSUASIVE 2014, LNCS 8462, pp. 1–12, 2014.
© Springer International Publishing Switzerland 2014

1.1   Subliminal Priming

Since subliminal stimulation may covertly influence behavior without entering consciousness, unconscious information processing represents one of the most long-standing topics in many disciplines. As a matter of fact, early seminal experiments on subliminal perception date back to the late nineteenth century, and the scientific literature on these phenomena is vast. In 1898, Sidis performed a basic experiment in which participants were shown cards containing either a letter or a digit. The distance between participants and card was such that they reported they did not see anything more meaningful than a blurred spot. Nonetheless, when they performed a forced-choice task, participants were able to guess above the chance level if the grapheme was a letter or a digit [1]. These results have been interpreted as the proof of subliminal perception.

Since then, scientists have been adopting several psychophysical methods that allow a systematic study of human mental activity under subliminal stimulation. Indeed, there are a number of conditions under which the visual perception can be systematically manipulated to obtain unconscious perception: binocular rivalry [2,3], visual masking [4], visual crowding [5,6,7,8,9], motion-induced blindness [10], inattentional blindness [11,12], change blindness [13,14], and attentional blink [15].

Within all of these subliminal techniques, visual masking has been applied over a variety of search fields, such as psycholinguistics [16], emotions [17,18], social perception and stereotypes [19,20], as well as persuasion through the application of masking to subliminal priming [21] and cueing paradigms. The subliminal priming consists in a facilitatory effect in terms of faster reaction times and/or greater accuracy in a task performed on a target stimulus when the latter is perceptually or semantically congruent to the subliminal preceding stimulus (i.e., the prime). The subliminal cueing through masked stimulus consists of biasing the user selection behavior between different alternatives, and is the specific technique applied by the present study.

1.2   Covert Persuasion

The main goal in the design and implementation of persuasive technologies is to give machines the ability to influence and/or change users' behavior. As defined by B. J. Fogg [22], "Persuasive technology is fundamentally about learning to automate behavior change." When persuasion is achieved without awareness, it is considered *covert persuasion*. Hogan and Speakman [23] defined this concept in their book as "to persuade others with such skill that your efforts are literally not observable." By bringing together these two definitions, the concept of *covert persuasive technology* can be defined as the aim to automate users' behavior change in an unobservable manner. Extensive work has addressed human-to-human covert persuasion [23], machine-to-human covert persuasion being still a young field of study. Previous work in the field comprises subconscious persuasion for energy-consumption awareness [24] and modification of drivers' behavior through subliminal tactile feedback [25]. The use of subliminal stimuli in human-computer interaction settings can therefore be included in this field, as the designed system aims to influence users' behavior in an unobservable manner. In a virtual environment, covert persuasion can prevent the overload of users when a large amount of data needs to be explored or remembered [26,27]. Examples of research include subliminal cueing in support of online help in a desk-top-computer text editing task application [28], just-in-time memory support using subliminal cues delivered in a head-mounted display [27], application in a tutoring system [29], and aid for visual search tasks [30,31].

1.3   Study Overview

In the present study we want to detect and face the challenges of influencing users' behavior through subliminal cues in a realistic task. Virtual environments allow the researcher to simulate realistic environments and therefore to design realistic, task-based studies. The objective of the present study is to evaluate subliminal cueing in an interactive application, simulating a task, while investigating the challenges of apply-ing subliminal cueing as covert persuasion. Specifically, it is studied whether subli-minal priming is a suitable mechanism to covertly persuade participants and bias their selection behavior. A simplified virtual kitchen was implemented using the game engine Unity3D. The kitchen consisted of a fridge and a table. The virtual environment was designed in order to be naturalistic and familiar to the user. To enhance the user engagement with the scenario, multiple different objects populated both the fridge and the table (see Figure 1). Covert persuasion in a virtual scene has proved to be especialy interesting for applications such as virtual product experience [32] or in domains such as serious gaming for wellbeing. A direct application of covertly persuading users in such a setting is, for instance, to influence uers' selection-decision towards the healthiest item.

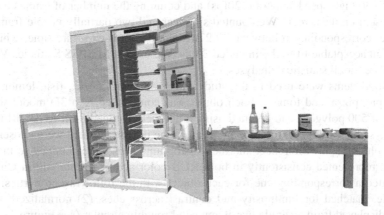

Fig. 1. Virtual kitchen scene populated with multiple objects

We designed a study based on a series of trials of forced-choice selection task be-tween two objects. Additionally, and according to standards in this research field [33], in order to determine if the cueing effect is genuinely subliminal, the subjects were required to perform a subsequent visibility test consisting of a forced-choice discrimi-nation task on the masked stimulus. We first aim to show that there is a genuine persuasive effect, that is, the frequency in which subliminally cued items are selected is higher than expected by chance. Then we discuss the implication of results, directions for future work as well as ethical issues in covert persuasive technologies.

2   Method

2.1   Participants

Participation was voluntary and participants were informed that they could withdraw from the experiment at any time. Informed consent was collected prior to participation, after the goals of the study and the procedure were outlined to them. Nine females and seven males participated in the experiment. The overall mean age was of 36.69 years (SD = 8.14). A mean of 7 hours (SD = 2.52) was assessed when self-reporting the duration of computer use per day. The participants were academic and administrative staff at Teesside University and were rewarded with the equivalent of $30 vouchers.

2.2   Apparatus

The experimental software was implemented in Unity3D (version 4.0.1f2) and was run on a Dell Precision T7600 computer (CPU: Intel Xeon E5-2609 2.40GHz; 32GB RAM; GPU: NVidia GeForce GTX 680; OS: MS Windows 7 Enterprise 64-bit) with a 24-inch' Dell U2412M monitor (60Hz refresh rate, 1920x1200 resolution). The timing of cue presentation was checked by recording presentations with a Panasonic Lumix TZ30 high-speed camera (220fps) and counting the number of frames the cues were present on the screen. We counted six clear and two partially visible frames for each cue, corresponding to between 27.27ms and 36.36ms exposure time, which we deemed an acceptable fit to the intended 33ms. We used IBM SPSS Statistics Version 20 software for all statistical analyses.

Ten food items were used in the study: apple, burger, cheese, fish, lemon, pear, pepper, pie, pizza, and tomato. Each object was constructed as a 3D model with an average of 500 polygons and detailed using a uniquely mapped 8-bit RGB diffuse and 8-bit grayscale specular texture. Colors used in the diffuse textures were chosen from real-life photographic reference, and their histogram levels were clamped so that they could be represented consistently in both RGB color and grayscale within Unity3D. We created a corresponding cue for each object with the following properties: (1) in grayscale, matched for luminosity and contrast across cues, (2) normalized in size, and (3) displayed from an angle that it appeared roughly circular (see Figure 2). These properties allowed for using the same masks for each target object, thereby avoiding possible confounds attributable to mask properties. The masks were created in Adobe Photoshop CS6 by overlaying the deconstructed, contrast-equalized images of the cues after using a Perlin noise mask for each cue (see Figure 3).

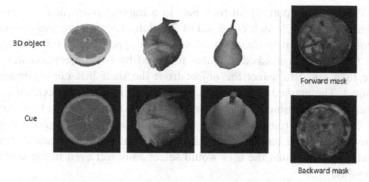

Fig. 2. Examples of 3D items, their corresponding cueing images, and masks. The cues are in grayscale, normalized for contrast and size, and roughly circular to allow for using the same masks. The 3D objects are matched in size and rotated for presentation only.

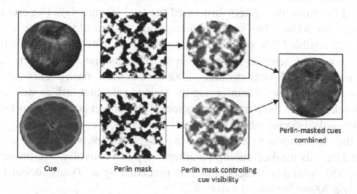

Fig. 3. Process of creation of masks, for two cue images. First, a separate Perlin mask is used to control the alpha channel of each cue. Then, these are combined in order to produce the masks. The masks used in the experiment were created including cues and separate Perlin masks from four objects each.

2.3 Design and Procedure

In order to study participants' selection behavior, a forced-choice selection task was designed. The full kitchen scene was presented to the users at the beginning of each of the three phases of the experiment. Then the camera zoomed in, presenting a front view of the empty fridge. The participants were then shown two different objects on the shelves of the refrigerator. They were asked to pick one of the items and to drag it to an adjacent table. In each trial, preceding the presentation of the objects on the shelves, a masked object was shown, while one of the two objects was subliminally cued. The participants were then asked to pick the item corresponding to the masked object. All of the participants took part in the same condition. Participants worked individually in a computer lab. The three successive phases involved in the experiment are explained below.

Training Phase. Every participant took part in a training phase at the beginning of the experimental session, which consisted of 30 trials. The training was carried out in order to ensure that the participants understood the experimental task. In each trial, they were first shown a masked stimulus followed by two objects on the shelves. They were then asked to select the object from the shelf that corresponded to the masked object. The masked object was clearly visible in eighty percent of the trials. In this case, the object stimulus was shown for 500ms followed by a backward mask shown for 200ms. In the remaining twenty percent of the trials no object stimulus was shown, only forward and backward masks were presented (200ms each). These trials were included to ensure that the user would select an object even in the absence of a visible stimulus.

Masked-cueing Phase. As in the training phase, at the beginning of each trial, the participant was presented the empty refrigerator and a white cross in the cueing area. The instructions "click on the crosshair when ready" were shown. When the participant clicked the cross, the system structured the trial (Figure 4a). The cross remained on the screen for 300ms. The system selected one of the following two conditions to trigger: clearly-visible (10% of trials) or short-exposure (90% of trials). If the clearly-visible condition was selected to be triggered, stimulus presentation was the same as in the training phase (500ms stimulus, 200ms backward mask). This condition was included with the purpose of reinforcing the trained selection task as well as to subsequently check whether the participants selected the object according to the cued stimulus. The masked-cueing phase comprised mainly short-exposure trials.

When the short-exposure condition was triggered, the subliminal stimulus was shown for 33ms, as masked-cueing paradigms typically involve cue presentation below 50ms [18]. Stimulus presentation was preceded by a 200ms forward mask and followed by a 200ms backward mask.

For each trial in both clearly-visible and short-exposure conditions, the system randomly selected the following parameters: the object to be cued (one out of ten), the object to be shown together with the cued object (one out of the nine remaining objects) and the position of both objects on the shelves (upper or lower shelf, one out of two possible combinations). The target object and the other object (filler) appeared on the shelves in the refrigerator after cue presentation, with the on-screen instructions "select an item and drag it to the table." After the participant dragged an object to the table, the trial ended and the next trial started (see Figure 5). The masked-cueing phase lasted until at least 100 trials in the short-exposure condition were logged.

Visibility Phase. This phase was included at the end of the experiment, after the masked-cueing phase, in order to avoid underestimating visibility due to familiarity with the presentation conditions [33]. Participants were shown subliminal cues in the same way as in the masked-cue condition. They were presented each object 6 times, for a total of 60 trials. Selection of objects and conditions was randomized. After one-second-long delay of the cue presentation [34], the name of an item from the complete list of items was presented on the screen with a question mark (e.g., "pear?").

The name was randomly selected to be congruent with the cued object (50% chance). The participants were required to assess by clicking on the corresponding "yes" or "no" boxes. The boxes were placed at the same positions as the objects in the masked-cueing phase.

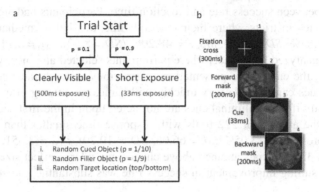

Fig. 4. Structuring of experimental trials in the masked-cueing phase (a), and cue presentation in the short-exposure trials (b)

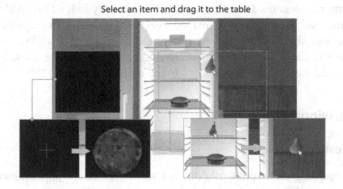

Fig. 5. Screen-layout of the training and experimental trials. The background image is a screen-shot taken as a participant moves an object to the table. Each trial begins with a request for the user to click the crosshair in the cueing area, which triggers a cue presentation (blue frame). The user is then asked to select an item from the refrigerator and drag it to the table (orange frame).

3   Results

Participants were explicitly instructed to select objects from the refrigerator that were congruent with the cued images. The success rate on the clearly visible trials was 100% for 12 participants and between 94% and 97% for the remaining four partici-pants, which indicates that they carried out the selection task according to the instruc-tions in the masked-cueing phase. A one-sample *t*-test concluded that the average success rate (M = 53.01%, SD = 7.60) was not significantly different from expected by chance (50%), $t_{(15)} = 1.59$, $p = .13$, $r = .38$ (medium[1]). Success rate was significantly non-normally distributed, $D_{(16)} = .30$, $p < .001$; and the distribution had a significant positive skew ($z = 2.28$), which indicates a build-up of low scores.

We performed a median split on the basis of reaction time by subjects to explore the relationship between success rate and reaction time. Participants had significantly higher success rates in trials where their reaction time was below median reaction time: $M_{below} = 57.83\%$ ($SD = 8.43$), $M_{above} = 48.20\%$ ($SD = 8.52$), $t_{(15)} = 5.14$, $p < .001$. Furthermore we analyzed those trials where participants selected an object within one second following the end of cue presentation, as previous research indicates that effect of masked cues can degrade very quickly with time, and cueing effects can decrease significantly if the subliminal cues are not acted upon in the first second or so [33,35,36]. For the amount of 222 trials with response time smaller than 1 second, success rate improved by 13.05% ($M = 66.06$, $SD = 19.70$), $t_{(13)} = 3.051$, $p = .009$, which represents 32% of trials attained above chance and a large effect size ($r = .65$). Therefore, the resulting improvement in success rate was substantial and statistically significant.

A genuinely subliminal cueing effect cannot be asserted without assessing the visibility of cues. We included 60 visibility trials in the experimental protocol to assess the objective visibility of masked cues. Using signal-detection theory [37], the hit rate and false-alarm rate was used to calculate the d' sensitivity index [38]. Although several participants had close to zero d' and the average d' was low in magnitude, objective visibility was significantly non-zero: average $d' = .45$ ($SD = .38$), $t_{(15)} = 4.69$, $p < .001$. These findings suggest that participants may have seen the cues, but only in a few trials, while they did not see the cues in the majority of trials.

4   Discussion

4.1   Implication of Results

The results regarding the overall data did not show significant improvement in success rate respect to chance level. Nevertheless, as previous literature suggests that the cueing effect might degrade quickly after the subliminal presentation [33,35,36], reaction time was used to analyze in depth the results. When considering only within one-second reaction time trials though, the success rate was significantly above chance level, and the observed effect size was large. Therefore, we believe that one of the major challenges when designing subliminal cueing based systems is the minimization of reaction time.

The fact of participants having seen few cues could be seen as an explanation for the recorded subliminal cueing effect on selection behavior. Nevertheless, the nearly perfect (99%) mean success rate on the clearly-visible trials, as opposed to the substantially lower (55%) mean success rate on short-exposure cueing trials, together with the moderate correlation between d' and success rate, indicate that objective

---

[1] Cohen's effect-size conventions are used: .10 – small, .30 – medium, .50 – large [39].

visibility alone cannot account for participants' performance. On the other side, it is important to recall that the participants were asked to look at a specific area of the screen in order to identify the subliminally cued object. Therefore, in more natural conditions, it is expected that the cues would mostly go unobserved. However, further studies should consider collecting subjective measures of visibility as well.

The present study goes further in the application of covert persuasive technologies to realistic human-computer interaction settings. Subliminal cueing can impact a realistic task in a virtual environment by guiding the user in a simulated operation of the product and, for instance, preventing overload of the user. A direct health-oriented application can be implemented exploiting the same system as the one of the present study. In the scenario, the user would be asked to select food items in order to prepare a meal. The system would systematically present subliminal cues related to the healthiest items, biasing the user's decision towards a healthiest meal.

4.2   Limitations and Directions for Future Work

The present work aimed to study the effects of subliminal cueing on a realistic task in a realistic environment. Virtual Reality implemented in a powerful game engine allowed the task specification to be very much realistic. Nevertheless, we consider the interaction with the system still far from being lifelike, as the setup was based on a standard desktop screen-mouse interaction. For instance, the participants were asked to click on a white cross in order to trigger the beginning of each trial. When aiming to more naturalistic tasks, these sorts of conditions are a must-avoid. The results need therefore to be replicated especially under more naturalistic setups before being able to draw final conclusions regarding the application of subliminal priming to realistic environments. Additionally, even though two almost equal sized gender groups participated in the study, each group was not large enough for statistical analysis of gender effect on subliminal cues. Nevertheless, when replicating the results, we encourage studying such effect, as gender difference in perception of subliminal stimuli has previously been reported [40].

Eye tracking technology is getting widely spread among the human-computer interaction community, while both its intrusiveness and economical cost decrease. The presentation of the subliminal stimuli at the exact gaze-location point is one of the possible applications of such technology, in order to make the interaction more natural. Additionally, such devices can also help in the above-mentioned criticality of reaction time. Eye tracking can be used to present the subliminal stimuli in the users' field of view, just before they perform an action, which, most probably, is going to decrease substantially the reaction time. Therefore, we suggest future research to address the integration of eye tracking technologies in such systems.

Gesture tracking as well as immersive displays such as large screens would also lead to more realistic interaction paradigms. Nevertheless, when including more degrees of freedom in the interaction with the system, the researcher will face several additional challenges when aiming to apply subliminal cueing paradigms. The combination of realistic human-computer interaction settings with eye tracking, gesture tracking and immersive displays need to be further explored to face the challenge of bringing covert perception technologies through subliminal cueing to more realistic and natural setups. An extended discussion around these can be found in Aranyi et al. publication [41].

4.3   Ethics

Besides technical challenges, a major challenge when in the field of persuasive technologies, especially in the domain of covert persuasion, is the definition and preservation of ethical standards. Even though some researchers have addressed the matter [42,43,44], surprisingly, ethical concerns in the field have not had a large impact so far [45]. The present study shows that it is possible to influence users' behavior by subconscious cognitive processes, which raises a variety of ethical issues: What is the final goal of covertly influencing users' behavior? Is users' subliminal persuasion strictly on behalf of the final users (e.g., to decrease their cognitive load)? Should the users be aware of the system using subliminal cueing paradigms? Recently, Smids discussed voluntariness of behavioral changes as being a mainstay of ethical standards in the domain of persuasive technologies [43]. Even though subliminal persuasion is commonly associated with manipulation, coercion or deceit, it is by no means the sort of persuasion approached by the present research. This study addresses covert persuasion as a mechanism to facilitate users' interaction within a human-computer interaction setting. We strongly believe that users always need to be aware of the persuasion techniques employed by such systems. Consequently, subliminal information cannot influence behavior in a way that is inconsistent with the participants' goals and intentions. In this way, covert persuasion is then used as a mechanism to supply users with extra information to help them in a task, rather than subliminally persuade them to adopt unwanted behaviors or to carry out unsolicited actions.

References

1. Sidis, B.: The psychology of suggestion. D. Appleton, New York (1898)
2. Fox, R., Herrmann, J.: Stochastic properties of binocular rivalry alternations. Perception & Psychophysics 2, 432–436 (1967)
3. Almeida, J., Mahon, B.Z., Nakayama, K., Caramazza, A.: Unconscious processing dissociates along categorical lines. Proceedings of the National Academy of Sciences of the United States of America 105, 15214–15218 (2008)
4. Breitmeyer, B.G., Ganz, L.: Implications of sustained and transient channels for theories of visual pattern masking, saccadic suppression, and information processing. Psychological Review 83, 1–36 (1976)
5. Bouma, H.: Interaction effects in parafoveal letter recognition. Nature 226, 177–178 (1970)
6. Levi, D.M.: Crowding–an essential bottleneck for object recognition: a mini-review. Vision Research 48, 635–654 (2008)
7. Pelli, D.G., Tillman, K.A.: The uncrowded window of object recognition. Nature Neuroscience 11, 1129–1135 (2008)
8. Whitney, D., Levi, D.M.: Visual crowding: a fundamental limit on conscious perception and object recognition. Trends in Cognitive Sciences 15, 160–168 (2011)

9. Kouider, S., Berthet, V., Faivre, N.: Preference is biased by crowded facial expressions. Psychological Science 22(2), 184–189 (2011)
10. Bonneh, Y.S., Cooperman, A., Sagi, D.: Motion-induced blindness in normal observers. Nature 411, 798–801 (2001)
11. Neisser, U.: The control of information pickup in selective looking. In: Pick, A.D. (ed.) Perception and Its Development: A Tribute to Eleanor Gibson, pp. 201–219 (1979)
12. Simons, D.J., Chabris, C.F.: Gorillas in our midst: sustained inattentional blindness for dynamic events. Perception 28, 1059–1074 (1999)
13. Rensink, R.A., O'Regan, J.K., Clark, J.J.: To See or not to See: The Need for Attention to Perceive Changes in Scenes. Psychological Science 8, 368–373 (1997)
14. Simons, D.J., Levin, T.: Change blindness. Trends in Cognitive Sciences 1, 261–267 (1997)
15. Raymond, J.E., Shapiro, K.L., Arnell, K.M.: Temporary suppression of visual processing in an RSVP task: an attentional blink? Journal of Experimental Psychology: Human Perception and Performance 18, 849–860 (1992)
16. Humphreys, G.W., Evett, L.J., Taylor, D.E.: Automatic phonological priming in visual word recognition. Memory Cognition 10, 576–590 (1982)
17. Kunst-Wilson, W.R., Zajonc, R.B.: Affective discrimination of stimuli that cannot be recognized. Science 207, 557–558 (1980)
18. Faivre, N., Berthet, V., Kouider, S.: Nonconscious influences from emotional faces: a comparison of visual crowding, masking, and continuous flash suppression. Frontiers in Psychology 3, 129 (2012)
19. Bargh, J.A., Chen, M., Burrows, L.: Automaticity of social behavior: direct effects of trait construct and stereotype-activation on action. Journal of Personality and Social Psychology 71, 230–244 (1996)
20. Devine, P.G.: Stereotypes and prejudice: Their automatic and controlled components. Journal of Personality and Social Psychology 56, 5–18 (1989)
21. Strahan, E.J., Spencer, S.J., Zanna, M.P.: Subliminal priming and persuasion: Striking while the iron is hot. Journal of Experimental Social Psychology 38, 556–568 (2002)
22. Fogg, B.J.: A behavior model for persuasive design. In: Proceedings of the 4th International Conference on Persuasive Technology, vol. 40. ACM (2009)
23. Hogan, K., Speakman, J.: Covert Persuasion: Psychological Tactics and Tricks to Win the Game. Wiley (2006)
24. Ham, J., Midden, C., Beute, F.: Can ambient persuasive technology persuade unconsciously?: using subliminal feedback to influence energy consumption ratings of household appliances. In: Proceedings of the 4th International Conference on Persuasive Technology, vol. 29. ACM (2009)
25. Riener, A.: Subliminal persuasion and its potential for driver behavior adaptation. IEEE Transactions on Intelligent Transportation Systems 13(1), 71–80 (2012)
26. Riener, A., Kempter, G., Saari, T., Revett, K.: Subliminal Communication in Human-Computer Interaction. Advances in Human-Computer Interaction (2011)
27. DeVaul, R.W., Pentland, A., Corey, V.R.: The memory glasses: subliminal vs. overt memory support with imperfect information. In: Proceedings of the Seventh IEEE International Symposium on Wearable Computers (ISWC 2003), pp. 146–153 (2003)
28. Wallace, F.L., Flanery, J.M., Knezek, G.A.: The effect of subliminal help presentations on learning a text editor. Information Processing & Management 27(2), 211–218 (1991)
29. Chalfoun, P., Frasson, C.: Subliminal cues while teaching: HCI technique for enhanced learning. Advances in Human-Computer Interaction 2011, 2 (2011)

30. McNamara, A., Bailey, R., Grimm, C.: Improving search task performance using subtle gaze direction. In: Proceedings of the 5th Symposium on Applied Perception in Graphics and Visualization, pp. 51–56 (2008)

31. Bailey, R., McNamara, A., Sudarsanam, N., Grimm, C.: Subtle gaze direction. ACM Transactions on Graphics (TOG) 28(4), 100 (2009)

32. Pizzi, D., Kosunen, I., Viganó, C., Polli, A.M., Ahmed, I., Zanella, D., Cavazza, M., Kouider, S., Freeman, J., Gamberini, L., Jacucci, G.: Incorporating subliminal perception in synthetic environments. In: Proceedings of the 2012 ACM Conference on Ubiquitous Computing (UbiComp 2012), pp. 1139–1144. ACM (2012)

33. Kouider, S., Dehaene, S.: Levels of processing during non-conscious perception: a critical review of visual masking. Philosophical Transactions of the Royal Society B: Biological Sciences 362(1481), 857–875 (2007)

34. Vorberg, D., Mattler, U., Heinecke, A., Schmidt, T., Schwarzbach, J.: Different time courses for visual perception and action priming. Proceedings of the National Academy of Sciences 100(10), 6275–6280 (2003)

35. Dupoux, E., Gardelle, V.D., Kouider, S.: Subliminal speech perception and auditory streaming. Cognition 109(2), 267–273 (2008)

36. Greenwald, A.G., Draine, S.C., Abrams, R.L.: Three cognitive markers of unconscious semantic activation. Science 273(5282), 1699–1702 (1996)

37. Macmillan, N.A., Creelman, C.D.: Detection theory: a user's guide, 2nd edn. Lawrence Erlbaum Associates, Mahwah (2004)

38. Stanislaw, H., Todorov, N.: Calculation of signal detection theory measures. Behavior Research Methods, Instruments, & Computers 31(1), 137–149 (1999)

39. Cohen, J.: Statistical power analysis for the behavioral sciences. Lawrence Erlbaum Associates, London (1998)

40. Winkielman, P., Berridge, K.C., Wilbarger, J.L.: Unconscious affective reactions to masked happy versus angry faces influence consumption behavior and judgments of value. Personality and Social Psychology Bulletin 31(1), 121–135 (2005)

41. Aranyi, G., Kouider, S., Lindsay, A., Prins, H., Ahmed, I., Jacucci, G., Negri, P., Gamberini, L., Pizzi, D., Cavazza, M.: Subliminal cueing of selection behavior in a virtual environment. Presence: Teleoperators and Virtual Environments (in press, 2014)

42. Fogg, B.J.: Persuasive technology: using computers to change what we think and do. Ubiquity 5 (2002)

43. Smids, J.: The voluntariness of persuasive technology. In: Bang, M., Ragnemalm, E.L. (eds.) PERSUASIVE 2012. LNCS, vol. 7284, pp. 123–132. Springer, Heidelberg (2012)

44. Spahn, A.: And Lead Us (Not) into Persuasion...? Persuasive Technology and the Ethics of Communication. Science and Engineering Ethics 18(4), 633–650 (2012)

45. Torning, K., Oinas-Kukkonen, H.: Persuasive system design: state of the art and future directions. In: Proceedings of the 4th International Conference on Persuasive Technology, vol. 30. ACM (2009)

Designing a Mobile Persuasive Application to Encourage Reduction of Users' Exposure to Cell Phone RF Emissions

Stefano Burigat and Luca Chittaro

Human-Computer Interaction Lab
Department of Mathematics and Computer Science
University of Udine
via delle Scienze 206, 33100, Udine, Italy
{stefano.burigat,luca.chittaro}@uniud.it

Abstract. The International Agency for Research on Cancer classifies radiofrequency (RF) electromagnetic emissions of cell phones as possibly carcinogenic to humans [1] and suggests the use of hands-free devices such as earphones to reduce direct exposure of the brain to such emissions. In this paper, we present the design of a mobile application that exploits persuasive principles to encourage the use of earphones during cell phone calls. We propose different notifications and visualizations aimed at informing the user about her behavior with respect to earphone use and discuss the results of a user study that was aimed at investigating aspects such as understandability, emotional impact, and perceived usefulness of the proposed solutions. Results of the study are used to inform the design of the application. To the best of our knowledge, this is the first investigation of persuasive technologies applied to the reduction of user's exposure to cell phone RF emissions.

Keywords: mobile persuasion, mobile phones, behavior change, health, RF emissions, earphones.

1 Introduction

Today, the positive effects of the availability of cell phones on our quality of life are undeniable. However, there is also concern about the potential negative impact of cell phone use on health even if the subject is controversial. In particular, currently available research has not provided complete evidence of a relationship between cell phone use and adverse health effects. However, pending more definitive answers, in 2012 the International Agency for Research on Cancer (IARC) changed the classification of radiofrequency (RF) electromagnetic emissions of mobile phones from level 4 (probably non-carcinogenic) to level 2B (possibly carcinogenic) [1]. To reduce user's exposure to radiofrequency energy, organizations such as the IARC, the Federal Communication Commission, and the Food and Drug Administration recommend pragmatic measures such as using cell phones only for shorter conversations and using hands-free devices which place more distance between the phone and users' head.

A. Spagnolli et al. (Eds.): PERSUASIVE 2014, LNCS 8462, pp. 13–24, 2014.

In this work, we explore persuasive technology as a way to foster awareness on the possible risk of RF emissions and recommend the use of earphones. In recent years, persuasion principles have been applied to the design of mobile applications aimed at such diverse goals as increasing user's physical activity [2] or encouraging the use of green transportation [3]. In our case, the cell phone is the ideal medium through which to convey the considered persuasive message. First, the cell phone is directly related to the target behavior, hence making it possible to convey messages at the most appropriate time. Second, users can be often reminded that they are trying to change their behavior since they take cell phones with them anytime, anywhere. Third, the cell phone is typically a personal object, not shared with others, which makes it ideal as a way to convey health-related messages.

In the paper, we illustrate the design of BrainSaver, a mobile application for Android smartphones that monitors call behavior and gives feedback about how the user is behaving with respect to the use of earphones. To determine the most appropriate stimuli to help the user improve her behavior while avoiding to annoy her with invasive and unsuitable messages, we created different notifications and visualizations based on persuasive principles and evaluated their effect with a user study. The study focused on aspects such as understandability of the messages, emotional impact of the visualizations, and perceived usefulness of the notifications.

2   Related Work

Some persuasive mobile applications have recently used the phone screen wallpaper to provide mobile users with feedback about specific behaviors, mapping them into metaphoric visualizations. In UbiFit Garden [2], the user is persuaded to maintain a certain level of physical activity through a wallpaper that displays weekly progress in the form of flowers (representing different performed activities) and butterflies (representing achieved goals). UbiGreen [3] was instead designed to make the user more conscious about her consumption of CO_2 through a wallpaper that displays a tree or a polar scenario with bears and icebergs whose state depends on the level of CO_2 consumption. In EcoIsland [4], users are mapped into virtual characters on an island, and positive behaviors are rewarded by allowing users to decorate their environment, while negative behaviors lead to flooding of the island. While some studies suggest to use only positive reinforcement to prevent users to feel frustrated when they do not achieve their goals [5], the evaluation of EcoIsland and UbiGreen pointed out that people were encouraged also by the negative feedback received by seeing the negative consequences of their actions on the visualization.

Changes in the wallpaper have the dual function of giving the user feedback on her actions and to remind her that she is trying to change her behavior since often this is not her main thought [6]. The reminder function is crucial to convey the message at the most appropriate time, i.e., immediately preceding or following the triggering of the unwanted behavior [7]. The message must also be presented in the most aesthetically pleasing and less intrusive way [8]. Moreover, since the message pertains to the private life of an individual, it must be presented in an abstract way so that other people who happen to see the user's phone could not easily understand the meaning of the visualization.

Besides providing feedback through the wallpaper visualization, the mobile application should build trust in the recorded data from which the visualization is derived. This can be achieved both by showing the user a history of how she behaved in the past in a truthful but neutral way, and also by giving the possibility to change behavior data if the application cannot determine data correctness [3][5][7]. To keep the user involved, the application can include an element of fun [9] or aim at establishing an emotional bond with the visualization, e.g. using a virtual animal whose fate is determined by user's behavior [3][10].

3   Considered Visualizations

In line with [2,3,4], we propose to use the phone wallpaper as the main way to provide users with feedback about their behavior. More specifically, the wallpaper should be updated each time the user makes or receives a call, based on whether earphones were used or not. To investigate different design choices, we created two wallpapers based on two different subjects, a cartoon dog and a skeleton. The cartoon dog was inspired by the use of virtual animals in the persuasive technology literature as a way to establish an empathic connection with the user [3][10]. The other character was aimed at testing the effect of a less cartoony approach that did not directly show emotions. It was introduced because a first informal test of the cartoon dog indicated that male acceptability of a "cute" emotional virtual character as phone wallpaper could be low. Starting from an initial neutral image, we designed 10 negative variants and 10 positive variants of the basic image (Fig 1). In the skeleton wallpaper, negative variants show a brain in the skull that progressively becomes more visible by turning red (simulating heating), while the positive variants show more and more cloth accessories being added to the character. In the dog wallpaper, the animal becomes sadder in the negative variants while it becomes happier in the positive variants. To keep consistency with the skeleton design, and always remind the user of the goals of the application, the state of the brain is clearly shown in the negative levels of the dog wallpaper.

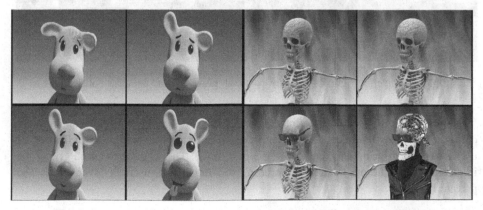

Fig. 1. A sample of images from the dog and skeleton wallpaper progressions

Unlike the previously mentioned mobile persuasive applications, which rely only on updating the wallpaper to convey their message, we also designed four alternative notifications to inform the user about the wallpaper change right after the end of a call without earphones (Fig. 2).

- The text-only notification (Fig. 2 upper left) displays a simple message reminding the user to use earphones the next time she makes or receives a call. The message uses an eye-catching red background which seems to be appropriate to convey important messages related to health [11].
- The pre-post-call notification (Fig. 2 upper right) displays the same message used in the text notification, and also shows a comparison of the state of the wallpaper before and after the last call. This notification provides a direct connection to the wallpaper, making users aware of how it changed as a consequence of the last call.
- The pie chart notification (Fig. 2 lower left) shows a graph summarizing the amount of calls with and without earphones in the last week. This notification allows the user to have a more global view of her behavior, which should encourage her to change it if considered negative.
- The bar chart notification (Fig. 2 lower right) shows a graph of the number of minutes users spent with and without earphones during calls for each day of the last week. In this way, the user can see trends in her behavior, which can serve as positive reinforcement if the data shows some progress over time.

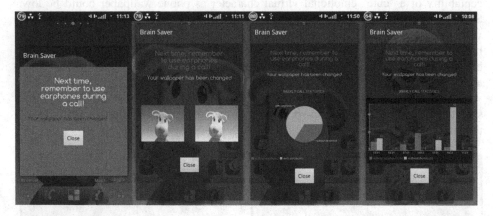

Fig. 2. From left to right, the text, pre-post-call, pie chart, and bar chart notifications

None of the proposed notifications (as well as the wallpapers) provides quantitative data about the last call (e.g., how long it lasted) but only a qualitative indication of user's behavior during such call (or in the past days). This is done to avoid giving the impression that the application is intruding too much into users' conversations and private life.

We designed the wallpapers and the notifications based on the following persuasive principles and techniques:

- *Reminder*: since users tend to forget that they are pursuing a specific objective, a message should be shown each time they should remember to use earphones. Also, the wallpaper should be changed to make the user aware of the goal even when she is doing other actions with the cell phone [6][12].
- *Feedback*: the user should be given immediate feedback about the action she has just performed. This is important to make the user immediately aware of the consequences of her actions and also to keep the user aware that the application is accurately monitoring her actions, thus increasing its credibility [4][7][13].
- *History/Trend*: the user should be offered the possibility to review the history and trends related to the last week of use of the application, to allow her to better monitor her behavior over time [12].
- *Positive/Negative reinforcement*: changing the wallpaper is a way to manage both positive and negative reinforcement with respect to user's actions, following an operant conditioning paradigm [7].
- *Empathy*: one of the two wallpapers uses a cartoon dog to exploit the possible empathic connection that could be established between the user and the virtual animal, as in [3][10].
- *Interoception*: visualizing the state of the brain in the negative sequences of wallpapers aims to give users a sense of the physiological condition of the body (interoception), making them perceive the possible changes in their brain due to the lack of earphones use. This idea was inspired by recent work on persuasion which is exploiting biomarkers (e.g. obtained through actual medical imaging of parts of the patient body [14]) to encourage health behavior change.
- *Fun and Engagement*: to maintain user's interest, the state of the virtual characters changes in a fun and engaging way [9].

4   User Study

To evaluate the effects of the considered visualizations on users, we carried out a lab study that investigated wallpaper preference and understandability, emotional impact of characters, and usability of post-call notifications. Wallpaper understandability was evaluated using card sorting: users were provided with paper cards depicting each wallpaper variant and were asked to separate negative variants from positive variants and then order all variants from the most negative to the most positive. Wallpaper preference, emotional impact of characters, and usability of post-call notifications were instead evaluated by showing users mock-up versions of the wallpapers and notifications on an actual mobile device and asking users to fill questionnaires for each considered aspect.

4.1   Participants

Sixteen users (9 male, 7 female) participated in the study. Their age ranged from 20 to 28 (M=26, SD=2.3). The average number of daily cell phone calls per user was 1.79 (SD=1.32), 50% of users made more than one call per day and 12.5% made more than 3 calls. Half of the users said they never use earphones during calls, mainly because they consider earphones uncomfortable or do not have them at hand when needed; 37.5% of the users claimed to use earphones only while driving or when needing their hands free.

4.2   Procedure

The study did not involve coercion or deceit and did respect applicable professional code of conduct. Users first filled a questionnaire to collect demographic as well as phone call statistics and earphone usage data. Participants were then briefed about the nature of the study. Then, they carried out the following 5 tasks:

- Grouping: users were handed two decks of paper cards depicting all wallpaper variants (one deck for each wallpaper) and asked to separate positively and negatively perceived variants. Half users started with the dog and half with the skeleton variants. The order of cards for each wallpaper was randomly generated for each user to avoid possible order effects. At the end of the task, users were asked to explain the criteria they used in separating variants. As a measure of user's success, we noted the number of errors users made compared to the correct grouping of variants.
- Ordering: users were handed two decks of cards (with a randomly generated order) and asked to order all variants from the most negative to the most positive for each wallpaper. As in the grouping task, at the end users explained the criteria they had used to complete the assignment. In this task, we measured the distance between positions indicated by users and the correct positions of variants in the card order.
- Preference: users were shown the two neutral conditions of the wallpapers as images on an actual mobile device (Android smartphone with 4.3" screen) and were asked to express their preference for the wallpapers on a 5-levels Likert scale (1=not at all; 5=very much). Users could move between the two images by a simple swiping gesture on the screen.
- Emotional impact: users were shown the two most extreme variants (-10 and 10) of the wallpapers on an actual mobile device and were asked to fill a questionnaire aimed at determining what emotions users felt while looking at the images. Questions were statements of the form "This character conveys a sense of happiness" and users could answer on a 5-levels Likert scale (1=not at all; 5=very much). We specifically considered the following set of emotions derived from the relevant literature on emotion measurement [15]: happiness, enthusiasm, enjoyment, nervousness, anger, fear, sadness, shame, and guilt.

- Post-call notifications: users were shown each of the four post-call notifications on an actual mobile device and were asked to fill a questionnaire containing statements about the clarity, effectiveness, aesthetic pleasantness, and usefulness of the notifications. An example statement is "This notification is clear". Users could answer on the same 5-levels Likert scale used for emotional impact.

4.3   Results

For the grouping task, the Wilkoxon signed-rank test did not reveal a statistically significant difference in the number of errors for the two wallpapers (p=0.07, W=-36). Means are shown in Fig. 3 (left). However, users tended to consistently make more errors with the skeleton wallpaper and some of the users perceived all variants of the skeleton wallpaper to be negative, commenting that the skeleton did not convey to them any positive meaning.

For the ordering task, the Wilkoxon signed-rank test did not reveal any statistically significant differences between the means of the number of errors for the two wallpapers (p=0.36, W=-19). Means are shown in Fig. 3 (center). However, users made more serious errors with the skeleton wallpaper compared to the dog wallpaper, where errors typically consisted in inverting two adjacent variants.

The Wilkoxon signed-rank test revealed a statistically significant effect for subjective preference (p<0.01, W=67), with users highly preferring the dog wallpaper to the skeleton wallpaper (Fig. 3 right).

For the emotional impact task, Figure 4 shows mean ratings for both positive emotions (happiness, enthusiasm, enjoyment) and negative emotions (nervousness, anger, fear, sadness, shame, and guilt). Friedman's test revealed a significant effect for happiness (p<0.0001, F=43.96), enthusiasm (p<0.0001, F=42.07), enjoyment (p<0.0001, F=42.70), guilt (p<0.0001, F=34.17), sadness (p<0.0001, F=34.61), and fear (p<0.0001, F=20.64). For happiness, enthusiasm, and enjoyment Dunn's post-hoc test pointed out a statistically significant difference (p<0.01) between both negative variants (level -10) and both positive variants (level 10) of wallpapers, with positive variants conveying a higher level of happiness, enthusiasm, or enjoyment. The ratings for nervousness, anger, fear, and shame were very low regardless of wallpaper variant. For guilt, Dunn's test revealed a statistically significant difference (p<0.01)

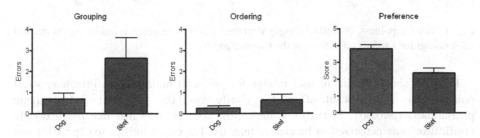

Fig. 3. Mean number of errors (with standard error bars) in the grouping (left) and ordering tasks (center) and mean preference (right) for the two wallpapers

between the negative variant of the dog wallpaper and both positive variants, with a higher score for the negative variant. For sadness, Dunn's test revealed a statistically significant difference (p<0.01) between the negative variant of the dog wallpaper and both positive variants, and between the negative variant of the skeleton wallpaper and the positive variant of the dog wallpaper, with a higher score for the negative variants. For fear, Dunn's test pointed out a statistically significant difference (p<0.01) between the negative variant of the skeleton wallpaper and the positive variant of the dog wallpaper, with a higher score for the negative variant.

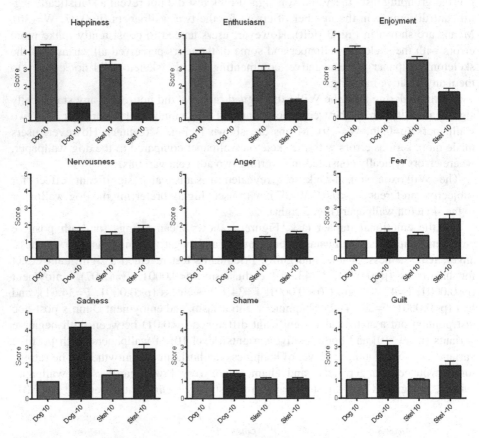

Fig. 4. Mean happiness, enthusiasm, enjoyment, nervousness, anger, fear, sadness, shame, and guilt ratings for variants -10 and 10 of the two wallpapers

Figure 5 shows means of user ratings for post-call notifications. Friedman's test pointed out a significant effect for clarity (p<0.05, F=10.07) and aesthetic pleasantness (p<0.001, F=18.32). Dunn's post-hoc test revealed that the text-only notification was perceived to be clearer than the bar chart notification (p<0.01) and that the pre-post notification was the most aesthetically pleasing (p<0.01).

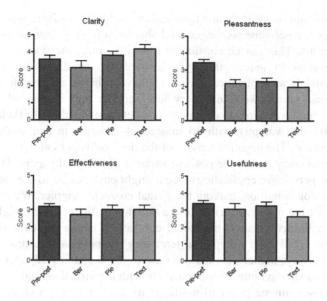

Fig. 5. Mean clarity, aesthetic pleasantness, effectiveness, and usefulness ratings for the post-call notifications

5 Discussion

The higher preference for the dog wallpaper compared to the skeleton wallpaper might be due to the stronger empathic connection users seem to establish with a virtual animal compared to other subjects as shown in other work in the literature [3][10]. It is interesting to note that females rated the skeleton wallpaper higher than males. On one side, this is possibly a general consequence of female tendency to give higher ratings in self-report scales dealing with emotions and preferences [16]. On the other side, males could have disliked the addition of cloth accessories to the skeleton in the positive variants of the wallpaper.

While we found no significant difference between the two wallpapers in terms of their understandability, some of the users had much more difficulty in interpreting the skeleton wallpaper than the dog wallpaper. In particular, there were users who considered all skeleton variants as negative. Additionally, from user's comments after the ordering task, we found that users tended to compare skeleton variants (especially in the positive group) based on a purely logical criteria, i.e., the number of accessories displayed on the character, while dog variants where compared based on more complex criteria, i.e., by considering the emotions displayed by the virtual character. These results, coupled with the higher global preference for the dog wallpaper, make us conclude that the skeleton wallpaper is less suitable than the dog wallpaper for our purposes.

The analysis of the emotional impact of wallpapers revealed that users associated positive wallpaper variants to positive emotions and negative wallpaper variants to negative emotions. However, while both types of positive wallpaper variants showed a connection to all the positive emotions we considered (happiness, enthusiasm, enjoyment), the emotional response to negative wallpaper variants was much more varied. Ratings for nervousness, anger, and shame were very low for both types of wallpaper variants. This can be considered a positive outcome since our wallpapers were not designed to induce this type of negative emotions, which could be counterproductive in an application aimed at behavior change and lead to abandon the application. Fear ratings were also very low and the only statistically significant difference we found was across wallpapers (i.e., between the negative skeleton variant and the positive dog variant), with no substantial variation in fear within the same wallpaper sequence. The negative variant of the dog wallpaper caused a high level of sadness and guilt compared to the positive variants of both wallpapers. This might be positive for the persuasive application since it might push people to use earphones just to improve the dog condition, making the virtual character happier. We did not find a similar effect for the negative variant of the skeleton wallpaper. This might be due to users feeling a limited (if any) emotional connection to the skeleton wallpaper. It should also be noted that, except for fear, user's emotional response to the dog wallpaper was always higher than the response to the skeleton wallpaper. Again, this might be due to a stronger empathic connection with the virtual animal.

The comparison among post-call notifications did not reveal a clear winner. The text-only notification reached a better score in terms of clarity of presentation, even if the difference was statistically significant only compared to the bar chart notification. Probably, this was a consequence of the limited amount of information available in the text-only notification, which made understanding easier. The pre-post-call notification was found to be the most aesthetically pleasing, with all three other notifications reaching a very low score on this aspect. In particular, users did not like the graphical complexity of the graph-based notifications and the graphical simplicity of the text-only visualization. The pre-post notification also reached a better score in terms of perceived effectiveness and usefulness even if there were no significant differences with the other notifications and, in general, all notifications obtained an average score on these aspects.

Overall, from these results we can draw the following conclusions and implications for the design of the persuasive application:

- The skeleton wallpaper does not seem to provide any significant advantage over the dog wallpaper. Inclusion of the dog wallpaper might instead lead to better user acceptance of the persuasive application and stronger emotional connection with the virtual character, thus possibly producing a more engaging and effective experience.
- Users can correctly understand the positivity/negativity level of proposed wallpaper variants. Moreover, they associate positive emotions to the positive variants and negative emotions to the negative variants. This is especially true for the dog wallpaper, whose design seems thus appropriate to provide positive/negative reinforcement in a persuasive application.
- Since aesthetics play an increasing role in the acceptance of current persuasive applications, the pre-post-call notification seems the most appropriate for inclusion in the application. Yet, a more thorough longitudinal investigation would be needed to better understand its impact in terms of effectiveness. Statistics on earphone usage should be displayed only on user request.

6   Final Application

Based on the results of the user study, we implemented BrainSaver as an Android application that makes use of the dog wallpaper and pre-post-call notification. The application constantly monitors user's call activity, identifying whether the user has earphones connected whenever she makes or receives a call.

The application operates in different ways based on earphone use and length of calls. If a call lasts less than 20 seconds, the application does not take any specific action. Bothering the user with some persuasive message after these calls would likely be perceived as overly intrusive and annoying, reducing user's willingness to use the application and possibly producing psychological reactance. Moreover, studies in the literature show that the temperature of the tissues which are closest to the cell phone during a call increases only after prolonged calls. If a call lasts more than 20 seconds and the user does not use earphones, the application takes the following actions at the end of the call: (i) the image preceding the currently used one in the wallpaper sequence is selected as base image for the wallpaper; (ii) the wallpaper is changed, using the output of step (i) as image; (iii) the user is notified of the changes to the wallpaper and reminded to use earphones, using the pre-post-call notification presented above. If a call lasts more than 20 seconds and the user uses earphones, the application takes the following actions at the end of the call: (i) the image following the currently used one in the wallpaper sequence is selected as base image for the wallpaper; (ii) the wallpaper is changed, using the image selected at step (i). Statistics on earphone use can be requested at any time by accessing the application options through the notification area.

Like other mobile persuasive applications [3], BrainSaver resets the wallpaper to its initial condition (neutral image) at the beginning of a new week. This is to give a higher sense of progression (positive or negative) in those cases in which the user is stuck at the maximum positive or negative level during the week (because of several consecutive calls with or without earphones, respectively).

7   Conclusions and Future Work

To the best of our knowledge, our research is the first to propose a mobile persuasive application to encourage safe and healthy behaviors with respect to cell phone RF exposure. The paper has illustrated in detail the design of the mobile application, motivating the different decisions taken and the novel combination of persuasive techniques that range from classical solutions (such as reminders and behavior statistics) to more advanced ones (such as data visualization and encouragement of empathy and interoception through specific visualizations). The user study we carried out provided useful information about the appropriateness of different design choices. We are now planning an extensive longitudinal study, recruiting participants to get data on the regular use of BrainSaver. We will also distribute the application to the public, through Google Play, to collect data on usage and acceptability of the application from larger samples.

Acknowledgements. Valeria Marcon greatly helped in the development and evaluation of the prototype.

References

1. IARC. Agents classified by the IARC monographs,
   http://monographs.iarc.fr/ENG/Classi-fication/index.php
2. Consolvo, S., Klasnja, P., McDonald, D.W., Avrahami, D., Froehlich, J., LeGrand, L., Libby, R., Mosher, K., Landay, J.A.: Flowers or a robot army?: encouraging awareness & activity with personal, mobile displays. In: 10th International Conference on Ubiquitous Computing, pp. 54–63. ACM Press, New York (2008)
3. Froehlich, J., Dillahunt, T., Klasnja, P., Mankoff, J., Consolvo, S., Harrison, B., Landay, J.A.: Ubigreen: investigating a mobile tool for tracking and supporting green transportation habits. In: 27th International Conference on Human Factors in Computing Systems, pp. 1043–1052. ACM Press, New York (2009)
4. Shiraishi, M., Washio, Y., Takayama, C., Lehdonvirta, V., Kimura, H., Nakajima, T.: Using individual, social and economic persuasion techniques to reduce CO2 emissions in a family setting. In: 4th International Conference on Persuasive Technology, pp. 13:1–13:8. ACM Press, New York (2009)
5. Consolvo, S., McDonald, D.W., Landay, J.A.: Theory-driven design strategies for technologies that support behavior change in everyday life. In: 27th International Conference on Human Factors in Computing Systems, pp. 405–414. ACM Press, New York (2009)
6. Jafarinaimi, N., Forlizzi, J.: Breakaway: An ambient display designed to change human behavior. In: 23rd International Conference on Human Factors in Computing Systems, pp. 1945–1948. ACM Press, New York (2005)
7. Fogg, B.J.: Persuasive technology: using computers to change what we think and do. Morgan Kaufmann, San Francisco (2003)
8. Choe, E.K., Kientz, J.A., Halko, S., Fonville, A.A., Sakaguchi, D., Watson, N.F.: Opportunities for computing to support healthy sleep behavior. In: 28th International Conference on Human Factors in Computing Systems, pp. 3661–3666. ACM Press, New York (2010)
9. Nawyn, J., Intille, S.S., Larson, K.: Embedding behavior modification strategies into a consumer electronic device: a case study. In: 8th International Conference on Ubiquitous Computing, pp. 297–314. ACM Press, New York (2006)
10. Dillahunt, T., Becker, G., Mankoff, J., Kraut, R.: Motivating environmentally sustainable behavior changes with a virtual polar bear. In: Pervasive 2008 Workshop on Pervasive Persuasive Technology and Environmental Sustainability (2008)
11. Gerend, M.A., Sias, T.: Message framing and color priming: how subtle threat cues affect persuasion. Journal of Experimental Social Psychology 45(4), 999–1002 (2009)
12. Klasnja, P., Consolvo, S., McDonald, D.W., Landay, J.A., Pratt, W.: Using mobile and personal sensing technologies to support health behavior change in everyday life: lessons learned. In: Annual Conf. American Medical Informatics Association, pp. 338–342 (2009)
13. Intille, S.S.: A new research challenge: persuasive technology to motivate healthy aging. IEEE Transactions on Information Technology in Biomedicine 8(3), 235–237 (2004)
14. Shahab, L., Hall, S., Marteau, T.: Showing smokers with vascular disease images of their arteries to motivate cessation: a pilot study. Br. J. Health Psychol. 12(pt. 2), 275–283 (2007)
15. Izard, C.E.: Human emotions. Plenum Press, New York (1977)
16. Eisenberg, N., Strayer, J.: Empathy and its development. Cambridge University Press (1987)

Opportunities for Persuasive Technology to Motivate Heavy Computer Users for Stretching Exercise

Yong-Xiang Chen[1], Siek-Siang Chiang[1], Shu-Yun Chih[2], Wen-Ching Liao[1],
Shih-Yao Lin[3], Shang-Hua Yang[3], Shun-Wen Cheng[1], Shih-Sung Lin[3],
Yu-Shan Lin[3], Ming-Sui Lee[3], Jau-Yih Tsauo[2], Cheng-Min Jen[4],
Chia-Shiang Shih[4], King-Jen Chang[5], and Yi-Ping Hung[3]

[1] Department of Computer Science and Information Engineering, National Taiwan University,
Taipei, Taiwan
[2] Division of Physical Therapy, Department of Physical Medicine and Rehabilitation,
National Taiwan University Hospital, Taipei, Taiwan
[3] Graduate Institute of Network and Multimedia, National Taiwan University, Taipei, Taiwan
[4] Hwacom Systems Inc., Taipei, Taiwan
[5] Chung-Kang Branch, Cheng-Ching General Hospital, Taichung, Taiwan
d96922029@ntu.edu.tw, hung@csie.ntu.edu.tw

Abstract. Reducing the negative effects of extended computer use is becoming increasingly important and it has been demonstrated that appropriate stretching yields benefits. We investigated the opportunities of motivating heavy computer users to stretch by incorporating mobile and sensing technologies into a 1-on-1 social competition game. We implemented the "Social Persuasion System for Stretching" (SP-Stretch) and conducted a 4-week study with 25 heavy computer users. Based on the quantitative and qualitative results, we identify a number of design considerations, and provide suggestions for future research.

Keywords: Heavy Computer User, Stretching Exercise, Competition Game.

1 Introduction

As computers are popular in modern life, musculoskeletal soreness, stiffness and pain are common among the computer users. The symptoms are most often the results of sustained static working postures (even awkward postures) and repetitive upper extremities movements persisting over extended periods of time. Researchers have revealed the negative effects associated with extended computer use, manifest in musculoskeletal discomfort and disorders (MSDs), such as muscle pain and tendonitis [6].

Stretching exercises are meant to lengthen soft tissue to increase range of motion and flexibility as well as reduce discomfort due to sustained working postures and repetitions. A stretching regime introduced by Marangoni contributed to a significant decrease in musculoskeletal pain associated with working at a computer workstation [9]. Though many are aware that stretching can prevent discomfort, knowing is not the same as doing. It is a challenge to motivate heavy computer users for stretching.

A. Spagnolli et al. (Eds.): PERSUASIVE 2014, LNCS 8462, pp. 25–30, 2014.
© Springer International Publishing Switzerland 2014

Recently, researchers are increasingly exploring the applications of technology to support behavior changes in domains such as health and sustainability. For example, mobile and sensing technologies have been used to encourage people for healthy behavior, track progress over time, trigger target behavior, and help people set and meet health-related goals [2, 8]. These persuasive technologies could be incorporated into games, and may be a potent motivator. The Social Cognitive Theory (SCT) provides the foundation for promoting behavior change by games. In SCT, game elements may enhance behavior change through aspects of intrinsic motivation [10].

In this study, we investigated the opportunities of motivating individuals to stretch by incorporating mobile and sensing technologies into a 1-on-1 social competition game. The game pairs players and mediates competitions by mobile technology, along with the proposed asynchronous competition mechanism. The game ensures a fair competition by adopting sensing technology to detect stretching exercise. A RGB-D camera and a ring sensor are involved in our detection module.

2   Related Work

Persuasive technology solutions to promote physical activity have been studied from various perspectives. For helping reduce the risk of physical inactivity and promote healthier computer use, Wang and Chern developed a time-scheduled delivery of health-related animations for heavy computer users. However, their intervention did not have a meaningful impact on the participants' behavior intention [11].

Many studies have investigated the use of social power and game competitions to increase motivation for performing target behavior. In Yee's study, the desire to challenge and compete with others is an important motivational factor of game-play [13]. The NEAT-o-Game study found that competition game appeared to increase the players' engagement [5]. However, the Fish'n'Steps study reported that team-based competition game did not have a significant effect while compared to a single-user equivalent [7]. Recently, Xu et al. found that deploying a group-based competition does not automatically lead to cooperative behavior [12]. In this study, we investigated the opportunities of designing a 1-on-1 competition game for motivating individuals to stretch.

For design competition game, maintaining fairness is another issue that should be highlight. For example, in above NEAT-o-Game and Fish'n'Steps cases, the physical activity of the users was quantified by the number of user's steps captured by a pedometer and then manually fed into the system. The self-report feature harms game fairness during competition and might decrease user's motivation to use the system. The study of Duh and Chen examined how virtual community is affected by cheating behavior and denoted the importance of fairness in gaming [3].

3   Design the 1-on-1 Competition Game for Stretching

For investigating the opportunities of motivating individuals to stretch, our research team includes two experts in physical therapy domain to select seventeen stretching movements. The seventeen movements are categorized into five types, upper back stretches, trunk stretches, upper extremity stretches, hip stretches and lower extremity stretches. The duration of performing five types of stretching exercise is between 3 to 7 minutes.

We designed a 1-on-1 social competition game and supposed that the challenge and competition with peers in the game might trigger one to stretch more, as considering that trigger is one of important factors for promoting target behavior [4]. Besides, the efficacy of stretching depends on the quality of practice, that is, correct stretch position and sufficient hold time [1]. Therefore, one of the design requirements was promoting qualified practices. Based on this idea, the result of each competition round was determined according to the quality of the stretching exercises performed by the competitors.

Adopt Multiple Sensors for Ensuring Fair Competition: This study adopted multiple sensors for the detection of stretching movements to ensure a fair evaluation method in the 1-on-1 competitions. A ring sensor (TI eZ430-Chronos) and a RGB-D camera (Microsoft Kinect) were selected to collaboratively detect the stretching movements. The ring sensor includes an accelerometer to detect fine motor movement such as wrist rotation, while the RGB-D camera detects gross poses. When a user begins practice, a monitor displays stretching multimedia for guiding stretch, and the sensors keep detecting user's movements during the practice. After the practice, the detection module generates a quality rank (Between A to D) of stretching to the user. The rank is calculated based on the similarity between user's pattern of stretch and the ground truth of stretch pattern performed by a specialist.

Design Asynchronous Mechanism of Competition for Motivating Stretching: This study designed a 1-on-1 competition game between peers, as outlined in Fig. 1. For participating the competition, all participants first installed a specifically developed App on their smart phones to receive competition invitations. Each competition collocates two participants with a type of stretch exercise. The competitions went as follows: when a competition was created by one participant (the proposer), the host returned a list of all legal competition pairs (available responder, stretching types) for selection. After selecting a competition pair, the proposer would begin practicing the stretching exercise. Once the proposer's practice session, the host displayed the rank to the proposer only. After the responder's practice session was finished, both the results of proposer and responder were displayed. The host also sent the results to the stretching App on the competitor's smart phones.

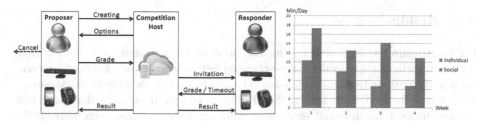

Fig. 1. The Mechanism of 1-on-1 competition   **Fig. 2.** Average daily duration of stretching

The asynchronous mechanism provides flexibility for beginning practice session to responders. The default setting of time limit for each competition was three days, to cover weekends. To promote balance and diversity of full body stretching, repetitive challenges of the same stretching type were limited.

4   Method

In order to determine whether participants responded positively to the effects of 1-on-1 competition game, this study compared the user experience with two types of stretching assist systems: "Multimedia System for Stretching" (M-Stretch) and "Social Persuasion System for Stretching" (SP-Stretch). The SP-Stretch includes all of the design features mentioned above and in the M-Stretch system, participants used a smart phone with guiding stretching multimedia without other sensors. The participants in the M-Stretch system cannot compete with other participants by our 1-on-1 competition mechanism. We designed a two-period cross over study and invited volunteers by word-of-mouth. Prior to enroll eligible participants in our study, we explained the study in great detail and answered questions to them. Participants were recruited into the study after signed the written informed consent forms. The consent provided the information about the safety and effectiveness of the evidence-based exercise intervention, along with mitigation procedures for pain or discomfort. 25 graduate students heavy computer use (normally worked more than 5 hours a day in front of a computer [11]) were recruited to participate in the 4-week stretching program. Eight of the participants were female, and seventeen were male. Each participant was randomly assigned a sequence of using both stretching assist systems. Twelve of the subjects used the SP-Stretch for the first two weeks followed by the M-Stretch for the remaining two weeks. The other thirteen subjects participated in the reverse order. All participants owned and regularly used a smart phone. We collect system logs for quantitative analysis, along with collect qualitative results by conducting semi-structured interview to twenty participants at the end of 4-week study. Interview questions focused on their experiences during the study, their use of SP-Stretch and M-Stretch, and how, if at all, they believed SP-Stretch motivated them and impacted their awareness for stretching. Five participants withdrew from this study. Participants were awarded a lottery ticket each day that they reached the recommended daily goal of 20 minutes stretching. The tickets were then entered into a post-experiment lottery to win $30 on average.

5   Results

For investigating whether detection module prevents cheating and unfair competition, we asked participants to evaluate their cheating behavior under two kinds of interventions in the post-study interview session. The result showed cheating in the M-Stretch system is 46%, and 0% cheating in the SP-Stretch system. It indicates that the stretch sensing method we designed tends to prevent cheating and maintains fairness for competition game. After removed the cheating records of stretching, Fig. 2 lists a global view of average weekly stretching time. Overall, the difference of stretching time between using M-Stretch (Individual) and using SP-Stretch (Social) reached significance (p<0.01). This result indicates that the SP-Stretch may have motivated the participants for stretching. Consistently, most of the participants agreed that social persuasion had a positive effect on their performance. They expressed appreciation for the 1-on-1 competition mechanism. Most participants described this mechanism as a useful reminder to perform stretching exercises, and they preferred such reminders to those provided by alarms due to the fact that they felt an obligation to respond to other participants' competition invitations.

Several subjects mentioned that they enjoyed the competitions and actively sought to earn more points by winning competitions, even without the incentive of a material prize for doing so. Furthermore, the SP-Stretch system was used not only as a reminder to stretch, but also as a guide to ensure the quality of stretching. Several participants described how the competition prompted them to pay attention to the quality of practice in order to obtain extra points.

Nonetheless, five of participants did not perceive the benefits of the competition mechanism, due to their tight schedules and workloads. One participant described the invitations of competition as additional pressure which he already had enough.

All participants agreed that the sensor-based evaluation of stretching quality was fair and not easy to get benefit in competition game by cheating. However, a number of participants were unsure why they lost competitions and would like to have a review function to observe and correct their movements.

Many participants reported that the asynchronous mechanism of competition is easy to understand and interesting. The tendency was to compete with people they know, especially their friends. After competing with friends, they often discussed the competition when they met outside the office.

6   Discussion and Conclusion

Our findings illustrate the effects of a 1-on-1 competition mechanism using social persuasion to promote stretching exercises among individuals heavily involved in computer-related activities. Most of the participants agreed that the system effectively promoted stretching; however, a number of shortcomings were noted. In the design of similar 1-on-1 competitions, we suggest that the system automatically assigns pairings in the beginning stages to expand the range of competition beyond already established social pairings. Furthermore, some participants mentioned that the reason why they stop challenging others more is because their competitors responded rarely. Thus, how to maintain certain amount of responses is also a challenge issue in the future. We also recommend that the image-based sensors can be augmented with a playback feature which provides a summary report outlining incorrect movements to facilitate correction, thereby to increase the usability and overall effectiveness of the similar system.

Although this preliminary result of the study presented opportunity of designing persuasive technologies to motivate stretching exercise for heavy computer users, there are many limitations existed in this study due to time, sample size, geographical, and institutional constrains. The experience gained from this study can be used to design related social persuasion systems for promoting health, especially for physical exercise which requires performing the movements appropriately and maintaining the specific position, for example, Yoga and Tai-Chi.

Acknowledgments. This work was supported in part by the National Science Council, Taiwan, under grants NSC 101-2622-E-002-005-CC2 and NSC 102-2627-E-002-006.

References

1. Armiger, P., Martyn, M.A.: Stretching for function flexibility. Philadelphia. Lippincott Williams and Wilkins (2010)
2. Consolvo, S., McDonald, D.W., Toscos, T., Chen, M., Froehlich, J.E., Harrison, B., Klasnja, P., LaMarca, A., LeGrand, L., Libby, R., Smith, I., Landay, J.A.: Activity sensing in the wild: a field trial of ubifit garden. In: Proc. of CHI 2008. ACM (2008)
3. Duh, H.B.L., Chen, V.H.H.: Cheating behaviors in online gaming. In: Ozok, A.A., Zaphiris, P. (eds.) OCSC 2009. LNCS, vol. 5621, pp. 567–573. Springer, Heidelberg (2009)
4. Fogg, B.J.: A behavioral model for persuasive design. In: Proc. of Persuasive 2009 (2009)
5. Fujiki, Y., Kazakos, K., Puri, C., Buddharaju, P., Pavlidis, I., Levine, J.: NEAT-o-Games: Blending physical activity and fun in the daily routine. ACM Computers in Entertainment 6(2) (2008)
6. IJmker, S., Huysmans, M., Blatter, B.M., van der Beek, A.J., van Mechelen, W., Bongers, P.M.: Should office workers spend fewer hours at their computer? A systematic review of the literature. Occup. Environ. Med. 64, 211–222 (2007)
7. Lin, J.J., Mamykina, L., Lindtner, S., Delajoux, G., Strub, H.B.: Fish'n'Steps: Encouraging physical activity with an interactive computer game. In: Dourish, P., Friday, A. (eds.) UbiComp 2006. LNCS, vol. 4206, pp. 261–278. Springer, Heidelberg (2006)
8. Mamykina, L., Mynatt, E., Davidson, P., Greenblatt, D.: MAHI: Investigation of social scaffolding for reflective thinking in diabetes management. In: Proc. of CHI 2008, pp. 477–486 (2008)
9. Marangoni, A.H.: Effects of intermittent stretching exercises at work on musculoskeletal pain associated with the use of a personal computer and the influence of media on outcomes. Work 36(1), 27–37 (2010)
10. Ryan, R., Rigby, C., Przybylski, A.: The motivational pull of videogames: a self-determination theory approach. Motivation and Emotion, 347–363 (2006)
11. Wang, S.Y., Chern, J.Y.: Time-scheduled delivery of computer health animations: "Installing" healthy habits of computer use. Health Informatics Journal 19(2), 116–126 (2013)
12. Xu, Y., Poole, E.S., Miller, A.D., Eiriksdottir, E., Kestranek, D., Catrambone, R., Mynatt, E.D.: This is not a one-horse race: understanding player types in multiplayer pervasive health games for youth. In: Proc. of CSCW 2012 (2012)
13. Yee, N.: Motivations for play in online games. Cyber Psychology & Behavior 9(6), 772–775 (2006)

Changing User's Safety Locus of Control through Persuasive Play: An Application to Aviation Safety

Luca Chittaro

Human-Computer Interaction Lab
University of Udine
via delle Scienze 206
33100 Udine, Italy
http://hcilab.uniud.it

Abstract. Virtual risk experiences have been proposed in persuasive technology as an approach to change people's attitudes and behaviors concerning safety topics. This paper advances the investigation of virtual risk experiences in different directions. First, we extend the study of their effects to safety locus of control, which is an important predictor of an individual's attitudes and behaviors with respect to risky situations. Second, we explore a design that relies much more on play than previous virtual experiences of risks in the literature. Third, we extend the investigation of persuasive technology to a topic in aviation safety (i.e., assuming a proper brace position during an emergency landing) that has never been approached before with an interactive system and we analyze if a novel game-based approach can be effective in fostering awareness of this fundamental safety action. Our study shows that the proposed persuasive game produces noteworthy results in terms of learning safety knowledge and improves players' attitudes towards aircraft accidents, increasing their internal safety locus of control and decreasing the external one.

Keywords: safety, persuasive games, virtual risk experiences, locus of control, aviation safety, brace position.

1 Introduction

Virtual risk experiences [5,6,18,31] have been proposed in persuasive technology as an approach to change people' attitudes and behaviors with respect to safety topics. This approach could be effective in persuading people to change because it enables them to observe the link between cause and effect [11], it can provide immediate feedback by showing the positive consequences of recommended behaviors and the negative consequences of dangerous behaviors [5], and those consequences can be simulated in vivid ways that can contribute to make them more memorable [18].

Studies of virtual experiences of risk carried out so far focused on measuring effects on attitudes towards risks deriving from threats such as climate change [18], floods [31] structure fires [6] and aircraft evacuations [5]. In this paper, we aim at

A. Spagnolli et al. (Eds.): PERSUASIVE 2014, LNCS 8462, pp. 31–42, 2014.

advancing the investigation of virtual risk experiences in different directions. First, we extend the study of their effects to safety locus of control, an important predictor of an individual's attitudes and behaviors with respect to risky situations. Second, we explore a design that relies much more on play than the previously cited virtual experiences of risks. Third, we consider a topic in aviation safety (i.e., assuming a proper brace position during an emergency landing) that has never been approached before with an interactive system and we analyze if a novel game-based approach can be effective in fostering awareness of this fundamental safety action.

The paper is organized as follows. In Section 2, we discuss previous work in persuasive technology for aviation safety and how the present research differs from it. Section 3 motivates and illustrates the importance of the safety locus of control construct. In Section 4, we present in detail the persuasive game application we created. Section 5 and 6 respectively illustrate the experimental evaluation and the obtained results, while Section 7 concludes the paper and introduces future work.

2   Related Work

The primary purpose of aviation safety education is to provide aircraft passengers with accurate cabin safety knowledge and cultivate positive passengers' attitudes to appropriately affect their behavior when an emergency occurs. As shown by the study in [4], the level of aviation safety education an aircraft passenger has does affect her knowledge, attitudes and behaviors. Safety awareness can lead passengers to efficient behaviors and being responsible for their own safety; therefore, improving passenger safety education increases the probability of their survival in an emergency [20,26].

Current approaches to passenger education are based on the safety card in the seat pocket and the flight attendant presentation to which passengers are exposed after boarding the aircraft. Unfortunately, as discussed in reports of the US Federal Aviation Administration (FAA) [7] as well as other papers in the literature [20,26], passenger attention to safety cards and briefings is poor at best, and the few passengers who pay attention have little knowledge and understanding of the information received. Reports conclude that safety and survival information needs to be presented and made available in substantially improved and creative ways [8,20].

Persuasive technology is a natural candidate to address this problem, but to the best of our knowledge the only study to date of persuasive technology for aviation safety was the one we described in [5]. In that work, a simple 3D world allowed users to partially experience a specific pre-scripted evacuation scenario, which started with an in-flight announcement that an emergency landing was going to be attempted and ended when the player got out of the plane. Progress in the scenario was determined at some choice points in which the player had to choose an action (for example, retrieving his/her luggage or leaving it on the plane). Choosing the right action made the scenario progress, otherwise the player was left where (s)he was and the question was asked again. The negative consequences of wrong choices were described by a very brief text, and not simulated with graphics and sound to avoid scaring the player. The way users chose actions was very basic too: a text menu appeared on the screen and the player had to push keys on the computer keyboard to choose an option.

The study conducted on 26 participants showed that playing the game (which required 2-3 minutes to complete) improved to some extent knowledge of the evacuation procedure and also self-efficacy (the participants' belief in their ability to carry out the evacuation procedure). Finally, the study checked if living the virtual experience had effects on the perception of vulnerability and severity of aircraft evacuation risks. While vulnerability did not change, an undesired decrease in severity was found, probably due the fact that the virtual experience was specifically designed not to be scary and did not show any kind of damage and adverse effects on the players' avatar.

The present project differs from the previous research in a number of ways. From the point of view of aviation safety, we focus on educating passengers about how to accurately perform a specific action (assuming a brace position), while the previous study focused on an abstract procedure in which complex actions such assuming the brace position reduced to simply choosing a single menu option. From the application point of view, we aim at creating more playful dynamics, in which the user does not simply choose options from a menu but can actively play with his/her avatar body, posing it in a wide range of different postures and seeing how this affects it in an accident. We also aim at providing much richer feedback. First, unlike the previous application that did not show any negative consequences, we fully simulate and show them to players with realistic graphics and sound. Second, after showing the possibly scary consequences, we provide hints to help the player avert them. Since our aim is to make the game available for public campaigns, we devoted particular care to obtaining a graphic and audio quality higher than typical research prototypes. Finally, we extend the study of the game effects to locus of control, an important construct in psychology and in safety, which we introduce and discuss in the next section.

3   Locus of Control and Safety

Locus of control, a construct originated from Rotter's social learning theory [22], can be defined as the degree to which a person perceives that the outcomes of the situations (s)he experiences are under his/her personal control. With respect to a given situation, an individual's locus of control can have an internal orientation (the individual perceives that she can exert control over the outcome of the situation) or an external orientation (the individual perceives that the outcome of the situation is due to external factors, such as fate, chance or the actions of other persons).

The importance of locus of control in safety was highlighted by several studies, which showed that it is a predictor of safety-relevant attitudes and behaviors. In particular, an internal orientation is usually associated with safer attitudes and behaviors. For example, in the domain of road safety, Hoyt [12] found that car passengers with an internal locus of control are more likely to wear seat belts, while Montag and Comrey [19] related drivers' internal locus of control with safer driving. Interestingly, a recent study [13] showed that drivers' locus of control can be influenced by training and by observer feedback, and the changes in drivers' locus of control can predict change in driving behavior. This suggests that the simulations people can live in a virtual risk experience and the feedback the application can provide users with are worth of study as possible techniques to change users' locus of control, in addition to improve their knowledge about the considered risky situation.

Wuebker [29] focused on locus of control in the industrial safety domain, proposing the Safety Locus of Control Scale. The results of her study indicated that externally oriented employees had significantly more accidents than employees with internal safety control beliefs. Moreover, accidents and injuries suffered by externally oriented employees were more serious than those of internally oriented employees. Jones and Wuebker [17] focused on hospital workers, confirming the relation of the Safety Locus of Control Scale with occupational accidents in that domain too.

Hunter [14] adapted the Safety Locus of Control Scale to measure aviation safety locus of control in pilots and found that civil aviation pilots with a more internal orientation were involved in fewer hazardous events. A study of airline pilots by You et al. [30] reinforces these findings, showing that locus of control influences safe operation behavior. Hunter and Stewart [15,16] extended the investigation of locus of control to U.S. Army aviators, developing the Army Locus of Control Scale and finding significant associations which are consistent with research conducted on civil aviation pilots. In particular, aviators with a more internal control orientation experienced fewer accidents than aviators who were low on that construct.

Improving safety locus of control seems to be particularly important also in the domain of air passengers' safety. Indeed, it is known that passengers tend to look at aviation emergencies with attitudes that are consistent with an external rather than an internal orientation, e.g. shifting the responsibility and capability of their safety to the cabin crew [20] or falsely believing that most aircraft accidents are unsurvivable [25]. This way of thinking is dangerous for the negative effects that an external orientation has on safety attitudes and behavior, and it is also unfounded for different reasons. First, in an emergency, the crew cannot provide individual assistance to every passenger, due to the workload and time constraints of the evacuation. Moreover, crew members could be injured or incapacitated, and this would require passengers to take an even more active role to survive. Second, passengers' pessimistic beliefs about survivability are contradicted by facts: a survey of commercial jet airplanes accidents conducted by Boeing [1] indicates that the majority of them is survivable, and a recently released FAA report [3] confirms and reinforces that conclusion.

Therefore, persuasive applications aimed at passengers, in addition to informing them about the correct actions and emergency procedures, have to address explicitly the issue of changing passenger's attitudes towards his/her role in the emergency and his/her actual possibility of exerting control on the outcomes. The goal of the study in the present paper is to determine if a playful virtual risk experience and the feedback that it provides can, as we hypothesize, be effective in changing users' locus of control as well as improving their knowledge about the considered risky situation.

4   The Persuasive Game

A fundamental action that passengers can take to contribute to their survival in aircraft accidents is to assume an appropriate "Brace for Impact" position. This is an action in which passengers pre-position their bodies against whatever they are most likely to be thrown against, significantly reducing injuries sustained [25]. The purpose of our persuasive game is to allow players to become familiar with the action of assuming a brace position in all of its details as well as improve their locus of control with respect to the risk posed by an emergency landing. The game is meant to be used in public campaigns conducted on the Web, so that users can conveniently play it on their computers, to familiarize with the brace position well before boarding a plane.

In designing the application, we organized gameplay in four steps. First, the player poses a 3D virtual passenger. In particular, the player sees the passenger seated in the cabin of a flying aircraft, from a third-person perspective. As shown in Figure 1, four distinct icons are associated to different body parts of the passenger. The player can freely drag each icon with the mouse to easily move the corresponding body part and pose the 3D character. The rationale for choosing this interface was that it supports a "puppeteer" metaphor in which the user pulls the strings connected to the head, hands and feet of the virtual passenger to pose it. Such kind of metaphor should be immediately familiar to users. Moreover, the point-and-click interaction technique (through which users move the icons to "pull the strings" in the game) is typical of many computer applications and should thus require no learning effort. The application invites the player to pose the passenger in a position (s)he believes to be safe for an emergency landing, but the player is allowed to pose the character in any position, including the most dangerous ones.

Second, when the player has finished posing the character, a hard emergency landing is simulated in real-time, after the user clicks the "Crash" button in Figure 1. The simulation is not pre-scripted: it is physically based so each player's try can have slight or major differences from a previously seen one, depending on the initial body position of the virtual passenger. The aim of the simulation is to vividly show the consequences of assuming a wrong position on the passenger's body as well as allow the player to discover experientially which positions do not produce such negative consequences. Figure 2 shows two instants in a specific simulation.

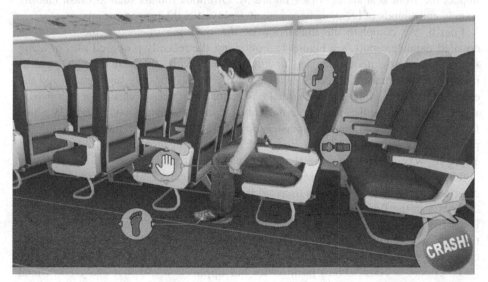

Fig. 1. Posing the virtual passenger

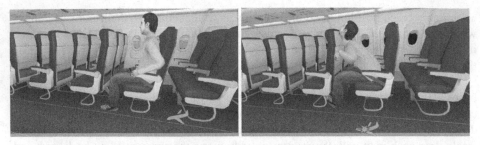

Fig. 2. Real-time crash simulation

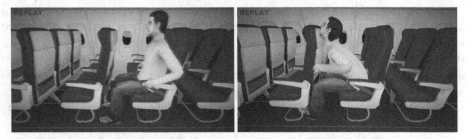

Fig. 3. Slow-motion replay with damage highlight

Third, since the impact in the real-time simulation occurs in a very short time as in real life, a slow-motion replay (similar to those shown in the media for car crash tests) is also presented to allow players appreciate details that cannot be noticed in a real-time simulation. To make the slow-motion replay more dramatic, we show it in greyscale and use color red to highlight the parts of the body which get injured as they impact the front seat surfaces (see Figure 3). Ominous sounds such as crash landing sounds and sounds of breaking bones are also played at the proper instants.

Fourth, we complete the illustration of the outcome of each game try with a detailed damage report (see Figure 4). Following the recently proposed idea of using visualizations of internal damage to human body parts obtained through medical imaging for persuasion purposes (see e.g. [24]), we do not only highlight in red the externally visible damage in the virtual passenger body but we enrich the report with x-ray visualizations that show internal damage in the affected body parts. We also follow fear appeals strategies of persuasion [21,23,28] that highlight how scaring the participant is a good tactic as long as the intervention also presents a simple and effective way of averting the depicted negative consequences. To do so, after highlighting each negative consequence on the passenger's body, we provide a short, clear and simple hint about how to avoid it (as shown in the left part of Figure 4 and described in the figure caption). This is meant to educate and reassure the player but is also an implicit incentive to retry again the game to see if one can do better next time. A prominent "Retry" button is displayed to conveniently restart from the character-posing phase.

To choose a correct brace position for our application, we first analyzed official normative information about brace positions [27], which derived from dynamic impact tests conducted in the 80's and 90's. We then considered the latest research conducted in 2013 by the FAA [25], after the injuries sustained by passengers in several recent commercial airline accidents (e.g., US Airways flight 1549) highlighted a need to review brace position effectiveness to determine if the recommended positions were still appropriate for today's passenger seats. As a result, we adopted the optimized brace position recommended by that research.

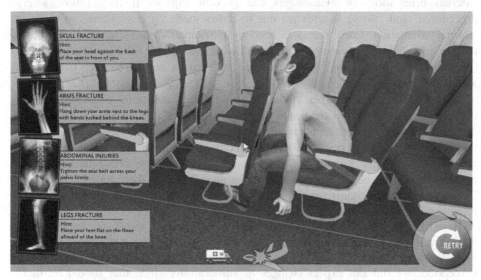

Fig. 4. Damage report and hints. The four hints in this scenario are (from top to bottom): (a) "Place your head against the back of the seat in front of you", (b) "Hang down your arms next to the legs with hands tucked behind the knees", (c) "Tighten the seat belt across your pelvis firmly", (d) "Tuck your feet firmly on the floor behind your knees".

5   Method

5.1   Participants, Design and Measures

We recruited 24 participants (11 male, 13 female) through personal contact. Participants were volunteer university students and people from various occupations who received no compensation. Their age ranged from 19 to 55 (M=30.50, SD=13.51).

We assessed video game use by asking participants to rate their frequency of video game use on a 7-point scale (1=never, 2=less than once a month, 3=about once a month, 4=several times a month, 5=several times a week, 6=every day for less than an hour, 7=every day for more than one hour). Mean rating was 3.38 (SD=1.86). Frequency of air travel was assessed by asking participants for their number of flights in the last two years. Answers ranged from 0 to 10 (M=2.63, SD=3.28).

To measure participants' knowledge about the brace position, we used 4 questions that asked them to describe where and how to position (i) hands, (ii) feet, (iii) safety belt, (iv) head. To avoid suggesting possible answers (e.g., as a multiple-choice questionnaire would do), participants were asked to answer orally the 4 questions and the answers were recorded.

To measure participants' locus of control with respect to emergency landing situations, we created a 12-item questionnaire, adapting items from the Aviation Safety Locus of Control Scale [14] by changing the context from the pilot's to the passenger's one. The items we used include statements such as "Surviving is a matter of luck, chance or fate" and "Most injuries and deaths are inevitable" to measure external orientation, or "Passengers can prevent injuries if they follow safety procedures" and "Some injuries are due to errors made by passengers" to measure internal orientation. Each item was rated by participants on a 7-point Likert scale (1=strongly disagree, 7=strongly agree). Answers to items for internal orientation (resp. external orientation) were averaged to form a reliable scale, Cronbach's alpha=.78 (resp .77).

We also measured risk perception by using the 6 questions employed by [9], changing the name of the risk into "emergency landing": vulnerability to risk was assessed by having respondents rate their vulnerability on 3 items (e.g., "how high do you believe your risk of being involved in an emergency landing is?") and severity of risk on the 3 other items (e.g., "how harmful would the consequences of an emergency landing be?"). Ratings were given on a 7-point Likert scale (1=not at all, 7=very). Answers to items for vulnerability (resp. severity) were averaged to form a reliable scale, Cronbach's alpha=.75 (resp .94).

Based on the considerations we described in Sections 3 and 4, we hypothesized that playing the game should increase player's knowledge about the brace position, increase his/her internal safety locus of control and decrease the external one. For risk perception, we did not expect changes in vulnerability since that should be more related to the traveling habits of participants. However, considering the vivid and possibly scary visualization of bodily damage to the player's avatar which is central to the studied game, we did expect an opposite trend with respect to [5]: playing the game could increase perception of risk severity, and we were interested in exploring to what extent this increase might occur.

5.2   Procedure

The study does not involve coercion or deceit and respects applicable professional code of conduct. Participants were told they were going to try a video game meant to illustrate the brace position passengers should assume during an emergency landing. They were told that they could use the game for as much time as they wanted without minimum or maximum limits. First, participants filled the demographic, locus of control, risk perception questionnaires, and answered the knowledge questions. Then, they played the game on a 15.6 inches LCD monitor with stereo speakers, without receiving any previous training or illustration of the game from the experimenter (this was done to check that the user interface was intuitive and immediately usable as planned). All the instructions for playing the game were contained in a brief text displayed as a starting screen. The text said: "You are going to face an emergency landing! Click and drag the 4 yellow icons with the mouse to choose a position you think is safe. When you're done, press CRASH!". When participants decided to stop playing, they filled the locus of control and risk perception questionnaires and answered the knowledge questions for the second time.

6   Results

The means for number of correctly answered knowledge questions are shown in Figure 5. Differences were analyzed with a non-parametric Wilcoxon test and confirmed our hypothesis: after playing the game, there was a statistically significant (Z=-4.40, p<0.001) and noteworthy increase in the number of correct answers which reached a value extremely close to the best one, moving from 1.08 (SD=.58) to 3.92 (SD=.28). In particular, 22 out of 24 participants reached the maximum number of correct answers (4), while the number for the remaining 2 participants was 3.

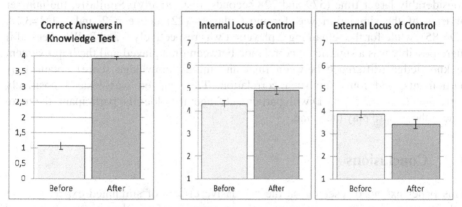

Fig. 5. Number of correctly answered knowledge questions and locus of control, before and after play. Capped vertical bars denote ±1 SE.

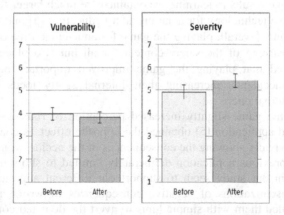

Fig. 6. Risk perception: vulnerability and severity, before and after play. Capped vertical bars denote ±1 SE.

Figure 5 also illustrates the means for locus of control. Differences were analyzed with ANOVA and confirmed our hypothesis: after playing the game, there was a statistically significant (F(1,23)=17.05, p<0.001) increase in internal orientation, which rose from 4.30 (SD=.80) to 4.91 (SD=.77). Consistently, there was a statistically significant (F(1,23)=7.58, p=0.01) decrease in external orientation, which moved from 3.88 (SD=.98) to 3.42 (SD=.98). In other words, participants felt the outcomes of an emergency landing were more under their personal control after playing the game.

The means for risk vulnerability and severity measures before and after the experience are shown in Figure 6. The obtained differences confirmed our hypothesis: after playing the game, there was no significant change in vulnerability perception, while there was a statistically significant ($F(1,23)=5.40$, $p<0.05$) although small increase in severity, which rose from 4.92 (SD=1.59) to 5.42 (SD=1.43).

Most participants (22) played the game for a time that varied between 145 and 389 seconds (M=241.38, SD=71.84). The remaining 2 participants played instead for a considerably larger time (579 and 728 seconds, respectively). Similarly, the number of tries of the simulation was for most players (22) between 2 and 5 (M=3.18, SD=.85), while for the remaining 2 players it was respectively 6 and 8. We checked if there possibly was a significant correlation between time played and the improvement in knowledge (difference between final and initial knowledge score) obtained by participants, and found no such correlation. Time played was instead positively correlated ($r(24)=.57$, $p<.01$) with participants' age: the older the participant, the more time (s)he took to play the game.

7 Conclusions

This paper extended research on the persuasive effects of simulated experiences of risk for aviation safety education in different directions. First, the experiment showed that a persuasive game that simulates a risk experience can be a very effective educational tool: the results in learning we obtained are much larger than the previous study on persuasive technology for aviation safety education [5] and extremely close to the ideal outcome. Overall, playing the game for an average time of just 4 minutes resulted in full learning of the safety content for all but two players. Second, the experiment showed that playing the game improved important players' attitudes towards aircraft accidents, increasing their internal safety locus of control and decreasing the external one.

The fact that the game slightly increased perception of risk severity, while the previously studied application [5] obtained the opposite effect, is consistent with our design choice of vividly showing the consequences of the accident on the passengers' body, while the previous application deliberately omitted to show them. The better results obtained in our study seem to support our different approach. We showed possibly scary visualizations of negative consequences of wrong actions, but we always accompanied them with simple hints to avert the depicted consequences. We illustrated the details of the recommended action with a simple interface that all participants were able to use immediately and provided clear simulations that highlight the effectiveness of right player's choices. The fact that all but two players fully learned all those details is an indication that we have likely succeeded. Moreover, the change in safety locus of control towards a more internal orientation indicates that participants felt more control over the outcome of an emergency landing after going through a sequence of virtual risk experiences with the game.

The results we have obtained go in a positive and opposite direction with respect to the previously mentioned limitations of traditional solutions, i.e. safety cards and briefings. We are anyway working at repeating the study with a group that is exposed to a traditional approach instead of the novel persuasive application, to precisely determine how large the differences between traditional and persuasive solutions to aviation safety education can be.

Another limitation of the study is that it considered only short-term effects. A longitudinal study aimed at measuring retention of knowledge and attitudes is needed.

After a few minor cosmetic improvements, our application has now entered a public beta-testing phase on Facebook (http://apps.facebook.com/learntobrace). Public accessibility of the game will also allow us to conduct remote evaluations that could possibly involve large, international and varied samples of players and to study their behavior in more naturalistic ways than laboratory studies.

Acknowledgements. This research is partially supported by a grant of the US Federal Aviation Administration (FAA).

We are grateful to Mac McLean (FAA Civil Aerospace Medical Institute) for his precious feedback and encouragement.

Nicola Zangrando (HCI Lab, University of Udine) carried out 3D modeling and computer programming activities for the development of the game.

References

1. Boeing: Statistical summary of commercial jet airplane accidents. Boeing, Seattle (2011), http://www.boeing.com/news/techissues/pdf/statsum.pdf
2. Chang, Y., Yang, H.: Cabin safety and emergency evacuation: Passenger experience of flight CI-120. Accident Analysis and Prevention 43, 1049–1055 (2011)
3. Cherry, R.G.W.: A Study Analyzing the Trends in Accidents and Fatalities in Large Transport Airplanes. Technical Report DOT/FAA/TC-13/46, Federal Aviation Administration, Washington, DC (2013)
4. Chang, Y., Liao, M.: The effect of aviation safety education on passenger cabin safety awareness. Safety Science 47, 1337–1345 (2009)
5. Chittaro, L.: Passengers' Safety in Aircraft Evacuations: Employing Serious Games to Educate and Persuade. In: Bang, M., Ragnemalm, E.L. (eds.) PERSUASIVE 2012. LNCS, vol. 7284, pp. 215–226. Springer, Heidelberg (2012)
6. Chittaro, L., Zangrando, N.: The Persuasive Power of Virtual Reality: Effects of Simulated Human Distress on Attitudes towards Fire Safety. In: Ploug, T., Hasle, P., Oinas-Kukkonen, H. (eds.) PERSUASIVE 2010. LNCS, vol. 6137, pp. 58–69. Springer, Heidelberg (2010)
7. Corbett, C.L., McLean, G.A., Cosper, D.K.: Effective Presentation Media for Passenger Safety I: Comprehension of Briefing Card Pictorials and Pictograms. Final Report DOT/FAA/AM-08/20, Federal Aviation Administration, Washington, DC (2008)
8. Cosper, D., McLean, G.: Availability of passenger safety information for improved survival in aircraft accidents. Technical Report DOT/FAA/AM-04/19, Federal Aviation Administration, Washington, DC (2004)
9. de Hoog, N., Stroebe, W., de Wit, J.B.F.: The processing of fear-arousing communications: How biased processing leads to persuasion. Social Influence 3(2), 84–113 (2008)

10. Floyd, D.L., Prentice-Dunn, S., Rogers, R.W.: A meta-analysis of research on protection motivation theory. Journal of Applied Social Psychology 30, 407–429 (2000)
11. Fogg, B.J.: Persuasive Technology: Using Computers to Change What We Think and Do. Morgan Kaufmann, San Francisco (2003)
12. Hoyt, M.F.: Internal–external control and beliefs about automobile travel. Journal of Research in Personality 7, 288–293 (1973)
13. Huang, J.L., Ford, J.K.: Driving locus of control and driving behaviors: Inducing change through driver training. Transportation Research Part F: Traffic Psychology and Behaviour 15, 358–368 (2012)
14. Hunter, D.R.: Development of an aviation safety locus of control scale. Aviation, Space, and Environmental Medicine 73, 1184–1188 (2002)
15. Hunter, D.R., Stewart, J.E.: Locus of Control, Risk Orientation, and Decision Making Among U.S. Army Aviators. Technical Report 1260, U.S. Army Research Institute for the Behavioral and Social Sciences, Fort Rucker, AL (2009)
16. Hunter, D.R., Stewart, J.E.: Safety Locus of Control and Accident Involvement Among Army Aviators. International Journal of Aviation Psychology 22, 144–163 (2012)
17. Jones, J.W., Wuebker, L.J.: Safety locus of control and employees' accidents. Journal of Business and Psychology 7, 449–457 (1993)
18. Meijnders, A., Midden, C., McCalley, T.: The Persuasive Power of Mediated Risk Experiences. In: IJsselsteijn, W.A., de Kort, Y.A.W., Midden, C., Eggen, B., van den Hoven, E. (eds.) PERSUASIVE 2006. LNCS, vol. 3962, pp. 50–54. Springer, Heidelberg (2006)
19. Montag, I., Comrey, A.L.: Internality and externality as correlates of involvement in fatal driving accidents. Journal of Applied Psychology 72, 339–343 (1987)
20. Muir, H., Thomas, L.: Passenger education: past and future. In: Proceedings of the 4th Triennial International Aircraft Fire and Cabin Safety Research Conference (2004)
21. Rogers, R.W.: Cognitive and physiological processes in fear appeals and attitude change: A revised theory of Protection Motivation. In: Cacioppo, J.T., Petty, R.E. (eds.) Social Psychophysiology: A Sourcebook, pp. 153–176. Guilford Press, New York (1983)
22. Rotter, J.B.: Social Learning and Clinical Psychology. Prentice-Hall, Englewood Cliffs (1954)
23. Ruiter, R.A.C., Abraham, C., Kok, G.: Scary warnings and rational precautions: a review of the psychology of fear appeals. Psychology and Health 16, 613–630 (2001)
24. Shahab, L., Hall, S., Marteau, T.: Showing smokers with vascular disease images of their arteries to motivate cessation: a pilot study. British Journal of Health Psychology 12, 275–283 (2007)
25. Taylor, A., Moorcroft, D., DeWeese, R.: Effect of passenger position on crash injury risk. In: Proceedings of the 7th Triennial International Fire & Cabin Safety Research Conference, Philadelphia, USA (2013)
26. Thomas, L.J.: Passenger Attention to Safety Information. In: Bor, R. (ed.) Passenger Behaviour, Ashgate, UK (2003)
27. U.S. Department of Transportation, Federal Aviation Administration: Advisory Circular AC 121-24B (1999)
28. Witte, K., Allen, M.: A meta-analysis of fear appeals: Implications for effective public health campaigns. Health Education and Behavior 27, 591–616 (2000)
29. Wuebker, L.J.: Safety locus of control as a predictor of industrial accidents and injuries. Journal of Business and Psychology 1, 19–30 (1986)
30. You, X., Ji, M., Han, H.: The effects of risk perception and flight experience on airline pilots' locus of control with regard to safety operation behaviors. Accident Analysis & Prevention 57, 131–139 (2013)
31. Zaalberg, R., Midden, C.: Enhancing Human Responses to Climate Change Risks through Simulated Flooding Experiences. In: Ploug, T., Hasle, P., Oinas-Kukkonen, H. (eds.) PERSUASIVE 2010. LNCS, vol. 6137, pp. 205–210. Springer, Heidelberg (2010)

What's Your 2%? A Pilot Study for Encouraging Physical Activity Using Persuasive Video and Social Media

Drew Clinkenbeard[*], Jennifer Clinkenbeard, Guillaume Faddoul, Heejung Kang, Sean Mayes, Alp Toygar, and Samir Chatterjee

Claremont Graduate University, 150 E 10th St.
Claremont, CA 91711
{drew.clinkenbeard,jennifer.clinkenbeard,guillaume.faddoul,
heejung.kang,sean.mayes,alp.toygar,samir.chatterjee}@cgu.edu

Abstract. The purpose of this study is to observe the response of a group of subjects towards a message persuading them to include   physical activities into their daily routine in order to improve and maintain their overall health. Our message, based on previous scientific studies, is in the form of short movie emphasizing that exercising during 2% of the day, or 30 min, is sufficient to remain in good health. The slogan, "What's Your 2%?" is appealing because "2%" is perceived as such a tiny fraction, yet it accurately reflects the 30-minute daily exercise goal as recommended by experts. This study uses persuasive techniques applied to a group of subjects composed of members of our personal Facebook networks, and this social network platform as way to communicate with them. We were able to demonstrate that changing a person's short-term exercise behavior is possible by using persuasive technology.

Keywords: physical health, two percent, exercise, persuasive messaging, social media, behavior change.

1   Introduction

"I'd really like to work out more, but I just don't have the time and energy." Does this sound familiar? Even at the best of times we often feel overextended between work, family, school, friends, and life in general. Many people agree that healthy behaviors are important, including "working out" on a regular basis. However, one of the major deterrents to engaging in these healthy behaviors is the perception that we just can't spare the time and energy necessary to do so.

The Mayo Clinic states that as a general goal, adults aged 18-64 should aim for at least 30 minutes of physical activity per day [10]. Although the Department of Health and Human Services identifies more specific objectives, most experts agree that 30 minutes per day is a healthy level of physical activity for this group irrespective of gender, race, ethnicity or income level. The exception to the rule is individuals with

---

[*] Corresponding author.

A. Spagnolli et al. (Eds.): PERSUASIVE 2014, LNCS 8462, pp. 43–55, 2014.
© Springer International Publishing Switzerland 2014

specific medical conditions limiting mobility [5] A recent study by the Center for Disease Control reports that 80% of American adults do not get the recommended amounts of exercise, potentially setting themselves up for years of health problems [1]. Major health problems linked to physical inactivity include obesity, Type II diabetes, and heart disease. A 2012 study linked physical inactivity to more than 5 million deaths worldwide per year--more than are caused by smoking [1]. Broadly speaking, we hope to increase physical activity among a pilot user group to healthy levels as recommended by the Mayo Clinic. Specifically, our goals are to:

1) Reframe the context and time commitment for healthy levels of physical activity;
2) Provide a trigger mechanism using the modern technology of digital video and social media;
3) Evaluate the efficacy of the trigger among a pilot user group.

To accomplish these goals, we design an intervention using a combined approach of digital video and daily messaging for three days. We use Facebook as the platform for both disseminating the video and sending the daily messages. We respected professsional code of conduct by confining the study to voluntary adult participants who participated in good faith, willingly and without coercion. Our study asks that users watch the video and fill out a short survey immediately following the viewing. Then, we encourage users to "like" the Facebook page, which will then include them in our pilot user group for daily messaging for three days. At the end of these three days, the pilot user group is given a post-survey.

Our project is centered around a slogan, similar to the hugely successful "got milk" campaign of the 1990s and 2000s [3]. We express the recommended amount of exercise (30 minutes daily) as a percentage of minutes in a day (24 hours x 60 minutes = 1440 minutes). Since 30/1440 =.02083, 30 minutes is roughly equivalent to 2% of a person's day (30 minutes a day equals to 2%). Based on this calculation, we coined the phrase, "What's Your Two Percent?" This slogan is intended to reframe the amount of time and energy necessary for healthy levels of physical activity in the user's mind, as well as to personalize the user's experience. The slogan is appealing because "2%" is perceived as such a tiny fraction, yet it accurately reflects the 30-minute daily exercise goal as recommended by experts. We use this slogan ubiquitously through all stages of our study.

We define our target audience as adults aged 18-64 without mobility or other health restrictions that self-identify as thinking that exercise is important (motivation present), but that they do not have the time/energy (low ability and missing trigger). Targeted users either 1) do not consciously engage in physical activity at all; or 2) engage in physical activities sporadically, but do not consistently exercise for 30 minutes per day on a regular basis. The targeted behavior is that for the three days watching the video and "liking" the page, the user will engage in 30 minutes per day or equivalent of moderate physical activity.

Physical activity is defined as any bodily movement produced by skeletal muscles that require energy expenditure [7]. World Health Organization identifies that for adults aged 18–64, physical activity includes physical activity for pleasure (for example: walking, dancing, gardening, hiking, swimming), transportation (e.g. walking or cycling), occupational (i.e. work), household chores, play, games, sports or planned exercise, in the context of daily, family, and community activities [7]. It is important to note that part of our first goal to is to reframe the perception of physical activity to include regular daily activities such as walking, chores, and play. Also, we do not measure the intensity level of the physical activity performed by the targeted user group; rather, the goal is for the user to engage in what he/she considers to be appropriate levels of activity.

In the next section, we review relevant literature. In particular, we study psychological variables, goal setting-considerations, and dissemination platforms associated with a persuasive technology based physical activity intervention.

2   Literature Review

We review papers about how persuasive technology can play a significant role in encouraging people with an inactive lifestyle to perform daily-life physical activity. First, in Lacroix et al. [6], we see that stressing that modern technology has a great advantage in persuasive behavior change interventions because it provides user-tailored interaction. The authors argue that, in order to produce tailored technology-based activity interventions in an effective way, it is significant to consider three cognitive variables that are key factors for the change and continuation of health behavior: 1) behavioral regulation, 2) types of motives, and 3) self-efficacy [6]. This argument is based on the result of their study which indicates that active individuals show "higher levels of self-determined behavioral regulation for daily-life activity," have "stronger motives to be active," and reach "higher levels of self-efficacy for physical activity" than inactive individuals [6]. Regarding the different result between inactive and active individuals on the cognitive variables, our video is designed to show a clear contrast between them and lead inactive individuals to generate and internalize the three cognitions that are important for the realization of daily physical activity.

In their paper "Goal Setting Considerations for Persuasive Technologies that Encourage Physical Activity", Consolvo et al. contend that goal-setting can be a useful strategy in persuasive technology that focuses on motivating individuals to have an active lifestyle [11]. Lock and Latham's goal-setting theory explains the way to establish goals to encourage behavior change by paying much attention to "the relationship between conscious performance goal and level of task performance". According to Lock and Latham, there are two elements that mainly influences goal performance: (1) the significance of goal achievement to the individual and (2) self-efficacy. Thus, when applying goal-setting theory to persuasive technologies whose aim is to encourage regular physical activity, the target audience should consist of the individuals who consider being physically active important [11]. Physical activity recommendations should propose specific and unambiguous goals. The goal should be something realizable and achievable to the individuals. Incentives or feedback should be offered to the individuals when they attain or exceed their goals. As an example of the use of goal-setting in technology-based physical activity interventions, the authors introduce another study in which the daily assigned goal for the individuals is to get at least seven "lifestyle points" each day by "doing 10 minutes of moderate physical activity" [11].

The key phrase, "What's Your Two Percent?" conveys that achieving a healthy level of daily exercise is a reasonable goal. The small amount of time necessary for "your two percent" is key to a person's belief that they can attain the goal. Behavioral psychologists Locke & Latham identify this as one of the two key factors that facilitates goal commitment [12].

In Serapio et al's literature, we found an effective way to distribute our video to target audience and provide them with feedback [2]. According to the authors, popular social networks such as Facebook can be powerful distribution environments for a video campaign. In their case study on a month video campaign of a popular consumer food brand (the CFB) distributed through Facebook, the authors found that the CFB campaign achieved a 1.5% clickthrough rate on Facebook. The rate was much higher than an average 0.37% clickthrough rate from a sample of 20 campaigns distributed through non-Facebook, non-social network websites. The success of CFB campaign resulted from the multiple tunnels that Facebook produced when a user join the campaign. First, a one-line notice appeared on the Facebook profile and the Facebook homepages functioned as a link to the CFB's video campaign. Second, the Invite tool led users to send a video link to their Facebook friends. Third, the CFB's Facebook application allowed users to save CFB campaign boxes to their Facebook profiles. For these reasons, Serapio et al argue that designers should consider social networks as an effective video distribution channel and make use of their beneficial features of "such tunnel maximization or entry-point maximization"[2]. For these reasons, we decided to take advantage of Facebook as a distribution channel for our video. In the next section, we describe the steps that we took to address the problem identified in Section 1.

3   Methods

In this section, we describe our solution to the problem identified in Section 1 and its implementation with a combination of a persuasive video and daily messages using Facebook.

First, we filmed a video for the purpose of promoting it to friends and family via Facebook. The video can be viewed at http://www.youtube.com/watch?v=dwX 5wnCsXLc&feature=youtu.be. The video begins by showing a "lazy" character going about her daily business, while avoiding physical activity by parking as close as possible to the store and ignoring the stairs in favor of an elevator. It then cuts to this character at home sitting on her couch, having a conversation with a friend about how a "2% off sale" is not very significant. Her friend notes that the amount of time necessary to exercise each day is just thirty minutes, or two percent of her day. She responds that she just doesn't have the time and energy to work out. As her friend tries to convince her that minor changes to her behavior can make a big difference in her health, a "doctor" in a lab coat shows up at the door and corroborates her friend's information. While he is explaining that 30 minutes of daily exercise is all it will take for her to be healthier, a superhero-type man in a cape comes to the door. He introduces himself to the flabbergasted character as "the two percent!" and encourages her to find simple ways to "get her two percent." The lazy character then notices that her house is full of people, and says she will consider it but that they all need to go. The video then cuts to clips of her incorporating exercise into her daily routine, such as taking the stairs and parking at the back of a large lot. The video ends with the "lazy" character and her friend having a conversation about how much better she feels and how easy it was for her to fit in short exercises into her daily routine. They discuss the importance of physical activity, citing a popular celebrity's recent announcement of

Type II diabetes. As they leave to go on a hike together, they wonder together who the doctor and the guy in the cape were.

After the video was complete, the members of the research team each posted a status update to their own personal Facebook page asking family and friends to participate in a small study at Claremont Graduate University. In this post, a link to the page with the video and immediate survey was given, as well as directions for participants and reassurance that the information provided would be confidential and used only for this project. The link takes the user to the Facebook page "What's Your Two Percent?" where the video is posted along with four follow-up questions (see Appendix I). At the bottom of the page, the user is encouraged to "like" the page or provide their email address for three days of daily messages and a follow-up survey. We promoted the page on Wednesday, November 6, 2013, starting at about 10:00 am.

During the following three days, the CGU team posted one message per day to the Facebook page. For users who had "liked" the page, this message showed up in their personal news feed (see Appendix I). The messages are as follows:

1) Today is the first day of the 2% challenge! You can do it!
   (Posted Thursday, November 7, 2013 at 9:20 am)
2) Did you get your 2% today? One more day left in the challenge. Finish strong!
   (Posted Friday, November 8, 2013 at 5:20 pm)
3) Today is the last day of the challenge. How will you get your 2% today?
   (Posted Saturday, November 9, 2013 at 8:50 am)

We deliberately chose to vary the times that the messages were posted in the hopes that as different people checked their news feeds at different times, we would reach as many people as possible with each post. On Sunday, November 10, at 12:45 pm, we posted a link to the follow-up survey, asking participants to take the survey and complete the challenge. The survey was 10 questions long and included several Likert-style questions, "check all that apply" questions, and a free-response (see Appendix I). This link was also sent via email to those who had chosen to provide email addresses.

The completion of the follow-up survey ended the "challenge" for the user. Although we hope that participation in the study will have a long-term effect on users, our study was complete at this point. In the next section, we analyze the methods presented here within the context of theories, techniques, and best practices for persuasive technologies.

4   Analysis of Methods

After our group had identified the problem, we took into account the theories, techniques, and best practices associated with persuasive technology in order to design and implement the methods described in the previous section. We identified the desired outcome as response-changing [8]. We want to replace the belief that the user is too busy to exercise with the belief that the user has the ability to do so. This ties in with Fogg's B=MAT theory [9]. We targeted users with medium to high motivation who think that the behavior is too difficult or time-consuming to do.

The desired behavior is defined as 30 minutes per day of physical exercise for the three days of the study. This corresponds to a "green span" or purple span" behavior in Fogg's behavior grid [9]. The motivation is the desire to be healthier. In the targeted user group, this motivation already exists at a medium to high level. However, the ability and trigger are at a low level. The ability is addressed by the constant reframing of the requirements of healthy levels of physical activity, emphasizing that two percent of a person's day is not very much at all. The trigger comes in the form of the video, the immediate survey, encouraging the user to "like" the page to participate, the daily messages, and the follow-up survey three days later. We intentionally posted consistently throughout the study time period, but limited posts to once per day in order to not "turn off" users or annoy them. By increasing ability and providing consistent triggers for a group that already had at least medium motivation, we help the user to perform the desired behavior.

Although we did not limit anyone from participating, we identify our target user group by the following questions/responses on the immediate survey below. We will assess the behavior of this group in the following section.

Targeted Users	
Question	**Response**
Are you between the ages of 18 and 64?	Yes
Do you want to exercise, but feel you don't have the time or energy?	Somewhat agree Strongly Agree
Are you already getting your 2% exercise on a regular basis?	No, never Once in a while Sometimes Usually

Fig. 1. Targeted Users

As we designed the tools for this target group, we considered the functional triad [9]. First, we considered the framework as a tool. We employed tunneling by putting the immediate survey on the same page with the video. We also utilized reduction by making it easy to "like" the page and therefore receive the messages and participate in the study. We tailored the suggestions for our target user group. For example, an avid exerciser would not necessarily be swayed by the focus on day-to-day activities or on the short amount of time required. Similarly, a person with no pre-existing motivation would not be affected, because they would have not identified exercise as important to their health. Second, we chose Facebook as the medium because it is a familiar communication platform with a significant social aspect. The user did not have to engage in any new behavior in order to participate in the study, because they are already Facebook users. Third, we addressed social acting in our methods. We chose to use humor and relatability as psychological cues in the video. In the surveys and daily messages, we considered social dynamics by keeping the surveys short, sending encouraging (positive conditioning) and short messages, and signed the messages "CGU team." Because it was our family and friends participating in the study, this was an especially important dimension to address because the user was partially motivated to participate because of his/her existing relationship with the researcher.

During the three days of the study, we are helping to move a person from the "preparation" stage to the "action" stage in the trans-theoretical model [9]. After the study, it is the user's responsibility to maintain the behavior. However, we hope that engaging in healthy behaviors even for a short period of time will help to induce replacing the attitude of inability with one of empowerment. Although the process of attitude change happens over a much longer span of time than our study allows for, we designed our slogan, "What's Your Two Percent?" to be short and catchy in the hopes that the user will remember it at opportune times and self-motivate in the future.

5   Limitations of the Study

It is important to note that there were significant limitations associated with this study. First, due to time constraints, we were not able to validate the measures used in the survey. Second, all data was self-reported. Problems inherent to self-reported data may include exaggeration, under-reporting, or biases such as social desirability bias. Third, we used a convenience sampling of family and friends that were willing to participate in the study, rather than true random sampling methods. We did this in order to reach as many people as possible. We also did not "exclude" people from participating based current motivation levels or current activity levels for the same reason. However, we do separate the data associated with the users that are not part of the intended target audience in the data analysis section.

We were not able to actually monitor the activity levels of participants, nor did we inquire as to the intensity of the exercise they completed. When we asked people about their exercise levels on the days of the study, they had a binary choice of "Yes, I got my 2% today" versus "No, I did not get my 2% today." We considered asking follow-up questions of participants who indicated that they did not "get their 2%" to find out if they exercised 10 or 20 minutes, rather than the full 30. However, we did not have a way of asking this question only of some users and not others, and we felt it could distract from our goal of continually reinforcing the mental reframing that 30 minutes of exercise daily is a reasonable and attainable amount.

In the interest of keeping the questionnaires positively oriented and non-invasive, we did not ask about the control for other factors that could have happened during the time of the study that might have influenced the user's behavior. Therefore, any results simply show a correlation (not cause-and-effect relationship) between the time period that the user was participating and the user's reported behaviors.

Finally, we also acknowledge that any results are based on reporting over a very short duration of time. Although it would have been preferable to study the subjects over a longer period of time, even a short-term behavior change is a desirable outcome, as evidenced in Dr. BJ Fogg's Behavior Grid [13].

In the next section, we evaluate the pilot study described in Section 3 using quantitative and qualitative data analysis techniques.

6   Results

Reach:

Tool	Reach
Video	79 Views
Facebook page "What's Your Two Percent?"	51 "likes" 54 people talking about this
Immediate survey	61 Respondents
Daily Post Views	Thursday: 63 Friday: 58 Saturday: 51
Daily Post "Likes"	Thursday: 4 Friday: 4 Saturday: 4
Follow-up Survey	20 respondents

Fig. 2. Reach results

User Comments on Daily Posts:
- Teaching 4 yoga classes and hill walking.
- Already did it!
- Walked around Target carrying 15 pound Wyatt [baby] for one hour and then pushed Dylan [small child] on the swing so did mine.
- Walking my dog is how I get my 2% every day! He's my furry little exercise coach!

Do you want to exercise, but feel you don't have the time or the energy?

Do you already get your 2% exercise on a regular basis?

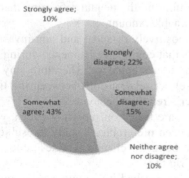
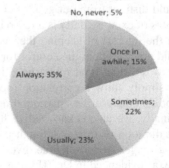

Fig. 3. Immediate survey results

Immediate Survey Results
Of the 61 respondents, 60 of them indicated that they were between the ages of 18 and 64. 58 of the 61 respondents pledged to get their 2% for the next three days. Of the 61 respondents, 30 of them fell into our target user category in both aspects described in Section 3.

Follow Up Survey Results
The follow-up survey questions were designed to assess the user's ability, motivation, trigger, and behavior during the three days of the study. Twenty people responded to this survey. The significant drop-off in participants is likely because the follow-up survey was only available for about 48 hours due to time constraints. 20 participants from the original 60 responded to the follow up survey.

Ability

Watching the 2% video helped me to mentally reframe the time and energy necessary for healthy levels of physical activity.	The daily Facebook messages were rewarding because they were positive and encouraging.

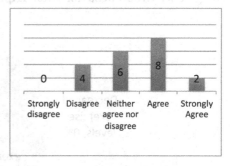

Fig. 4. Follow up survey: Ability results

Trigger	Motivation
The daily Facebook messages acted as a "trigger" for me to get out and get my 2% that day.	Watching the 2% video was a good reminder for me about the importance of daily exercise.

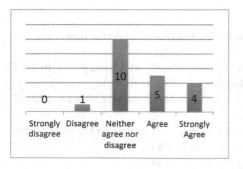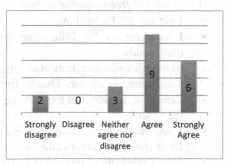

Fig. 5. Follow up survey: Trigger and motivation results

Behavior

Respondents in Targeted User Group: Reported less than 30 minutes daily exercise prior to study		Respondents not in Targeted User Group: Reported 30 minutes or more daily exercise prior to study	
10 respondents		10 respondents	
7 reported increase in exercise	3 reported maintaining exercise	1 reported increase in exercise	9 reported maintaining exercise

Fig. 6. Follow up survey: Behavior results

None of the twenty users reported a decrease in exercise behavior after viewing the video and receiving the Facebook messages. Of the targeted user group, 70% of them reported an increase in exercise after participating in the study.

Target User Group Behavior After Exposure to Video and Messages

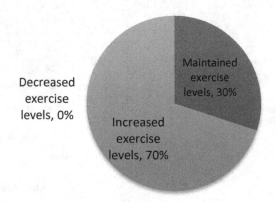

Fig. 7. Follow up survey: Targeted user group behavior results

User Comments in free response section
- I got my 2% by walking.
- Easy to get my 2%. I did more than the 30 minutes of exercise just doing my daily routine.
- My health is more important than my schoolwork so I always try to find some time to exercise. Thanks for the daily reminders though!
- I exercise already, but the messages gave me a better attitude about it. I loved the video!
- I was unable to exercise 30 minutes each day, but I parked in the back of the lot at shopping centers and took a walk after lunch on Friday.
- Now I think about the video when I'm in the elevator.
- I don't know if I hit 2%, but I parked farther away than I normally would.

7   Discussion of Results

Our results show a positive response to the combination approach of video and daily messaging via Facebook. By measuring the "reach" of the video and posts, we saw that a relatively large number of people viewed the video and posts. The positive comments and "likes" showed that in general, people responded positively to this study. We also saw a positive effect on the users in both the immediate survey and in the follow-up survey. In the immediate survey, almost everyone committed to "getting their two percent" for the next three days. Although the number of respondents was lower for the follow-up survey, the responses continued to be quite positive and showed a significant increase in exercise activity.

An interesting result in both surveys was the proportion of people that reported they were already exercising for 30 minutes per day or more. This was not consistent with the national reports that 80% of people do not exercise this much. There could be several reasons for this. First, because the data was self-reported, it is possible that people exercise less than reported. Second, it could have been a self-selecting group because it was optional to participate; people who did not exercise already may not have been as inclined to "take the challenge." Third, the survey was distributed over a short period of time to a generally relatively active group of people. In this sense, the convenience sampling may have skewed the results.

In general, the user responses to this project were very positive. Family and friends continue to reference "my two percent" and have indicated that they found the experience of participating in the study fun and enjoyable. Several people indicated that they thought it was a great slogan for a larger fitness ad campaign. Of all of the participants, no one decreased their exercise levels; and all of those identified in our target audience increased.

8   Conclusions and Future Work

By using a combination approach of digital video and daily messages disseminated via Facebook, we carried out a pilot study for the purpose of persuading people to engage in healthy levels of physical activity. We found that this approach had a positive effect on participant's short-term behavior. The main components of our approach were a simple and catchy slogan, a funny yet informative short digital video, encouraging people to "like" the page, and sending short messages via Facebook. The positive response, as evidenced in both our quantitative and qualitative data, shows that Facebook is a powerful platform for technology-mediated behavior change.

The findings of this study could be corroborated and refined through additional work. First, a larger post-survey sample would have allowed for more statistical analysis. Second, common research practices for large studies, such as random sampling, user monitoring, and a longer trial period, would help to strengthen the result. Finally, it would be interesting to study the effect of other mediums on the persuasive capacity of the slogan (advertisements, mobile app, Web site, etc). In the future, we plan to implement a Web site for this purpose, with more specific information tailored to the participant's currently reported level of physical activity.

References

[1] Jaslow, R.: CDC: 80 percent of American adults don't get recommended exercise, http://www.cbsnews.com (May 3, 2013)

[2] Serapio, N., Fogg, B.: Designing for video engagement on social networks: a video marketing case study, p. 1 (2009)

[3] Got Milk?, Wikipedia, the free encyclopedia (November 6, 2013)

[4] Chatterjee, S.: ACM Digital Library. In: Proceedings of the 4th International Conference on Persuasive Technology. ACM, New York (2009)

[5] Services, H.: Two Thousand Eight Physical Activity Guidelines for Americans: Be Active, Healthy, and Happy. Government Printing Office (2008)

[6] Lacroix, J., Saini, P., Goris, A.: Understanding user cognitions to guide the tailoring of persuasive technology-based physical activity interventions. In: Proceedings of the 4th International Conference on Persuasive Technology, New York, NY, USA, pp. 9:1–9:8 (2009)

[7] WHO | Physical activity, WHO, http://www.who.int/topics/physical_activity/en/ (accessed November 11, 2013)

[8] Dillard, J., Shen, L.: The Sage Handbook of Persuasion: Development in Theory and Practice, 2nd edn. Sage, Los Angeles (2013)

[9] Fogg, B.: Persuasive Technology: Using Computers to Change What We Think and Do. Morgan Kaufman Publishers, San Francisco (2003)

[10] Edward, R., Laskowski, M.D.: Exercise: How much do I need each day?, http://www.mayoclinic.com/health/exercise/AN01713

[11] Consolvo, S., Klasnja, P., McDonald, D.W., Landay, J.A.: Goal-setting Considerations for Persuasive Technologies That Encourage Physical Activity. In: Proceedings of the 4th International Conference on Persuasive Technology, New York, NY, USA, pp. 8:1–8:8 (2009)

[12] Locke, E.A., Latham, G.P.: Building a practically useful theory of goal setting and task motivation: A 35-year odyssey. American Psychologist 57(9), 705–717 (2002)

[13] Fogg, B.: Behavior Grid, http://www.behaviorgrid.org/ (accessed November 15, 2013)

Appendix I

A.1   Immediate Survey

1. Are you between the ages of 18 and 64?
   - o   Yes
   - o   No
2. Do you want to exercise, but feel you don't have the time or energy?
   - o   Strongly agree
   - o   Somewhat agree
   - o   Neither agree nor disagree
   - o   Somewhat disagree
   - o   Strongly disagree
3. Are you already getting your 2% exercise on a regular basis?
   - o   No, never
   - o   Once in a while
   - o   Sometimes
   - o   Usually
   - o   Always
4. Will you pledge to get your 2% for the next three days?
   - o   Yes
   - o   No

Please like this Facebook page or enter your email address below to take a follow up survey in three days.

A.2   Follow Up Survey

Thank you for participating in our project! We appreciate your time and effort. We had a tremendous amount of support from our friends and family, and we will put some summary data on the site soon so that you can see our results. We hope that you will continue to get your 2%! This survey is 9 questions long, and will take you about 5-10 minutes to complete. It is important to this study that you respond honestly. Your response will be kept confidential to the extent allowed by the law.

1. Watching the 2% video was a good reminder for me about the importance of daily exercise.
    - o Strongly agree
    - o Somewhat agree
    - o Neither agree nor disagree
    - o Somewhat disagree
    - o Strongly disagree

2. Watching the 2% video helped me to mentally reframe the time and energy necessary for healthy levels of physical activity.
    - o Strongly agree
    - o Somewhat agree
    - o Neither agree nor disagree
    - o Somewhat disagree
    - o Strongly disagree

3. The daily Facebook messages were a good reminder for me to get my 2% that day.
    - o Strongly agree
    - o Somewhat agree
    - o Neither agree nor disagree
    - o Somewhat disagree
    - o Strongly disagree

4. The daily Facebook messages were rewarding because they were positive and encouraging
    - o Strongly agree
    - o Somewhat agree
    - o Neither agree nor disagree
    - o Somewhat disagree
    - o Strongly disagree

5. The daily Facebook messages acted as a "trigger" for me to get out and get my 2% that day.
    - o Strongly agree
    - o Somewhat agree
    - o Neither agree nor disagree
    - o Somewhat disagree
    - o Strongly disagree

6. As a result of my participation, I have
    - o Completely stopped exercising
    - o Decreased my daily exercise levels
    - o Continued exercising as I did before
    - o Increased my daily exercise levels
    - o Begun exercising, which I did not do before

7. Which daily messages did you see in your Facebook news feed or notifications? Please check all that apply.
    - o Thursday: Today is the first day of the 2% challenge! You can do it!
    - o Friday: Did you get your 2% today? One more day left in the challenge. Finish strong!
    - o Saturday: Today is the last day for the challenge. How will you get your 2% today?

8. On which days that you saw the daily message did you exercise for at least 30 minutes? Check all that apply.
    - o Friday
    - o Saturday
    - o Sunday

9. (Free response) Please share any thoughts, comments, or additional information. For example, what did you do to get your 2% during these three days? How difficult was it for you to get your 2% each day? Were you able to exercise, but not for the full 2% (i.e., for 10 minutes per day)?

--Thank you from the CGU team!

The Effect of Credibility of Host Site Upon Click Rate through Sponsored Content

Martin Colbert, Adam Oliver, and Eleni Oikonomou

Computing and Information Systems, Kingston University London, Penrhyn Road,
Kingston upon Thames, United Kingdom
m.colbert@kingston.ac.uk, {adjamo,eco.eleni}@gmail.com

Abstract. This paper demonstrates the effect of website credibility upon the click rate through Sponsored Content. The study compares three versions of a live website - high, medium and low credibility – and collects quantitative data from traffic logs, and qualitative data from remote usability tests. The high credibility version of the website achieved a significantly higher click rate through sponsored Content, because the site's credibility encouraged visitors to explore the site for longer, and because the perception of the site overall 'rubbed off' on the perception of the Sponsored Content in particular (a halo effect). This finding is important, because it shows how site design and content creation may increase persuasiveness *without* impairing user experience – there is an alternative to Banners and Banner blindness! We hope the paper helps the on-going rethink of the design of online publications in relation to their underlying business models.

Keywords: advertisement, sponsored content, click through rate, traffic study, remote usability test, credibility, halo effect.

1   Introduction and Background

In the 'free content paid by ads' business model, visitors are attracted to content in online publications, shown advertisements, and the publisher then receives payment for each click through an advert. For this model to succeed, the publication must *both* persuade many users to click through adverts *and* provide a great user experience in appropriate balance. This way, it generates income and encourages visitors to return.

The kind of advert most commonly used to realise this model is perhaps the Display Advert. Display adverts, here, include 'Banners' - large, possibly animated images – and 'Text Ads' – title, snippet and destination URL. To include Display Adverts in a publication, a publisher defines the size, shape, and placement of adverts to be displayed on the page. An advertising network then programmatically selects and serves up particular adverts to display. Guidelines for the selection, design and placement of Display Adverts are widely available [1][2][3][4]. A well-known limitation of Display Adverts is 'banner blindness' - web users often find Display Adverts irrelevant, so they gradually learn to exclude them from conscious awareness [5][6][7]. Consequently, the Click Through Rate (CTR) for Banners and Text Ads

A. Spagnolli et al. (Eds.): PERSUASIVE 2014, LNCS 8462, pp. 56–67, 2014.

tends to be very low - typically, less than 1% [8][9][3]. Further, if excluding Display Adverts from conscious awareness requires too much effort from visitors, the overall user experience is also impaired – Banners are perceived as 'annoying' or 'intrusive' [10][11][12]. Developments in advertising technology are improving Display Advert performance by tailoring ads to the visitor. For example, in a lab test of a system that used behavioural targeting, Yan et al report a six-fold increase in CTR [13]. Also, Chen and Canny report a two-fold increase in CTR in a field test of an EBay recommender system [14]. However, although tailoring appears to increase CTR, its implications for user experience appear complex and context-dependent. For example, a recent structured interview study of American Internet users suggested that, while many perceive the benefits of tailored advertising, many also believe that notice and choice mechanisms do not necessarily reach visitors [15]. Another study suggested that users are in principle willing to share selected information about themselves for certain purposes and to devote effort to managing privacy and profile settings [16]. However, a survey by Purcell suggested most search engine users are 'not okay' with the collection personal information, for the purposes of personalizing search results and advertising[17].

Given these limitations, there is growing interest in other kinds of persuasive page element, including Sponsored Content, the focus of this paper. Sponsored Content is information paid for by a sponsor that is so relevant to a publication's 'organic' or 'editorial' content (the articles), and so informative for the visitor, that it may be embedded within the article. The Sponsored Content completes a coherent body of information. An off-line example is the Jamaica Shell Road Map [18]. This indexed, 1:250,000 scale map presents Jamaica's topography, natural parks, and parish boundaries, plus road information, tourist sites and civic buildings based on data from the island's Land Information Council. Additionally, it also marks the location of Shell petrol stations – relevant, helpful waypoints for tourists travelling by car.

On the Internet, Sponsored Content is most often encountered in sites affiliated with online marketplaces, such as Amazon and EBay. Often small, independent sites, affiliates refer their visitors to stores and auctions within the marketplace, and are paid per click. For example, an affiliate site may include an article about the life and works of designer and architect Charles Rennie Mackintosh. The article may include a list of Mackintosh reproduction items in manufacture today. Each item on this list links to a store within a marketplace that sells that item of furniture.

Affiliate marketing programmes are growing rapidly, so it is worth investigating some of the design challenges that Sponsored Content poses. One challenge is the optimization of the publication's articles, Sponsored Content and destination URL in order to achieve the most appropriate balance of CTR and user experience. Optimisation is important, because it is closely tied to revenue. Optimisation is also challenging, because the design of the Sponsored Content is highly constrained by the online publication in which it is embedded. The information provided in Sponsored Content must be highly relevant and informative with respect to the host article – this is an ethical precondition for embedding Sponsored Content within an article [1]. Also, and again for ethical reasons, the form of Sponsored Content must be visually distinct from editorial content [1]. However, provided this distinction is made,

Sponsored Content should also support the visual unity and coherence of the page, and so it is often visually similar to editorial content, to ensure consistency, and to cue relevance.

Given these somewhat tight constraints, what can a publisher do to enhance CTR and user experience? The form and content of Display Adverts can be adjusted, for example, to become more eye-catching, or to include the same words as the user's query [19], but for Sponsored Content, these options may be excluded by the constraints. The response explored in this paper is to change the *context* in which visitors interact with Sponsored Content, that is, to change what is around the advert (the surrounding page, the surrounding publication, the task context, the user context, etc.), rather than the advert itself.

1.1   Site Quality and Halo Effects

A first step in this response is to identify context factors with the potential to affect CTR without impairing user experience. A review of the literature identified the credibility of the website as one such factor. Credibility – trustworthiness and expertise – has emerged as a key quality of online information [25]. It may affect the performance of Sponsored Content, because of 'halo effects' - judgement biases, in which a user's global perception of an entity influences their perception of specific attributes [20][21]. This bias may occur without the user being aware of their bias, and even when the user has ample opportunity to observe specific attributes independently and accurately. Halo effects are widely applied in traditional marketing, for example, when an established brand is used to encourage sales of an unfamiliar product, and when a tarnished company uses sponsorship of a well-liked cause to rebuild relationships with clients [22]. In principle, halo effects may also occur online. For example, if a user perceives the overall website positively, then display adverts specifically might also be perceived positively, and so be clicked through more often. Such an effect has been recently demonstrated online in relation to Banners [11][23], and the credibility of electronic Word of Mouth systems has been shown to effects their persuasiveness [26]. However, the behavior that brings about these effects was not examined in detail. Also, the exact conditions under which halo effects arise, and the strength of any effect, remains a topic for debate [24], and the perception of online information may be unlike the perception of individuals. There is value, then, in demonstrating halo effects in relation to Sponsored Content, and focusing on credibility in particular.

2   Aim

The aim of this work is to demonstrate that website credibility can affect the CTR and user experience of Sponsored Content via halo effects. The work focuses upon website credibility – the more trustworthy and expert the site overall, the more these qualities will 'rub off' on the Sponsored Content in particular, and so CTR will increase. Greater credibility may also improve the user experience – it is certainly unlikely to reduce it.

3 Research Strategy

3.1 Method

We pursued these aims by studying the use of multiple versions of a live website developed for the purposes of this research. The study obtained quantitative data from traffic logs, and qualitative data from a remote usability test. The traffic log collected data unobtrusively, and in the context of everyday Internet use. This is important when studying discretionary, situated behaviours such as persuasion, engagement, and diversion. The remote usability tests provided a rich set of qualitative data about user perception and decision-making - video-recordings of interaction, plus a live, verbal commentary from the participant, followed by a survey of perceptions and feelings about the experience. This data gave insight into the mental processing that lay behind the user actions detected by the log, and so helped to interpret the log correctly.

The traffic log and remote usability test were conducted separately, and involved different participants. Separate tests had the benefit that the experience of the website remained 'natural' and 'free', and not interrupted by pop-up invitations to take part in usability tests, which would have distorted log data. Usability tests were conducted remotely, in order to recruit participants from around the globe, not just our locality.

The research involved the following stages:

i. build a website that includes Sponsored Content.

Then, for each study:

ii. create multiple versions of the site, as required;
iii. recruit visitors to the site;
iv. gather traffic data;
v. conduct a remote usability test. Observe user behavior, listen to user comments and develop explanations for traffic data;
vi. analyse video tapes. Quantify user behavior and perceptions to support explanations;

Our attempts to obtain feedback from actual visitors after the log study had been completed by using on-page polls and pop-up questionnaires and nominal incentives (an alternative phase (v)), were not successful. Visitor participation rates were less than 1%, and although such rates are not uncommon on the Internet, they were too low to collect enough data from our low volume research website.

3.2 Research Vehicle Website

Both studies concerned the same website - an online bicycle maintenance manual for everyday cyclists. The site comprised a home page, and ten article pages. Each article describes how to carry out one common bicycle repair task, step by step, using text and images (see Figure 1). The site normally attracts around 50 visitors per month.

On each repair page was a subsection called 'Buy Kit?'. The 'Buy Kit?' section contained one line of editorial text ('Tools you need for this fix.'), and then, embedded in the article, Sponsored Content about purchasing the tools required, comprising a picture of the tool, a sponsored link, and the shop's brand logo. The sponsored link comprised a title, such as 'Buy a pedal spanner', tag text - 'Comprehensive range of quality products' - and a destination URL e.g. www.wiggle.co.uk/pedal_spanners (a page showing the tool for sale from an actual online store). This content resembled traditional Sponsored Links, and the kind of page elements that can be created within affiliate advertising programs. The Sponsored Content is distinguished from editorial content by a different background colour and the heading 'Sponsored Links selected by Bike Fixer' ('Bike Fixer' is the author of the article).

The store brand logo was included to increase visitor recognition and reassurance, and so encourage clicks. A picture of the tool was included to clearly provide relevant information. The overall appearance of the Sponsored Content on the page 'tunneled' readers from the top of the article, down towards this section, without disturbing on-page search. The image of the tool, the shop logo, and the background colour increases the visual emphasis of Sponsored Content, but only gently. Also, the background colour does not grab user attention, or suggest that this section is somehow irrelevant to the article, or entirely separate from it.

3.3   Relationship between Sponsored and Editorial Content

Only content promoting the sale of the tools required to carry out the repair task described in the article was included. This ensured that Sponsored Content was always relevant, since, to comprehend the instructional article, and to carry out the instructions, it is necessary to comprehend the term for the tool - to comprehend the instruction, 'Loosen the spoke nut using a spoke key', it is necessary to comprehend the term 'spoke key'. High relevance was confirmed in a pilot study, by qualitative comments about Sponsored Content such as 'useful' and 'helpful'. Between one and three tools were featured in the article, as appropriate for the repair concerned.

The Sponsored Content was placed after the second step in the repair task. Placement after the second step defined a simple and consistent placement rule for the whole site, and ensured that most visitors would encounter the Sponsored Content. Placement here also fitted the rhetorical structure of task instructions [26]. In instructional articles, information about required tools is relevant in at least 3 places: i) before the start of the instructions (step 0 'Preparation'); ii) after the final instruction ('Enough Reading, Now Let's Do It'); or iii) as an aside, whenever the tool in mentioned in the instructions. After the second step was thought to be a simple approximation to option iii) and to achieve a reasonable balance of CTR and user experience.

3.4   Versions of the Site

Three versions of the online manual were created. Each version suggested a different level of credibility to visitors - high, medium and low. Each version of the site comprised the same information (articles and Sponsored Content) and the same architecture (structure, navigational scheme etc.). However, the 'decoration' around each article, and the superficial appearance of the article, was modified to suggest different levels of trustworthiness and expertise, in line with findings about the features of web sites that effect the perception of credibility [28, p64-65] and user feedback from a previous evaluation (see Figure 1). The high credibility site identified all sources of information in a verifiable way, took responsibility for the content, and was well-designed and published. Eight features of the site were modified to reduce credibility: 1. Inconsistent, 'clunky' styling. 2. Unnecessary requests for information. 3. Author not identified. 4. Search error message. 5. Blurred image. 6. Irrelevant information and inappropriate attitude. 7. Uninformative comments, rather than references, and information about the author. 8. Contact information and street address not present. The medium, and low credibility versions of the site were increasingly unclear and evasive about sources of information and made increasingly severe and obvious errors in design and publishing.

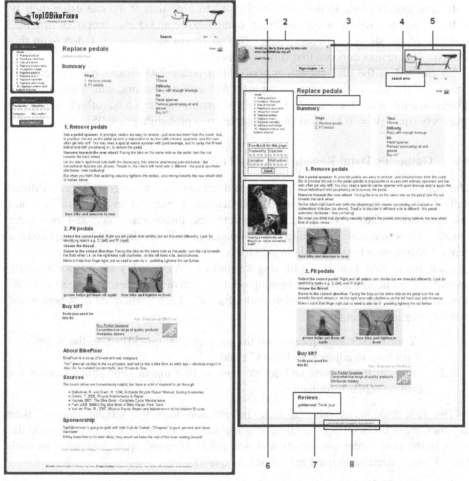

Fig. 1. 'Replace pedal' page from the research vehicle website, high credibility version (left) and low credibility version (right)

3.5   Gathering Data: Traffic Log

An online recruitment campaign attracted visitors from the UK to a landing page via Sponsored Links on a search engine results page (google.co.uk). 'Natural' traffic was not used, as the volume was too small to complete the study within a reasonable period of time. The landing page then redirected each visitor to a version of the website according to the final digit in their IP address. This redirection enabled data collection from an approximately equal numbers of visitors per condition in parallel. However, redirection also lost some visitor information from the data log. For example, the referring site for each visitor was no longer 'google.co.uk' but 'localhost'.

Traffic data was collected for approximately 13 weeks – from 19th March to 15th June, 2012 – and a preliminary data analysis carried out. The most important metrics were CTR (for persuasion) and time on site, pages per visit, total page views and bounce rate (for engagement and user experience).

In principle, because visitors were redirected to a version of the site using their IP address, return visitors using different computers could have accessed different versions of the site on different visits. So, all return visits are excluded from this analysis - the results concern first-time visitors only.

By the end of the data collection period, just under 200 visitors had visited each version of the site, giving a total sample of 578 unique visitors, which constitutes a discriminating test (for df $=2$, power>0.9, assuming any halo effect would be relatively small (w $= 0.15$), and an acceptable error probability of 0.05).

3.6   Gathering Data: Remote Usability Test

The remote usability test was planned and conducted in August 2012. Fifteen individuals participated in this test - five participants per condition (high, medium and low credibility sites). Of these five participants, three were male and two were female. Participants were recruited from a panel of individuals, who had expressed a general willingness to participate in user trials.

Each participant read the following scenario – "You and your partner recently bought second hand bikes and have adopted more active lifestyles. You need to know how to fix your bikes to travel safely and reliably". Each participant then performed two information seeking tasks:

1. "Your brakes are squeaky and do not stop you quickly. Use the website to learn how to adjust your brakes" ; and
2. "Browse the website and decide how well it meets your general needs for cycling repair information".

The first task seeks more specific information than the second task. Taken together, these tasks reflect the range of actual usage. Each participant performed the tasks in the same order (as above), and was asked to spend up to 5 minutes on each task. Finally, each participant answered four questions:

   i.   Overall, how trustworthy is this site?;
   ii.   Overall, how knowledgeable is this site?;

iii.   How trustworthy are the adverts on this site?; and
iv.   How knowledgeable are the adverts on this site?

These questions were selected to examine whether the perception of the site overall (questions i. and ii.) was rubbing off on the adverts in particular (questions iii. and iv.). Separate questions about trustworthiness and expertise were posed, because participants may not understand 'credibility' in the specific sense intended by the researchers. Each participant answered each of these questions using a 5-point rating scale, 5 being high, and 1 being low. The ratings for trustworthiness and expertise were then combined with equal weighting to produce a single rating for credibility.

Each session was self moderated, but guided by online instructions, and conducted from the participant's workstation. During analysis, responses to questions i. and ii., and to questions iii. and iv., were then averaged to give a rating for credibility for the site, and for the adverts respectively.

3.7   Expected Results

If halo effects were present, the high credibility site was expected to achieve the highest CTR, and the low credibility site the lowest CTR. If the high credibility site also achieved the highest credibility ratings, both for the site overall, and for the embedded display adverts in particular, then halo effects would be directly supported, and the test conditions would be verified as 'high, medium and low credibility' would be verified.

Also, the high credibility site was expected to achieve a user experience that was at least as good, if not better than, the medium and low credibility sites. This would be indicated by longer and deeper site visits, and fewer bounces.

4   Results

The high credibility site achieved the highest CTR per visitor (8.45%, see Table 1), the site intended to have medium credibility actually achieved the lowest CTR per visitor (3.68%), and the low credibility site achieved CTR of 5.31%. These differences in CTR between sites is statistically significant (chi2 test, p=0.003).

Table 1. Traffic data and ratings by credibility

Credibility of Host Site	New Visits	Time on Site (min: sec)	Pages per Visit	Total Page Views	CTR per visitor	CTR per page view	Rating Site	Advert
High	198	2: 22	3.94	839	8.45%	2.15%	4.4	3.375
Medium	182	2: 00	3.32	631	3.68%	1.11%	4.3	3.300
Low	198	2: 09	3.10	642	5.31%	2.15%	4.2	2.875

Bounce rates are similar for all sites (21.6% for the High and Medium sites, and 22.7% for Low site). In contrast, the time on site, pages per visit and total page views, are all somewhat elevated for the high credibility site – which confirms the suggestion that the high credibility site, indeed, provided a better user experience. However, any apparent difference is far from significant, and greater engagement with the high credibility version introduces the possibility that the increase in CTR per visitor may be due to longer duration of the visits alone - there may be no need to postulate halo effects. To confirm a halo effect, we need to also calculate CTR *per page view*.

The high credibility site again achieved the highest CTR per page view (2.15%) (see Table 1). However, the low credibility site achieved an identical CTR per page view (2.15%). Only the medium credibility site achieved a lower CTR (1.15%). The effect of credibility on CTR per page view, however, is still significant (chi2 test, p=0.017).

The remote usability test provided data about visitor perceptions of the site and the Sponsored Content. The trend in the data supports the assumption that the high credibility site was indeed perceived as the most credible version of the site (see Table 1).

5   Discussion

Taken together, these results confirm the presence of halo effects, and the idea that increased credibility will increase both CTR and user experience via perceived credibility and greater engagement.

This finding is important, because it shows how site design and content creation may increase persuasiveness without impairing user experience. There *is*, then, an alternative to Banners, Banner blindness and the apparent contest between persuasion and user experience in online publications (see Section 1). These criteria may be brought into better alignment and balance, even mutually support, provided the business model of the publication permits.

To be clear about the process that brought about this finding, much of the increase in CTR *per visitor* appears due to the effect of credibility on user experience (greater credibility encourages longer visits), rather than an induced decision bias. Encouraging a visitor to stay for longer, and view more pages, just creates more opportunities to click through Sponsored Content. The impact of credibility on CTR *per page view* is only around 1%, and appears more effective at the lower end of the scale i.e. a lack of credibility reduces clicks, but above a certain threshold (the medium condition in our experiment) additional credibility does not bias decision-making much further. So, credibility affects Sponsored Content CTR via engagement, as well as via halo-ing.

5.1   Implications for Site Optimisation

This paper confirms that the halo effect does indeed operate in relation to websites and Sponsored Content. One way of achieving higher levels of *both* CTR and user experience, then, is to increase the credibility of a website – make it feel more knowledgeable and trustworthy. Several authors have identified site features that may increase credibility [28] – we support those suggestions, and indeed applied them in this research.

This paper also reminds us that greater credibility also encourages visitors to stay for longer, and to explore more widely, and that this prolonged interactions itself creates more opportunities to attend to, and click through, Sponsored Content. To maximize the benefits of greater credibility, then, websites are also well advised to encourage engagement at the same time as they attempt to increase credibility, for example, by removing features that might trigger quitting the site, through disorientation; complex or illogical information architecture, or lack of convenient ways of saving a relevant page for investigation later.

5.2   Wider Applicability of the Findings

The Halo effect reported in this paper was observed when visitors accessed an online publication containing Sponsored Content from desktop devices. This effect will also arise in relation to other kinds of persuasive element, access device, and application domain. For example, embedding Sponsored Content more explicitly in the host article, might increase the Halo, because visitors may more readily perceive the Sponsored Content to be 'part of the site'. The Sponsored Content could also be made more informative, for example, by including information about the range of types of tool, or the article author's recommendations. Sleek and highly desirable mobile devices might also elicit stronger halo effects, as the positive device qualities rub off on the persuasive elements. However, this study cannot guarantee that its findings will generalize, because, as outlined in section 1, the strength of Halo effect, relative to other factors affecting CTR, appears to be context sensitive [24]. Further studies, then, are needed to confirm the possibilities identified above.

5.3   Methodological Issues

Before the findings of this paper are acted upon, there are a number of methodological issues to consider.

First, the participants in the traffic studies reported here were not representative of actual Internet users. Most Internet users say they never, or very rarely, click through Display Adverts[9]. However, all participants in this study were 'advert clickers', in that they comprised the server log category 'search traffic' i.e. visitors who found the test website by clicking on a Sponsored Link on a search engine results page. Actual Internet users also include referrals from all kinds of web site, and direct arrivals, who may be less prone to click through Display Adverts. That said, 'advert clickers' are no more prone to Halo effects than the majority of Internet users, we believe, so the Halo effect reported here should still generalize to the population as a whole. The mean CTR reported here, however, may be a slight over-estimate.

Second, the indicator of persuasion used in this research (CTR) is not ideal. Sponsors are increasingly concerned with the *quality* of traffic referred from affiliate sites, not just the number of referrals. Ideally, then, this work would have collected data about the behavior of visitors on the destination site, such as the number of tool pages viewed and the number of tools purchased. Future studies may want to collaborate with retailers and join affiliate advertising programs in order to consider the full impact of halo effects – which behaviours are affected, and how far down the conversion funnel? That said, the absence of information about traffic quality in this study does not undermine its findings about click through rate, so the Halo effect reported here should still generalize.

Third, and finally, the traffic log study did not verify the actual level of credibility perceived by visitors. An optional feedback poll about perceived trustworthiness and expertise was presented to visitors on the left-hand side of every article (see Figure 1). Unfortunately, almost no visitor ever responded to this poll. Credibility ratings in line with expectations were obtained in remote usability tests, but not enough to estimate a value for the population. However, there is uncertainty about the levels of credibility actually perceived by visitors to the medium and low credibility sites. For example, the medium credibility site date-stamped each article with a date one year earlier. In contrast, the low credibility site did not stamp any date on the article. But is it more credible to say nothing, than to state that content is one year old? Users may not notice the absence of a date stamp on brief visits. Similarly, is failing to state a content policy less credible than explicitly stating an *in*appropriate policy. Future studies need to find an effective technique for verifying actual credibility, perhaps by sending incentivised follow-up questionnaires to visitors who have signed in. That said, the high credibility condition complied with Fogg's guidelines for high credibility, and the high credibility condition certainly outperformed the other conditions. This study successfully demonstrated a halo effect, then, just not as clearly as it could have towards the bottom of the credibility scale.

Acknowledgements. This work was in part supported by a Google Research Award. We are also very grateful for the support and guidance of Robin Jeffries, Felix Portnoy and Nalini Edwards. This work was conducted according to professional codes of conduct.

References

1. American Society of Business Publication Editors Guide to Preferred Editorial Practices, http://www.asbpe.org/about/code.htm
2. EBay partner network, https://www.ebaypartnernetwork.com/files/hub/en-US/index.html
3. Adsense Help. Tips for Success, http://support.google.com/adsense/bin/topic.py?hl=en&topic=2 717009&parent=1250102&ctx=topic
4. Internet Advertising Bureau Guide to Online Display Advertising. Internet Marketing Handbook Series, http://www.iabuk.net/sites/default/files/publication-download/IABguidetoonlinedisplayadvertising.pdf
5. Benway, J.P.: Banner Blindness: The Irony of Attention Grabbing on the World Wide Web. Proc. Human Factors and Ergonomics Society Annual Meet. 42(5), 463–467 (1998)
6. Burke, M., Hornof, A., Nilsen, E., Gorman, N.: High-cost banner blindness: Ads increase perceived workload, hinder visual search, and are forgotten. ACM Transactions on Computer Human Interaction 12(4), 423–445 (2005)
7. Owens, J.W., Chaparro, B., Palmer, E.M.: Text advertising blindness: the new banner blindness. J. Usability Studies 3(2011), 172–197 (2011)

8. Dahlen, M.: Banner advertisements through a new lens. Journal of Advertising Research 41(4), 23–30 (2001)
9. Fulgoni, G.M., Moern, M.P.: How online advertising works: whither the click? comScore paper prepared for Empirical Generalisations in Advertising Conference for Industry and Academia, December 4-5. Wharton School, Philadelphia (2008)
10. Edwards, S.M., Li, H., Lee, J.H.: Forced exposure and psychological reactance: antecedents and consequences of the perceived intrusiveness of pop-up ads. J. Advertising 31(3), 83–96 (2002)
11. McCoy, S., Everard, A., Polak, P., Galletta, D.F.: The effects of online advertising. Communications of the ACM 50(3), 84–88 (2007)
12. Brajnik, G., And Gabrielli, S.: A Review of Online Advertising Effects on the User Experience. International J. of Human-Computer Interaction 26(10), 971–997 (2010)
13. Yan, J., Liu, N., Wang, G., Zhang, W., Jiang, Y., Chen, Z.: How much can behavioral targeting help online advertising? In: Proc. International World Wide Web Conference, WWW 2009, Madrid, Spain, April 20-24, pp. 261–270. ACM, New York (2009)
14. Chen, Y., Canny, J.F.: Recommending ephemeral items at web scale. In: Proceedings of Annual SIGIR Conference on Research and Development in Information Retrieval, SIGIR 2011, Beijing, China, July 24-28, pp. 1013–1022. ACM, New York (2010)
15. Ur, B., Leon, P.G., Cranor, L.F., Shay, R., Wang, Y.: Smart, useful, scary, creepy. In: Proc.Symposium on Usable Privacy and Security, SOUPS 2012, Washington, DC, USA, July 11-13, pp. 1–15. ACM, New York (2012)
16. Kern, D., Harding, M., Storz, O., Davis, N., Schmidt, A.: Shaping how advertisers see me: user views on implicit and explicit profile capture. In: Extended Abstracts on Human Factors in Computing Systems, CHI EA 2008, Florence, Italy, April 5-10, pp. 3363–3368. ACM, New York (2008)
17. Purcell, K., Brenner, J., Rainie, L.: Search Engine Use 2012. Pew Research Center, Washington, USA (2012)
18. Jamaica Shell Road Map. Macmillan International, London, UK (2007)
19. Clarke, C.L.A., Agichtein, E., Dumais, S., White, R.W.: The influence of caption features on clickthru patterns in web search. In: Proceedings SIGIR 2007, pp. 135–142 (2007)
20. Thorndike, E.L.: A constant error in psychological ratings. J. Applied Psychology 4, 25–29 (1920)
21. Nisbett, R.E., Wilson, T.D.: The halo effect: Evidence for unconscious alteration of judgments. J. Personality and Social Psychology 35(4), 250–256 (1977)
22. Dacko, S.G.: The Advanced Dictionary of Marketing: Putting Theory to Use. OUP, Oxford UK (2008)
23. Choi, S.M., Rifon, N.J.: Antecedents and Consequences of Web Advertising Credibility: A Study of Consumer Response to Banner Ads. Journal of Interactive Advertising 3(1), 12–24 (2002), American Academy of Advertising
24. Beckwith, N.E., Kassarjian, H.H., Lehmann, D.R.: Halo effects in marketing research review and prognosis. Advances in Consumer Research 05, Hunt, K. (ed.): Association for Consumer Research, Ann Abor, pp. 465–467 (1978)
25. Fogg, B.J.: Persuasive Technology: Using Computers to Change What We Think and Do. Morgan Kaufmann, San Francisco (2003)
26. Park, C., Lee, T.M.: Information direction, website reputation and eWOM effect:A moderating role of product type. Journal of Business Research 62, 61–67 (2009)
27. Vander Linden, K.: The expression of local relations in instructional text. In: Proc. Assoc. of Computational Linguisitcs, ACL 1992, pp. 318–320. ACM, New York (1992)
28. Fogg, B.J., Marshall, J., Laraki, O., Osipovich, A., Varma, C., Fang, N., Paul, J., Rangnekar, A., Shon, J., Swani, P., Treinen, M.: What Makes Web Sites Credible? A Report on a Large Quantitative Study. In: Proceedings of Annual Conference on Human Factors in Computing Systems, CHI 2001, Seattle, WA, USA, March 31-April 4, pp. 61–68. ACM, New York (2001)

Informing Design of Suggestion and Self-Monitoring Tools through Participatory Experience Prototypes

Nediyana Daskalova, Nathalie Ford, Ann Hu, Kyle Moorehead,
Benjamin Wagnon, and Janet Davis

Grinnell College, Department of Computer Science,
1115 8th Avenue, Grinnell, IA 50112
{daskalov,fordnath,huann,mooreheal,
wagnonbe,davisjan}@grinnell.edu

Abstract. We aim to design a persuasive technology to help college students, who are particularly susceptible to sleep deprivation, get better, longer, and more regular sleep. In order to gain the insights of our future users, we applied a participatory design approach that included experience prototypes, which aim to actively engage designers and participants with the functions that new technology might serve in the context of their daily lives. We deployed two experience prototypes: paper sleep logs and scripted reminders. We show how deploying low-technology experience prototypes as part of a participatory process can engender valuable insights into persuasive technology design.

Keywords: Experience prototypes, participatory design, persuasive technology, self-monitoring, reminders, sleep, college students.

1   Introduction

Beyond impacts on physical health, lack of sleep impairs cognitive achievement and memory [1]. College students are particularly susceptible to sleep deprivation because of the unfamiliar college environment, busy schedules, and minimal adult supervision. Over 70% of students report getting less than the average 8 hours of sleep required for young adults [2], which can cause a downward cycle of poor sleep leading to poor cognition, inefficient work and bad decisions, and even less sleep.

College students' sleep habits could be improved through persuasive technology, that is, technology intended to promote changes in users' behaviors or attitudes [3]. In particular, we aim to design technology that help college students obtain longer, better, and more regular sleep. Although several commercial technologies serve to monitor sleep quality, Choe et al. argue that sleep is under-explored in human-computer interaction [4]. They raise design questions about where, when, and how people interact with sleep technologies. We build upon these considerations in our design process aiming to support students in developing better sleep habits.

To help ensure our persuasive technology would be useful and appropriate [5], we engaged students in a participatory design process. Building on prior work [5,6],

A. Spagnolli et al. (Eds.): PERSUASIVE 2014, LNCS 8462, pp. 68–79, 2014.

we conducted a series of design activities to engage potential users and help them think critically about their needs and values, developing directions for design.

Our contribution is to show how experience prototypes [7] can inform persuasive technology design. Experience prototypes are defined by Buchenau and Suri as "any kind of representation, in any medium, that is designed to understand, explore or communicate what it might be like to engage with the product, space or system we are designing" [7]. Like paper prototypes [8], experience prototypes are interactive; participants engage actively rather than passively. Experience prototypes can be low-technology and low-fidelity, gaining the benefits of expedience and flexibility. However, our experience prototypes are designed for use in situ rather than in the laboratory. They aim to prototype not so much "look and feel" as the new roles that technologies can fulfill [7, 12]. We believe experience prototypes are well-suited to persuasive technology design because they can provide experience with persuasive strategies before investing in building new technologies.

In this work, we do not adopt a scientific approach in evaluating persuasive strategies. Rather, we propose the application of an established interaction design technique to persuasive technology. Although the technique resonates with Fogg's 8-step method for persuasive technology design [9], we are not aware of any prior work explicitly connecting Fogg's approach to experience prototyping. We address Davis's directions for future work by "selecting and tailoring [participatory] methods for each stage of persuasive technology design and reflecting on the methods' effectiveness" [6].

After an overview of our design process, we further explain our rationale for deploying experience prototypes. We then elaborate on the methods and results for two iterative deployments. We finally discuss benefits, limitations, and lessons learned.

2   Design Process Overview

We built on prior work applying a participatory design approach to persuasive technology [5,6]. Throughout our design process, we collaborated with potential future users of our technology through a series of design discussions and workshops. Through their partnership in the design process, we developed shared understandings of the design space; participants saw their influences manifested in the form of mock-ups and prototypes. We obtained informed consent from all participants.

To begin, we facilitated an asynchronous discussion of wellness concerns on campus, and met with key stakeholders. Once we had identified sleep as our area of focus, Fogg's 8-step method for persuasive technology design suggested we proceed by identifying an audience, a technology channel, and a concrete behavior to change [9]. After committing to Grinnell College students as our audience, we designed a short survey based on National Sleep Foundation (NSF) guidelines [10] to identify what students would most like to change about their own sleep habits. The behavior change that appealed to the most students (about 57%) was to make and follow through on plans for getting enough sleep. We also asked participants about their technology use to help us choose which technology channels to focus on.

With a direction established, we conducted participatory workshops to engage future users, promote mutual learning, and generate design ideas. Because Fogg argues that complex behavioral change is most successful when taken in small steps [9], the first workshop tasked participants with transforming NSF's sleep guidelines [10] into simple first steps for behavior change. Next, during the Mockups workshop, participants designed technologies to promote sleep and then altered them based on stakeholder and designer prompts [11]. While the Mockups workshop let participants explore one design idea in depth, the goal of the Inspiration Cards workshop was to generate diverse ideas through combinations and elaborations of cards illustrating relevant technologies and concepts [12].

From participants' designs, we identified two persuasive strategies of broad interest: self-monitoring and suggestions [3]. We designed and deployed experience prototypes to gain experience with these approaches. Participants saw their ideas embodied in these prototypes, and their experiences with the prototypes helped further our mutual understanding of the roles that new technologies could serve. After a two week deployment, we met with participants to learn about their experiences. During the fall semester, a new group of participants evaluated a revised experience prototype and mocked up new designs.

3   Why Experience Prototypes?

We decided to deploy experience prototypes because we and our participants lacked concrete experience with interventions to improve sleep. Experience prototypes help both users and designers experience what it may be like to interact with technologies that fill new roles in daily life. They emphasize "active participation to provide a relevant subjective experience," in contrast to approaches where participants must imagine the experience and give feedback from a more distant perspective [7].

We were also inspired by BJ Fogg's approach to persuasive technology design: Quickly testing many simple prototypes at low cost enables rapid exploration of persuasion tactics [9]. Experience prototypes fit Fogg's approach because they are informal, low-tech, and focus on function, lending themselves to rapid exploration, evaluation, and iteration. However, Fogg does not necessarily propose a participatory approach. Rather, designers learn from whether their experiments succeed or fail at influencing behavior. By contrast, we used experience prototypes as part of a participatory feedback loop. Prototypes communicate design ideas from the designers to the participants, who then draw on their first-hand experiences to collaborate with designers in critiquing and modifying those ideas.

We created two experience prototypes: paper sleep logs for self-monitoring and scripted reminder messages. Our aim was not to explore "look and feel" or technical implementation, but rather the role of such technologies in behavior change [13].

Why a sleep log? In many of the participants' designs from the Mockups and Inspiration Cards workshops, users would monitor their own sleep hours and related information. One group's mockup explicitly involved a sleep log, and the other two groups also used self-monitoring. In the Inspiration Cards Workshop, three out of the four groups used the "YawnLog" [14] technology card. Furthermore, although keeping a sleep log is one of the NSF's recommendations for improving sleep [10], none of the researchers had used a sleep log; neither had our participants. At the same time, a paper sleep log is a good match to the experience prototype paradigm: paper forms are easy to make and use, yet provide experience with recording objective and subjective data, as well as self-reflection. We hoped to learn how participants would respond to particular questions, but also how a sleep log fit into their daily lives.

Sleep logs were not the only idea we wanted to test. Many participants remarked that they tend to lose track of time and go to bed later than they intended. Four out of the five groups at the Mockups workshop included a suggestion or reminder in their design. Moreover, all groups in the Inspiration Cards workshop used the "Reverse Alarm Clock" technology card: an alarm clock which tells you not when to wake up but when to go to bed [15]. We therefore wanted to learn whether reminders were effective, and gain insight into message content and delivery.

As Buchenau and Suri suggest [7], we took part in the experience prototypes alongside participants. We wanted to directly share in our participants' experiences. Designer engagement with experience prototypes provides a subjective lens and greater empathy for people who may be affected by future designs. Participants and designers "explore by doing" and develop a common perspective [7].

4   Experience Prototypes: First Iteration

We deployed two iterations of experience prototypes. In the first iteration, during the summer, our main goal was to evaluate the approach and major features of sleep logs and reminders. We conducted the second iteration in the fall semester, with a new group of participants, to gain experience in the context of the academic term.

4.1   Method

We adapted a one-page sleep log from the National Sleep Foundation (NSF) [16]. As in the NSF sleep log, we asked participants for their actual bedtimes and wake times, what they were doing right before going to sleep, and if there were additional factors that might have affected their sleep. We also asked participants to retrospectively record when they had intended to go to bed and wake up, so that participants could see and reflect on any disparity in the actual and intended times. The sleep log also asked participants whether they felt tired the following day, because college students need to feel awake throughout the day to study effectively [2]. Finally, the NSF sleep log asks five specific questions about behavioral and environmental factors that might affect sleep quality, such as taking medications. Because we aimed to help participants allow enough time for sleep, we combined these questions into one, final, open-ended question. Based on the workshops, we suggested more college-specific factors, such as naps, alcohol, noise, and worries.

We also began thinking about ways to trigger students to go to bed. All students have access to email, and we learned from our survey that more than 98% of students have mobile phones. Thus, we explored both email and text messages, as well as desktop computing. We created an experience prototype that included email, text, and pop-up desktop messages to remind participants to go to bed. We used the UNIX `cron` program to automatically send emails and text messages. We also set up an AppleScript or Visual Basic script to display a pop-up reminder on participants' laptops; we scheduled the scripts using iCal for MacOS and Task Scheduler for Windows. We sent participants a different message each day to keep the reminders interesting and to experiment with a variety of persuasion tactics (Table 1).

Table 1. Reminder messages draw on persuasion tactics and sleep guidelines

Day	Reminder message	Rationale
1	Time to turn off your phone and computer and get ready for bed!	A basic suggestion or trigger [3,16]
2	Hello! It's time to brush your teeth and put your phone on silent! Good night!	Links new habit of silencing phone to existing habit of brushing teeth [17]
3	If you start getting ready for bed now, you will feel refreshed tomorrow!	Suggests a motivation [3,16]
4	It's time to charge your phone and get into PJ's!	Links preparation for bed to another nighttime habit [17]
5	It's time to go to bed. Listen to meditation music to relax: http://youtu.be/uRhoWQX2OF8	NSF suggests listening to relaxing music to promote sleepiness [11]. Provides a link to make this easier [3]
6	Watch these cute animals yawn and start getting ready for bed: http://youtu.be/B907 aaDw7Ec	Yawning is contagious - a social cue [3].
7	It's time to get ready for bed and listen to some relaxing white noise for a better night's rest: http://youtu.be/qorkD6n PYQM	NSF suggests that white noise helps people sleep better throughout the night [10].

Of the 23 participants who came to at least one of our workshops, twelve volunteered to engage with experience prototypes alongside the researchers. We collected information regarding participants' usual bedtimes and wake times, their phone number and carrier, and which operating system they use. During the first week with the experience prototypes, participants filled out a sleep log without reminders of any kind. Each day of the second week, each participant received a different reminder 30 minutes before their stated bedtime, and continued to maintain a sleep log.

At the end of the two-week deployment, nine participants met to share their experiences with the prototypes. The remaining three we interviewed individually via email or Skype. Discussion took place in two groups, of four and five participants; each included two researchers to facilitate discussion and take notes. Facilitators encouraged participants to converse about aspects of their experience they found surprising, problematic, or compelling. Prompts involved whether the reminders triggered participants to go to bed, what barriers to sleep they encountered, what they would change or keep the same about the sleep log, how they saw the prototypes fitting in their lives during the academic year, and how their sleep habits may have changed as a result of their experiences with the prototypes. Finally, if participants were comfortable sharing with us, we took photos of their sleep logs.

4.2   Results

Participants increased their awareness of the amount of sleep they were getting each night, and also observed trends over the two weeks. Reflecting on recent behavior was helpful for identifying personal barriers to sleep. Moreover, knowing to expect a sleep reminder helped some participants be more aware of their approaching bedtimes.

During the second week of the deployment, reminders prompted participants to go to bed 30 minutes before their intended bedtime. Some participants stopped what they were doing and started getting ready for bed, while others were distracted with people or entertainment. All participants paid less attention to their sleep reminders during the weekends. There was disagreement over the best time to send the reminders: some participants liked our default of 30 minutes before their intended bedtime, while others preferred an earlier reminder so that they could plan the rest of their evening. Participants paid the most attention to text messages, but predicted that desktop reminders would be more useful during the academic year when they are working on assignments late at night. Finally, the groups discussed the reminders' content. Reminders with links were especially problematic. For example, some were uninterested in listening to white noise (Table 1, Day 7). Others found that YouTube videos were a tempting distraction from going to sleep. As a solution, participants suggested that users should have the ability to choose or create their own reminder messages.

Reminders served as immediate prompts to go to bed, but sleep logs showed participants their sleep habits over time. Many participants found discrepancies between their actual and intended bed and wake times, which often correlated with their energy levels during the next day. Participants especially liked the question, "What were you doing/thinking before you went to bed?" because it helped them identify barriers to going to bed when they intended to. In particular, sometimes participants went to bed late because of friends who had inconsistent sleep schedules. At the same time, some participants felt social pressure to maintain a consistent schedule: they felt accountable to us and to others who may see their sleep logs. During weekends, participants often forgot to fill in their sleep log; one participant stopped logging altogether.

In reflecting on the sleep log, participants found they could easily see differences between their intended and actual sleep times and relate this to what they were doing before bed. Participants suggested that the sleep logs also ask "What would you change for tomorrow?" so that they could contemplate or commit to a behavior change in addition to reflecting on past behavior. Both groups also suggested that we address napping – based on the NSF recommendation to avoid sleeping after 4pm [10] – to help users consider napping as a reason for inconsistent sleep at night.

Overall, participants favored a quick and simple sleep log, but interaction with the sleep log varied from person to person. Some filled it in when they woke up, others in the mid-morning or afternoon, and others at night. Some started in the morning and completed the log at night. When the participants thought about their habits during the academic year, the answers changed again. "I wouldn't have time to fill it in the morning because I like to sleep as much as I can before class, but I can see myself filling it in after class," said one participant. Participants generally thought that sleep logs and reminders could help students improve their sleep habits during the academic year. Some were ready to continue sleep logging into the school year; others said they would not have started a sleep log on their own, but would use one if prompted.

A discussion of paper sleep logs versus a web or mobile app turned the conversation to privacy concerns. Although a paper log can be hidden from view, participants often found it convenient to leave it visible. We asked participants if they would feel comfortable sharing their sleep information in a web or mobile app. Several were happy to share that information and said privacy is no issue–unless we shared it with their mothers. Other participants felt this information was too private to share; they favored anonymized data. One participant explained he would feel comfortable sharing numeric data as long as his comments were kept private. Some participants felt that sharing could create positive social pressure to get enough sleep; however, several participants were concerned that sharing would perpetuate competitiveness in favor of being too busy to sleep.

5   Experience Prototypes: Second Iteration

We used participants' experiences in the summer to revise the experience prototypes for a second iteration during the fall semester.

5.1   Method

Based on participants' discussion of their experiences, we adjusted the second round of reminders in both content and delivery. We changed some messages that participants found unappealing. We also omitted any potentially distracting audio/visual links. For example, a reminder which included a link to relaxing music on YouTube (Table 1, Day 5), was replaced with, "It's time to go to bed. Take a few deep breaths and relax!" To address concerns about timing, the second iteration allowed for personalization. Participants could choose their own times for each day of the week, or retain the default of 30 minutes before their intended bedtime. This change allowed for differences between weekday and weekend schedules.

We also revised the sleep log based on participants' discussion. In the first iteration, the sleep log made participants more aware of their sleep habits and barriers to sleep. Our second iteration on the sleep log sought to go beyond awareness, to help participants set goals for sleep. Instead of asking "What time did you intend to go to bed?" and "What time did you intend to wake up?", the revised sleep log asks "How many hours of sleep do you want to get tonight?", "What time do you intend to go to bed tonight?" and "What time do you intend to get up in the morning?" Having participants plan their sleep and wake times gives them a goal to work toward and holds them accountable. These questions were moved to the end of the form so that participants could set goals based on their reflections about their sleep the night before.

Further, we drew on participants' experiences and reflections to add salient questions and remove uninformative questions. Because several participants suggested we address naps, we added a question: "Did you nap today? For how long? At what time of day?" To address other people as a barrier to sleep, we added the question "Who, if anyone, was with you [before going to bed]?" Some items on the sleep log were removed because they did not prove useful. We removed the question "Did you wake up before your alarm or did you need it?" because many participants always needed an alarm on weekdays or never used an alarm on weekends. We removed another question, "How did you feel when you woke up?" because some never felt refreshed in the morning regardless of how much they slept. However, the dichotomous question "Do you feel tired today?" was reworded as "Overall, how tired do you feel today?" with a scale from "not tired" (1) to "very tired" (5). We put this item first so that answers would be less influenced by questions about the previous night's sleep.

We deployed the revised experience prototypes over a two week period during the middle of the fall semester. We held two workshops with 17 new participants. In the first workshop, participants discussed barriers to sleep, as well as solutions. We also collected participants' intended bed and wake times during the week and weekends, their preferred bedtime reminder times, and their phone number and carrier. For those who brought their laptops, we set up the reminder scripts. Before leaving, participants took two copies of the sleep log, which they were to start filling out the next day. The daily email, text message, and desktop reminders began at the start of the second week. The researchers did not participate in this second deployment.

After the two-week deployment, we held three sessions of a debrief and mockups workshop: participants discussed their experiences with the prototypes and designed a technology of their own. Of the 17 participants, seven attended the first meeting, one attended the second, and nine attended the third. All participants brought their completed sleep logs.

5.2   Results

Consistent with what we learned over the summer, the experience prototypes helped participants become more aware of their sleep habits and causes of inadequate sleep. However, we gained more reliable insights into how users might interact with reminders and sleep logs while classes are in session.

Overall, participants liked having reminders to start preparing for bed. However, there were situations where it was easier to ignore the reminders than to follow them. Participants over the summer noted that the desktop reminders may be more useful during the academic term, but experiences in the fall did not support that prediction. Although more participants saw the desktop reminders, they tended to ignore the reminders if they were doing homework. Some participants found emails unhelpful because they were not seen until long after they were sent. Thus, text messaging was still the most favored medium.

For this iteration, participants were given the option to decide when, prior to their bedtimes, they would like to receive the reminders. Several took advantage of this option; most tended toward 1-hour reminders on weekends, suggesting our design needs to adapt to weekday and weekend schedules. However, the majority of participants defaulted to the 30-minute reminder.

As over the summer, participants during the academic year found the sleep log helpful. For many, it was useful to have salient information about how tired they felt during the day and how many hours of sleep they got the night before. This allowed them to think about what they could change or maintain for the following nights. As predicted, participants valued naps more during the academic term, and many appreciated the question about napping. Again, thinking about what they were doing before bed helped them identify specific barriers to sleep. However, some participants found it unhelpful to record who they were with: the answer was always the same. In general, there were more mixed responses to the questions in the second iteration, supporting the need for flexibility in our design to account for individual differences.

As in the first iteration, many participants were made aware of the disparity between their intended and actual bed times. In the second iteration, the sleep log asked participants to commit to particular bed and wake times. Throughout their discussions, participants questioned the usefulness of the "intended" bed and wake times. Participants raised concerns about whether these questions actually encouraged accountability. In particular, some participants were unsure whether to give realistic or ideal bedtimes. This uncertainty reveals a major barrier: In the context of all the work students want to do, or feel they must do, sleep is often not highly valued.

Because we added a mockup exercise to the debriefing session, participants were able to use their experiences and discussions to inform their own designs. Here, privacy manifested not so much as a concern but as a preference. To make the prototype more persuasive, several groups incorporated social sharing, so that others can strengthen the user's accountability in going to bed at the intended time.

6 Discussion

Experience prototypes provided important design insights in the context of our participatory design process. Our prototypes let participants (and designers) directly experience the potential functions of new technologies. Although participants incorporated self-monitoring and suggestion strategies in their workshop designs, they could speak only hypothetically about how effective these strategies might be. Experience prototypes changed that. When participants understand not just the purpose of a new technology, but the experience of using it in the context of their own lives, they can more aptly address concerns about practicality, meaning, and ethics. For example, participants told us that text messages were by far the most effective technology channel for reminders, contrary to their predictions. Participants found that some reminder messages were not effective, or even counterproductive. We worked with participants to develop sleep log questions that help them meaningfully reflect on their behavior; participants challenged our ideas about goal setting and identified other questions that were simply not useful. Through our discussions with participants, we learned that variability in how and when people use sleep reminders and sleep logs means that personalization is important to both strategies. And finally, participants varied widely in their views about how private sleep log data should be and what it would mean to share that information. Without directly engaging our participants in conversation and reflection, and without our own use of the experience prototypes, we would not have gained such a rich understanding of the potential range of experiences with the proposed technology.

We found that experience prototypes fit well into the middle stage of our participatory design process. Rather than eliciting values and generating ideas (as in the Inspiration Card and Mockup Workshops) or refining elements of more concrete designs (as in implementation or look-and-feel prototypes [13]), experience prototypes allowed us to evaluate persuasive strategies and tactics in the context of use. Workshops conducted beforehand allowed us to incorporate values and ideas put forward by participants, and the results allowed future workshops to be tailored around ideas which provoked participant response.

Like many prototyping techniques, experience prototyping enables low-cost testing and rapid iteration. In keeping with Fogg's [9] advice to build on success, we were able to incorporate feedback from the first deployment in the second deployment, while maintaining elements that participants liked and found effective. However, we remained focused on the role the technology would serve. We were able to revise sleep log questions, reminder messages, and reminder delivery times. Because our prototypes were relatively simple to assemble, we were able to easily move between iterations, and also test multiple strategies at once. Although participants interacted with our prototypes over multiple weeks–a much longer time than required for other design activities like storyboarding–our prototypes were much faster to produce than a software system prototype that would provide comparable experiences.

Given the limited capabilities of paper forms and computer scripts, we did not delve deeply into look and feel, usability, personalization, information displays, or sharing. Although there is much design left to do, we do not plan to conduct a third iteration of experience prototypes. After our second iteration, we believed a third iteration would have diminishing returns. We were starting to find more differences between people's experiences than similarities. The features we would have added to our experience prototypes, such as personalizing reminder messages, would have added too much complexity without much additional insight. Further design will require us to move forward with other kinds of prototypes.

7   Conclusion

Our work suggests that experience prototypes can fill a valuable niche for informing the design of persuasive technology. In contrast to more abstract prototypes, where designers and participants must imagine how new technologies will fit into everyday life, experience prototypes provide concrete, lived experience with the roles that persuasive technologies can serve. Beyond the implications for design discussed above, our process provides some support for the use of suggestion and self-monitoring strategies to improve sleep habits: reminders helped some participants go to bed on time, and sleep logs helped all of our participants reflect on their behavior. We learned all these valuable lessons at a relatively low cost. Iterating on the experience prototypes let us evaluate our proposed revisions in the real context of use.

Extending Fogg's 8-step method for designing persuasive technology [9], we recommend a participatory approach when applying experience prototypes of persuasive technology. Close interactions with our participants helped us gain better insight into their needs, values, and preferences regarding the final product, going beyond assessing the effectiveness of our prototypes in changing behavior. When both designers and participants engage with experience prototypes, they develop a shared perspective on the role that new technologies can play in shaping behavior.

Acknowledgments. We thank our participants for their time, enthusiasm, and insights. We thank Grinnell College for its support of this research through the Mentored Advanced Projects program.

References

1. Curcio, G., Ferrara, M., De Gennaro, L.: Sleep loss, learning capacity and academic performance. Sleep Med. Rev. 10(5), 323–337 (2006)
2. Lund, H., Reider, B., Whiting, A., Prichard, R.: Sleep patterns and predictors of disturbed sleep in a large population of college students. Journal of Adolescent Health 46(2), 124–132 (2010)
3. Fogg, B.J.: Persuasive technology: Using computers to change what we think and do. Morgan Kaufmann (2003)
4. Choe, E.K., Consolvo, S., Watson, N.F., Kientz, J.A.: Opportunities for computing technologies to support healthy sleep behaviors. In: Proceedings of the SIGCHI Conference on Human Factors in Computing Systems (CHI 2011), pp. 3053–3062. ACM, New York (2011)
5. Miller, T.M., Rich, P., Davis, J.: ADAPT: Audience design of persuasive technology. In: Extended Abstracts on Human Factors in Computing Systems (CHI 2009), pp. 4165–4170. ACM, New York (2009)
6. Davis, J.: Early experiences with participation in persuasive technology design. In: Halskov, K., Winschiers-Theophilus, H., Lee, Y., Simonsen, J., Bødker, K. (eds.) Proceedings of the 12th Participatory Design Conference: Research Papers (PDC 2012), vol. 1, pp. 119–128. ACM, New York (2012)
7. Buchenau, M., Suri, J.S.: Experience Prototyping. In: Boyarski, D., Kellogg, W.A. (eds.) Proceedings of the 3rd Conference on Designing Interactive Systems: Processes, Practices, Methods, and Techniques (DIS 2000). ACM, New York (2000)
8. Rettig, M.: Prototyping for tiny fingers. Communications of the ACM 37(4), 21–27 (1994)
9. Fogg, B.J.: Creating persuasive technologies: an eight-step design process. In: Proceedings of the 4th International Conference on Persuasive Technology (Persuasive 2009), vol. Article 44, 6 pages. ACM, New York (2009)

10. Healthy Sleep Tips, http://www.sleepfoundation.org/article/sleep-topics/healthy-sleep-tips
11. Yoo, D., Huldtgren, A., Woelfer, J.P., Hendry, D.G., Friedman, B.: A value sensitive action-reflection model: evolving a co-design space with stakeholder and designer prompts. In: Proceedings of the SIGCHI Conference on Human Factors in Computing Systems (CHI 2013). ACM, New York (2013)
12. Halskov, K., Dalsgård, P.: Inspiration card workshops. In: Carroll, J.M., Bødker, S., Coughlin, J. (eds.) Proceedings of the 6th Conference on Designing Interactive Systems (DIS 2006), pp. 2–11. ACM, New York (2006)
13. Houde, S., Hill, C.: What do prototypes prototype? In: Helander, M., Landauer, T.K., Prabhu, P. (eds.) Handbook of Human-Computer Interaction, 2nd edn. Elsevier Science B.V. (1997)
14. YawnLog, http://beta.yawnlog.com/
15. Reverse alarm clock, https://play.google.com/store/apps/details?id=org.example.alarmclocksleepeng
16. National Sleep Foundation Sleep Diary, http://sleep.buffalo.edu/sleepdiary.pdf
17. Fogg, B.J.: Tiny Habits, http://tinyhabits.com/

Persuasion in the Wild: Communication, Technology, and Event Safety

Peter de Vries, Mirjam Galetzka, and Jan Gutteling

University of Twente, Enschede, The Netherlands
{p.w.devries,m.galetzka,j.m.gutteling}@utwente.nl

Abstract. Recent disasters during major events have resulted in increased focus on influencing crowds, both during emergencies and under normal circumstances. In this exploratory study event experts were interviewed to uncover good practices regarding the use of technology to communicate with crowds.

They agree that, rather than using directive means and force, crowds can best be persuaded; proving relevant information enables them to decide for themselves what course of action to take. Some of the experts remain critical about use of social media at events; effectiveness depends on target group composition, visitors' engagement in the event, and reliability. Additionally, the abundance of information visitors have at their fingertips may reduce effectiveness of information emitted by organisers. Especially important in communicating with crowds is "communicating as one", not only pertaining to explicit messages but also to non-verbal communication.

Based on these results, implications for event safety are discussed.

Keywords: crowd control, crowd management, event safety.

1 Introduction

Large events pose considerable risks to the safety of its participants, as illustrated by Pukkelpop, 2011, in Hasselt, Belgium, and the Love Parade, 2010, in Duisburg, Germany. People may get crushed or trampled during ingress and egress, emergencies may cause panic and confusion, and sports events sometimes result in misbehaviour of its spectators. Fortunately, such calamities are relatively rare. Nevertheless, ensuring that events go as planned requires extensive preparations before (crowd management) and constant monitoring and intervention during an event (crowd control).

An important element of the crowd management and crowd control toolbox is communication with visitors. Especially in the interst of safety, visitors need to know how to get to and from an event location, what they are allowed to take with them, where they can find food stalls and toilets, which places have become crowded and are closed off, what to do to prepare for extreme weather conditions, etc.

Technological developments have both facilitated and complicated communication with crowds. On the one hand, the popularity and widespread use of smart phones has prompted event organisers to make apps available, allowing visitors to inform themselves of changes in and amendments to the schedule, the festival location layout, etc.

A. Spagnolli et al. (Eds.): PERSUASIVE 2014, LNCS 8462, pp. 80–91, 2014.
© Springer International Publishing Switzerland 2014

In addition, they may actively disseminate event-related information; using websites, Facebook, and Twitter accounts they may inform others about matters as congestion and safety issues. On the other hand, smart phones and social media enable visitors underway to or during events to look for relevant information themselves, instead of relying on what the organisers hand out to them, and communicate with and inform others.

Surprisingly, very little on communicating with event crowds is formally available in publications. The current study is a first attempt to record the knowledge of practitioners. Based on expert interviews, the current exploratory study aimed to uncover good practices about the use of technology to influence crowds at major events. These findings will be brought into accordance with insights from scientific literature, e.g. on crowd psychology. Specific attention will be devoted to the use of communication technology.

2   Theory

2.1   Mass Psychology and Communication

To many, the term "mass" to denote a large gathering of people, probably has negative connotations. Examples of mass events with disastrous consequences, such as the Love Parade and Pukkelpop, readily spring to mind. Mass behaviour has always had a reputation for being difficult to predict and control, earning crowds the epithet "mad, bad and dangerous to know" (Reicher et al. [1], p. 558). Consequently, crowds have long been regarded as irrational.

An early yet persistent view, put forward by LeBon in 1895, postulates that anonymity in crowds causes its members to lose the ability to think and reason, to decrease quality of judgement and personal responsibility, et cetera; cf. Reicher et al. [1]. In fact, this tradition views crowd behaviour as pathological and abnormal: once immersed in a crowd people give themselves to non-conscious and anti-social behaviour. According to some, this reductionist and mechanical view on crowds has legitimised repressive crowd control tactics and strategies [2].

Although the notion that anonymity decreases rationality and increases diffusion of responsibility has also been central to later theories in social psychology, such as the Deindividuation Theory [3, 4], many have come to regard this as a unnecessarily negative and little productive view on crowds and their behaviour [4, 5]. In addition, results of some studies actually contradict its central tenet that anonymity leads to anti-social and aggressive behaviour, and, rather, point in the opposite direction [6].

More recently, this view has been supplanted by the notion that crowd behaviour is normative and rational after all – or, at least, boundedly rational [7-9]. Crowd behaviour is seen as the result of a shift from individuals' personal identity to a social identity, rather than a loss of identity altogether [1]. In essence, norms and behaviour of the relevant group supersede those of the individual. Consequently, social identity has been argued to be the key to understanding crowds and dealing with them [1], cf. [10]. Social identity determines who influences others to perform certain behaviour, how others and their behaviour are viewed, and which behaviours are seen as normal [1, 11, 12].

This change in views on crowds corresponds to a shift in the way crowds are managed. Strategies aimed at influencing group processes have been adopted by police departments around the world and employed in settings as diverse as football matches and protesting crowds [11-16], and are argued to be suitable for handling emergency situations [17].

A more or less similar shift has emerged in the domain of risk and crisis communication. Parallel to the idea that people do not cease to be reasoning beings whenever they are immersed in crowds, research in this field has very recently started to focus on how to motivate citizens to help themselves and others prepare for or cope with extreme situations. The underlying idea is that, when faced with an emergency, the majority of citizens do not panic [18] or passively wait for whatever local governments or police instruct them to do. If given the right information, most citizens are perfectly able to decide for themselves what course of action to take before or after emergency situations [19]. Recent experiences with such situations indeed suggest there to be considerable numbers of people who are willing to assist professional emergency responders, so much so that these professionals often do not know what to do with these volunteers [20].

2.2 Social Media

Recent research has indicated that social media may play an important role in emergency situations. An analysis of the events following an outbreak of extreme weather at a Belgian music festival in 2011, for instance, show that one Twitter user was able to mobilise the nearby village of Hasselt. This resulted in inhabitants offering afflicted visitors a place to sleep, shower, food, drink, Internet access, etc. Intersetingly, some of these offering assistance appeared not to have been active on Twitter prior to these events [21]. Additionally, American research on Twitter use after disasters as the Tennessee River fly ash spillage [22], the Red River floods, and the Oklahoma grass fires [23] showed that Twitter users played an important role in spreading relevant information by re-tweeting messages from people involved in the disasters and from local media, and correcting wrong information.

That smart phones and social media offer great potential for crowd management and crowd control, for instance by proving realtime information to event visitors under normal circumstances and in case of (pending) emergencies, is acknowledged by many event organisers. Events such as Rock Werchter in Belgium, and Lowlands and North Sea Jazz Festival in the Netherlands routinely use apps to communicate line-ups, programming changes, etc. They also allow broadcasting messages to warn for crowded locations, weather conditions, etc. Recently, the city of Amsterdam created an app to be used on the Queen's Day celebrations. The app showed a map of the city, indicating crowdedness and points of interest, such as First Aid stations and public transportation stations (in the end, however, the crowding indicator had to be removed to prevent a mobile network overload).

A drawback to the omnipresent smart phone in combination with access to Internet and social media platforms, is that they unlock vast amounts of information, relevant as well as irrelevant, which may lead to overloading [e.g., 24]. An additional down side, particularly from the perspective of event organisers, may be the clutter that this causes. Specifically, the abundance of information that results from visitors actively searching for information on websites and social media, or from passive exposure to other people's contributions on social media, may well swamp the messages from organisers, which consequently lose their effectiveness.

A useful, new technique is so-called "cell broadcast" via mobile networks, in principle allowing each mobile phone in a specific area ("cell") to be reached by way of radiofrequencies, instead of text messaging or telephone frequencies, provided that these phones are suitable for receiving such signals. As such, it is impervious to overloading of these latter channels [25]. To our knowledge, however, this has not been put into practice at events.

A prerequisite of these services, however, is that their availability and necessity needs to be communicated to the public, and they will have to undertake some action in order for it to function, e.g., download an app, switch on Bluetooth, or subscribe to text message services.

3   Expert Interviews

The 16 interviewees in this project were all individuals with direct experience with crowd management and crowd control at large events. The selection was such that ten interviewees represented three different stakeholder groups involved in the organization and/or execution of five specifically selected events: they represented (commercial) organisers, municipalities, and the police organization. In addition, six experts represented more "general" experience; these came from the Dutch Police Academy, and from event safety consultancy firms. The five events were selected from a list of major Dutch events that are publicly accessible and are held each year or every two years. Several criteria were used to achieve variety in the number of visitors, location in urban or rural areas, hosted by large and small municipalities, duration, and free or paid admission. One event, the annual Queen's Day Celebration in Amsterdam, was added because during previous editions incidents occurred, such as rioting and visitors blocking railways. Table 1 presents an overview of the selected events, and the background and experience of the interview participants.

Professional code of conduct was followed while conducting these interviews. Participants were granted full anonymity and were fully informed about the research and, in particular, the topics that were addressed in the interviews, before consenting to take part. They were not in any way subjected to deception, coercion, or discomfort.

The interviews took place on location (face-to-face) or by telephone, and, on average, lasted about an hour. Each interview was recorded. As part of a more encompassing topic list, participants were, for instance, asked to list and reflect on the means of communications they had at their disposal, their use, and effectiveness, both before as well as during events. Specifically relevant to the current paper were questions about the use and effectiveness of technology, such as LED displays, Internet and social media, and smart phones. Directly after each interview, the recordings were used to create detailed (but not literal) descriptions of the expert's remarks. These were subsequently sent to the respective participants, to allow them to inspect our rendering of the interview and make corrections when necessary. After completion of all 16 interviews, all remarks were categorized and coded, and subsequently grouped based on their specific content.

Table 1. Background and experience of the experts interviewed

	Involvement				Experience (Work years)	Events					
	Organizer	Municipality	Police	Other		1	2	3	4	5	Other
Expert 1	■				11	■					
Expert 2		■			8	■					
Expert 3			■		10	■					
Expert 4				■	data missing		■				
Expert 5		■			5		■				
Expert 6			■		>8	■					■
Expert 7			■		10			■			■
Expert 8		■			4				■		
Expert 9			■		4	■		■			
Expert 10	■				>11				■		■
Expert 11			■		4				■		
Expert 12				■	>5	■	■		■		■
Expert 13				■	>5	■	■		■		■
Expert 14			■	■	30						■
Expert 15				■	4						■
Expert 16				■	40						■

Note:
Event 1: Vierdaagsefeesten (festivities surrounding Four Day Marches, Nijmegen); 2: 3FM Serious Request, Enschede; 3: Queen's Day Celebration Amsterdam; 4: Appelpop festival; 5: Zwarte Cross festival.

In the following paragraphs those interview results pertaining to the topics at hand are presented. Quantification is done either in the text or by numbers in parentheses. These represent the number of experts who made a particular remark. As most interviewees were highly experienced professionals, with work experience sometimes stretching decennia, several remarks were considered noteworthy results even though only one interviewee mentioned them.

3.1   Treatment of the Crowd

In conformance with the state-of-the-art of crowd psychology, none of the interviewees considered irrationality to be a relevant aspect of crowd behaviour. Many of them (5) advocate treatment of visitors as mature, sensible individuals. Consequently, crowds can best be influenced not by force, but by handing them relevant information so that they can decide for themselves what course of action to take (5). This is also reflected by the tendency of the police to decrease presence of personnel at events (4), leaving communication with the crowd to an increasing extent to municipalities and event organisers (1).

3.2   Use of Technology

The means of communication with event visitors range from the conventional flyers, LED-displays to messages in local or regional newspapers, radio and TV-stations, to digital media; respondents mentioned apps (1) specifically developed for events, events pages on Facebook, Twitter accounts (3); also text alerts may be used (3). Not surprisingly, every event has its own website.

With some events communication with the crowd is inextricably linked with monitoring and signaling (4). One particular event, for instance, makes use of a camera control room, in which camera streams on different locations are continuously monitored. When crowding exceeds a certain threshold, operators will start communicating with the public using LED displays, informing them that that the particular location has become too crowded. It is then left to the individual to act as they see fit. Because the crowding threshold is set at a level at which there is no immediate safety risk, as long as the fast majority decides to abstain from moving to this location, it is not problematic if individuals should decide to ignore this information. LED display messages (such as "Location X is crowded; please go to another location") therefore form the first line of defence against crowding at this particular event. If this fails, one of a handful of standard auditory messages, recorded on a CD and delivered to stage managers on all festival locations beforehand, is selected and subsequently broadcast. When other undesirable situations (a calamity, extreme weather, etc.) threaten to happen, a signal from the police will lead to the emission of identical standard messages to the public; not just the auditory messages mentioned before, but also messages via LED displays, text-alerts, and Twitter (2). As soon as the situation is back to normal, LED display are turned off again, in order to retain their "attention value" (1); overuse of LED displays may cause important messages to go unnoticed. A similar cycle of monitoring and intervening is implemented at other events (3).

Cameras, however, are not always the only means for monitoring purposes. Personnel "on the ground" are often valuable sources of information about crowdedness and crowd states, and sometimes the one is used to back-up the other as a double check (1).

3.3   Social Media

The majority of the events focused on in this study made use of social media as means of communicating with their visitors. Facebook, Whatsapp en Ping are deemed less suitable because of their selective availability. Twitter on the other hand is openly accessible and is often used (8). One of the experts interviewed indicated that a small study conducted during the event had established that Twitter messages managed to reach some 120 000 recipients. This, however, was greatly helped by a local TV-station re-tweeting the messages, a local newspaper reporting about them, and websites taking it up (1). This incidental study indicates that the reach of Twitter messages is increased when they combine with other media (1). These other media may also allow for communication with visitor groups who cannot be reached by Twitter alone.

The use of social media at events is by no means restricted to a one-way stream of information. In addition to providing information to event visitors, messages transmitted via social media also allow organisers to adapt to them. Not only may messages on social media be indicative of tensions in crowds, they may also make organisers aware that a part of the event location has become littered and that garbage containers and trash cans need to be emptied, for instance (2).

Despite these evident advantages, some of the experts (5) remain critical of the use of social media. First of all, events differ amongst each other in terms of the particular groups of people they attract, and even within events there may be widely varying groups of people simultaneously present. The effectiveness of social media, or of any other media for that matter, depends to no considerable extent on the composition of event crowds: social media may be effective with a relatively young crowd, whereas older people may prefer more conventional medias as TV or newspapers (2).

Second, one expert remarked that whereas social media may be effective before an event takes place, this may not necessarily be the case during events. When visiting an event, people may be busy enjoying themselves with performances and each other, or determining where they want to go next and how to get there. Thus being otherwise engaged makes it less likely that social media will be an effective means of communication, the occasional posting of pictures and clips aside (1). Other experts point to the limited reliability of telecommunication networks (5), and recommend the use of a media mix, i.e. not just social media but also more traditional means as LED displays, folders, and sound systems (1).

3.4   Communicating as One

Several interviewees stress the importance of "communicating as one" (6), to prevent spreading of contradictory information and increase message effectiveness. Communicating as one requires considerable effort. It involves not only explicit messages dissipated via many channels and with a vast array of potential senders, but it also requires bringing non-verbal communication in line (1). Several incidents involving crowd behaviour have been attributed to an incongruence in communication. For instance, one interviewee recalled an incident in the city of The Hague in the early nineties in which the police's intent, to divert the flow of a protesters, was not matched by their non-verbal communication, i.e., the presence of riot police in full combat gear (helmets, truncheons, shields, etc.). This resulted in a tumultuous course of events, including protesters clashing with riot police (1) – rather different from what was intended.

In addition, the official investigation into the so-called Project X riots in Haren (2012), a small town in the north of the Netherlands, stresses the negative effect of incongruent communication. In response to an accidental open invitation on Facebook, several thousand adolescents travelled to Haren ostensibly to celebrate a local girl's sixteenth birthday. Prior to and during this "event" local authorities and the police did their utmost to stem the flow of visitors using traditional and social media, but failed to communicate congruently and as one. Efforts focused on dissuading people to come to Haren by communicating that there would not be a party. A local government spokesperson, however, let it be known that an alternative party on one of the sports fields was under consideration. Likewise, explicit messages that visitors would be forced to turn back did not correspond with what they experienced on-site, as alcohol prohibition was not enforced. Especially the arrival of riot police sparked heavy rioting, resulting in considerable damage to adjacent homes and gardens, and the arrest of some 108 people.

Especially pregnant in this regard is the widespread use of social media by the many parties involved in events, such as the municipality, organising committee, and police. Each realise that social media could increase their means to actively communicate with the public. With so many parties involved, however, their use of Twitter accounts further increases the risk of one party explicitly or implicitly contradicting another.

For similar reasons, event organisers are wary of the presence of police helicopters and drones (2). Visitors noticing helicopters flying overhead might well conclude that something is going on – why else would police be watching from the sky? Similarly, the use of drones may be very desirable from a crowd monitoring perspective, but may also lead to undesirable perceptions among those being monitor. Not only might they infer that something is amiss, but they might also feel their privacy is being violated – an issue very much alive in Dutch media. Such deductions might be in stark contrast with what organisers or police want to convey, which is considered to possibly result in averse crowd states and behaviours.

Not surprisingly, many interviewees strive to create unity in the messages they transmit, not only within but also across organizations, i.e. incorporating the organizing committee, municipality, police, security personnel, public transportation organizations, etc. Preferably, these message are identical, not just content wise, but also on the actual word level (1). Usually, all those involved are enthusiastic participators, and may feel the urge to send out updates from their specific points of view, putting communication congruence at risk (2). One interviewee expressed the wish to replace individual Twitter accounts by one event-specific account, but realised this would probably be met with considerable resistance.

4   Conclusions and Discussion

The current study was part of a much larger project attempting to tap into the body of practical experience of experts in the field of crowd control and crowd management. Reported here are the findings specifically pertaining to technology as a means to communicate with event visitors.

One of the general findings is that, in line with insights in crowds psychology, virtually all experts interviewed acknowledge crowds and their behaviour to be (boundedly) rational, and that influencing crowds and crowd flow should be about providing information and advice, rather than forcing them or restricting movement. Information provision, for instance that one particular location has become crowded, may occur through LED displays at strategic locations. It is then left to the individual to act appropriately. Whether this stance is a direct result of developments in crowd psychology, or that it has come about through (accumulated) experience, is a question that cannot be answered on the basis of these data.

Smart phones and social media offer great potential for crowd management and crowd control. Consequently, they are much used means to inform visitors before and during events, in addition to undiminished use of more conventional means, e.g., LED displays, sound systems, local and regional media, etc. Interestingly, social media enable a bi-directional stream of information; event organisers may use them to optimise service provision, for instance, or get a feel for the general mood.

Several drawbacks can be derived from existing literature and the interviews, however. The availability of vast amounts of information, both relevant and irrelevant, may cause overloading [e.g., 24], or may cause information from organisers to lose effectiveness. In addition, effectiveness of social media depends on the composition of event crowds, and one could also object that perhaps, during an event people pay less attention to social media. Other experts point to the limited reliability of telecommunication networks, but this would apply to all technical means of communication.

Experts attach great importance to maintaining unity in communicating with the crowd. Communicating as one and information congruency are key to persuasion effectiveness. The more means of communication are at organisers' disposal and the more parties are involved in organising an attempt, the greater the risk may be that this unity is jeopardised. In addition, it is important to note that this applies to all communication, be it in text, speech, or behaviour, verbal or non-verbal. Also the use of police helicopters or drones for monitoring purposes may well conflict with what organisers want to communicate.

With regard to social media one could argue that a complicating factors is the change in popularity of the many platforms over time. According to Dutch research [26], Facebook and Youtube are currently the largest, followed by LinkedIn and Twitter. Although the growth of Facebook is momentarily diminishing, still about 80 % of 15 to 20 year olds still use it (50 % for Twitter). Based on these data Facebook may appear to be a safe bet for events targeting this particular age group, but in fact very little is known about social media use during events. If activity is limited to posting the occasional picture of one's favourite artist, this would argue against using Facebook as a means of communication during events.

The omnipresent smart phone, in combination with access of Internet and social media, could seriously hamper organisers in their attempts to manage crowds. For instance, accidents occurring during the event may start to lead a life of their own on social media, confronting organisers with the often difficult task to bring this back to the right proportions. In addition, with meteorological information being readily available, people may draw premature conclusions about the weather, deviating from that of a dedicated meteorologist who advices the event organiser. A very relevant question therefore would be how organisers can maintain or increase persuasion effectiveness in the face of a deluge of social media contributions, so as to ensure that all those present at an event take the right precautionary action or abstain from unnecessary ones. A recent first step in answering the question how crisis communication should be designed to be able to compete with Internet messages [27] suggests that incorporating action perspectives, i.e. informing people which actions they themselves can take to counter an emergency situation, reduces people's tendency to look for additional information elsewhere.

Similarly, one of the major challenges of persuasive technology in the field of event safety is uncovering how to compete with other available information. We have already seen signs of an evolution in the use of apps, from the dedicated apps at major events, such as Rock Werchter in Belgium, to the Amsterdam Queen's Day celebration app, which was developed to communicate all kinds of information, directly or indirectly linked to safety. For instance, the app showed a map of the city, indicating crowdedness at specific locations, where to find First Aid stations, toilets, and public transportation stations. However, as some of the apps functionality had to be discontinued prematurely to prevent a mobile network overload, we still lack any insight into its full potential. An important next step would therefore be to test effectiveness of safety apps, and relatedly, how to increase their impact. In other words, research should be dedicated to studying to what extent such apps remain standing in the barrage of competing information, and how their "competitiveness" could be increased. Subsequently, it will be up to designers to transform these findings into persuasive technology that appeals to users.

The interviews on which this paper is based were not transcribed verbatim. Although great care was taken to ensure adequate renderings of the participants' opinions, this should be noted as a limitation of the study.

The current study constitutes a first attempt to uncover good practices among event safety professionals. Although 16 experts generously allowed us to take a look in their world, we feel we have only scratched the surface concerning the role technology may have in crowd persuasion - we hope this study will motivate others to add onto it.

References

1. Reicher, S., Stott, C., Cronin, P., Adang, O.: An integrated approach to crowd psychology and public order policing. Policing 27, 558–572 (2004)
2. Durrheim, K., Foster, D.: Technologies of social control: Crowd management in liberal democracy. Economy and Society 28, 56–74 (1999)
3. Festinger, L.: Some consequences of deindividuation in a group. Journal of Abnormal and Social Psychology 47, 382–389 (1952)
4. Challenger, R., Clegg, C.W., Robinson, M.A., Leigh, M.: Understanding crowd behaviours. Supporting Theory and Evidence, vol. 2. Cabinet Office (2010)
5. Reicher, S.D., Spears, R., Postmes, T.: A Social Identity Model of Deindividuation Phenomena. European Review of Social Psychology 6, 161–198 (1995)
6. Lea, M., Spears, R., De Groot, D.: Knowing Me, knowing You: Anonymity effects on social identity processes within groups. Personality and Social Psychology Bulletin 27, 526–537 (2001)
7. Kahneman, D.: Maps of bounded rationality: psychology for behavioral economics. The American Economic Review 93, 1449–1475 (2003)
8. Simon, H.: Bounded rationality and organizational learning. Organization Science 2, 125–134 (1991)
9. Sime, J.D.: Crowd psychology and engineering. Safety Science 21, 1–14 (1995)
10. Van Hiel, A., Hautman, L., Cornelis, I., De Clercq, B.: Football hooliganism: Comparing self-awareness and social identity theory explanations. Journal of Community and Applied Social Psychology 17, 169–186 (2007)

11. Stott, C., Adang, O., Livingstone, A., Schreiber, M.: Variability in the collective behaviour of England fans at Euro2004: 'Hooliganism', public order policing and social change. European Journal of Social Psychology 37, 75–100 (2007)
12. Stott, C., Adang, O., Livingstone, A., Schreiber, M.: Tackling football hooliganism: A quantitative study of public order, policing and crowd psychology. Psychology, Public Policy, and Law 14, 115–141 (2008)
13. Adang, O.M.J.: Initiation and escalation of collective violence: an observational study. In: Madensen, T., Knutsson, J. (eds.) Preventing Crowd Violence. Lynne Rienner Publishers, Boulder (2011)
14. Holgersson, S., Knutsson, J.: Dialogue Policing: AMeans for Less Crowd Violence? In: Madensen, T.D., Knutsson, J. (eds.) Preventing Crowd Violence, vol. 26, pp. 191–216. Lynne Rienner Publishers, Inc., London (2011)
15. P.E.R.F.: Managing major events: Best practices from the field. Police Executive Research Forum, Washington, D.C. (2011)
16. Stott, C.: Crowd Dynamics and Public Order Policing. In: Madensen, T.D., Knutsson, J. (eds.) Preventing Crowd Violence, vol. 26, pp. 25–46. Lynne Rienner Publishers, Inc., London (2011)
17. Drury, J., Cocking, C., Reicher, S.: Everyone for themselves? A comparative study of crowd solidarity among emergency survivors. British Journal of Social Psychology 48, 487–506 (2009)
18. Leach, J.: Why people 'freeze' in an emergency: Temporal and cognitive constraints on survival responses. Aviation Space and Environmental Medicine 75, 539–542 (2004)
19. Ruitenberg, A., Helsloot, I., Balk, H.: Zelfredzaamheid van burgers bij rampen en zware ongevallen. Kluwer Academic Publishers, Dordrecht (2004)
20. Oberijé, N.: Civil response after disasters: The use of civil engagement in disaster abatement. In: 14th Annual Conference on TIEMS 2007 (Year)
21. Terpstra, T., Stronkman, R., de Vries, A., Paradies, G.: Towards a realtime Twitter analysis during crises for operational crisis management. In: Proceedings of the 9th International ISCRAM Conference, Vancouver, Canada (Year)
22. Sutton, J.N.: Twittering Tennessee: distributed networks and collaboration following a technological disaster. In: 7th International ISCRAM Conference. ISCRAM (Year)
23. Starbird, K., Palen, L.: Pass it on?: Retweeting in mass emergency. In: 7th International ISCRAM Conference. ISCRAM (Year)
24. Aldoory, L., Van Dyke, M.A.: The roles of perceived "shared" involvement and information overload in understanding how audiences make meaning of news about bioterrorism. Journalism & Mass Communication Quarterly 83, 346–361 (2006)
25. Wood, M.: Cell@lert, for Government-to-Citizen mass communications in emergencies; "it's about time". In: Proceedings of the 2nd International ISCRAM Conference, Brussel (2005)
26. Newcom: Social Media in Nederland 2013. Newcom Research & Consultancy (2013)
27. Verroen, S., Gutteling, J.M., De Vries, P.W.: Enhancing Self-Protective Behavior: Efficacy Beliefs and Peer Feedback in Risk Communication. Risk Analysis 33, 1252–1264 (2013)
28. Lorenz, J., Rauhut, H., Schweitzer, F., Helbing, D.: How social influence can undermine the wisdom of crowd effect. Proceedings of the National Academy of Sciences 108, 9020–9025 (2011)
29. Dalal, S., Khodyakov, D., Srinivasan, R., Straus, S., Adams, J.: ExpertLens: A system for eliciting opinions from a large pool of non-collocated experts with diverse knowledge. Technological Forecasting and Social Change 78, 1426–1444 (2011)
30. Hill, S., Ready-Campbell, N.: Expert stock picker: The wisdom of (experts in) crowds. International Journal of Electronic Commerce 15, 73–101 (2011)

Appendix: Interview Topic List

During interviews, participants were asked to list and reflect on the following:

- Their interviewee's role in activities leading up to events crowd management, in particular with respect to communication with various stakeholders and/or during critical incidents
- Planning of communication as part of crowd management
- Means of communication employed as part of crowd management
- Means of communication employed as part of crowd control
- The specific roles of LED displays, social media, Internet, mobile phone, etc.
- The extent to which these are an effective means of communication before and during events

Mitigating Cognitive Bias through the Use of Serious Games: Effects of Feedback

Norah E. Dunbar[1], Matthew L. Jensen[2], Claude H. Miller[1], Elena Bessarabova[1], Sara K. Straub[1], Scott N. Wilson[3], Javier Elizondo[3], Judee K. Burgoon[4], Joseph S. Valacich[4], Bradley Adame[5], Yu-Hao Lee[1], Brianna Lane[1], Cameron Piercy[1], David Wilson[4], Shawn King[1], Cindy Vincent[6], and Ryan Scheutzler[4]

[1] Department of Communication and Center for Applied Social Research, University of Oklahoma, 2 Partners Place, 3100 Monitor, Suite 100, Norman, OK 73072, USA
[2] Price College of Business and Center for Applied Social Research, University of Oklahoma
[3] K20 Center, University of Oklahoma. 3100 Monitor Ave., Suite 200, Norman, OK 73072, USA
[4] Center for the Management of Information, University of Arizona, McClelland Hall, 1130 E Helen St. Tucson, AZ 85701, USA
[5] Hugh Downs School of Communication, Arizona State University, P.O. Box 871205, Tempe, AZ 85287, USA
[6] Department of Communication, Salem State University, 352 Lafayette Street, Salem, MA 01970, USA
{ndunbar,mjensen,chmiller,ebess,sk_straub,scott.wilson, elizondoj,leeyuhao33,blane,cpiercy,shawn1}@ou.edu, {jburgoon,jsvalacich,rschuetzler}@cmi.arizona.edu, davewilsonmism@gmail.com, cindy.vincent@salemstate.edu

Abstract. A serious video game was created to teach players about cognitive bias and encourage mitigation of both confirmation bias and the fundamental attribution error. Multiplayer and single-player versions of the game were created to test the effect of different feedback sources on bias mitigation performance. A total of 626 participants were randomly assigned to play the single player/multiplayer game once or repeatedly. The results indicate the single player game was superior at reducing confirmation bias and that repeated plays and plays of longer duration were more effective at mitigating both biases than a control condition where participants watched a training video.

Keywords: Cognitive bias, Confirmation bias, Feedback, Fundamental Attribution error, Serious Games.

1 Introduction

In our daily lives, we are often challenged with making fast decisions, and to do so, we rely on heuristics. Chaiken's *Heuristic-Systematic Model* of information processing [HSM; 1, 2] defines heuristic processing as relying on mental shortcuts or simple decision rules arising from conventional beliefs, whereas systematic information

A. Spagnolli et al. (Eds.): PERSUASIVE 2014, LNCS 8462, pp. 92–105, 2014.

processing requires a careful consideration of all available evidence and is much more cognitively taxing [3]. Heuristics are beneficial because they facilitate faster solutions and minimize cognitive effort, but they also lead to insufficient consideration of relevant, diagnostic information. When heuristics are used repeatedly and without systematic thought, they can lead to cognitive bias and poor decisions.

Reported here is an experiment incorporating a cognitive bias serious game we developed called MACBETH *(Mitigating Analyst Cognitive Bias by Eliminating Task Heuristics)* that tested alternative game mechanics in order to identify designs which are most conducive to mitigating reliance on cognitive biases. Different feedback manipulations were tested (multiplayer versus single-player game, repetition, and duration) to uncover improved ways to teach players to decrease biased reasoning, be able to recognize certain cognitive biases, and rely less on heuristics during decision-making.

2   Using a Serious Game to Mitigate Cognitive Bias

2.1   The MACBETH Game

The MACBETH game is a learning system where players must counteract a fictional terrorist threat by using the intelligence data at hand. Through game play, the system highlights the use of a bias and then provides the player information on and opportunities to practice bias mitigation techniques based on the HSM theoretical model. The development of the MACBETH game is described more fully by (author citation removed for blind review).

MACBETH teaches players to identify and mitigate two specific cognitive biases, confirmation bias and the fundamental attribution error[1]. Confirmation bias (CB) is the tendency for people to favor information that confirms their prior beliefs, expectations, or initial hypotheses [4]. This bias leads people to selectively choose or misinterpret information and discount disconfirming evidence. Fundamental attribution error (FAE) is the tendency for people to over-emphasize stable, personality-based explanations for behaviors observed in others (known as dispositions) while under-emphasizing the role of transitory and situational influences on the same behavior [5]. Overlooking situation and context can lead to biased interpretations of others' behaviors.

2.2   Feedback

One of the most important factors in mitigating cognitive bias is giving decision-makers appropriate feedback on their faulty decisions. For example, in the deception-detection literature, scholars have lamented the use of bias and stereotypes by both professional and lay detectors and have pointed to a lack of timely and relevant

---

[1] The game also trains players to be more aware of their own bias, something known as the bias blind spot, but the results of BBS are reported elsewhere because of page limitations and because BBS mitigation used different design mechanics (author citation removed for blind review).

feedback as one of the primary causes of their failures to make accurate veracity judgments [6, 7]. Similarly, research indicates that simply playing a learning game does not produce learning [8]. Providing instructional feedback responsive to specific player actions is a key technique for teaching within a learning game [9]. Instructional feedback influences learning as it guides player perception, knowledge, and actions [10-12]. Feedback is an effective teaching tool when it provides players objective learning goals with clear criteria of successful achievement, methods for players to compare their performance to the goals, and an understandable course to achieve the goals [13-15].

Feedback is particularly crucial for new players of learning games. New players can be overwhelmed with game mechanics and lose focus on the training components of the game if specific guidance or instruction during the new task is not provided [16]. MACBETH incorporates feedback into game play in order to guarantee player usage. Despite potentially slowing down game play initially, Billings [17] finds that detailed feedback early in the learning process may lead to faster learning.

Shute [18] argues "formative feedback," or feedback telling players what they are doing correctly or incorrectly through suggestions or guidance in order to "modify thinking or behavior for the purpose of improving learning" (p. 154), leads to better learning than only receiving "outcome feedback" (e.g., score, grade, accomplishment list, etc.). Accordingly, MACBETH incorporates both formative and outcome feedback in the form of mentors who provide guidance on how to play as well as from other players or artificial intelligence computer agents (AI).

2.3   Alternative Feedback Sources

Cognitive bias can be minimized when making decisions with a group when compared to making decisions individually because you must be prepared to defend your reasoning to the group [19]. Even having a computerized "critic" question one's decisions can reduce the bias [20]. Further, Michael and Chen [21] posit that immersive collaborative virtual environments may increase students' understanding of abstract concepts. Multiplayer gaming environments encourage players to "communicate and collaborate to achieve individual and collective goals" [22]. Therefore, the construct of collaborative multiplayer gaming provides an opportunity to analyze alternative sources of feedback within serious games.

We believe a collaborative multiplayer game design has the potential to mitigate bias more than a single-player design. In a review of educational research, Johnson, Johnson, and Smith [23] note multiple studies indicating that cooperative learning improves learning outcomes relative to individual work. Application of their findings to serious games indicates the opportunity for players to actively interact and construct knowledge with another player, not simply having knowledge transmitted from a screen, should lead to higher levels of learning. We tested alternative feedback sources by creating a collaborative multiplayer game in which players received messages from other players in during play and shared a common goal, we compared this multiplayer game to a single-player game in which players only received information from the game after submitting a hypothesis (see section 3.1.1 below). We predict:

H1: The collaborative Multiplayer version of MACBETH is superior to the Single-Player version at mitigating CB and FAE.

2.4   Repeated Play and Duration

Learning a new game increases extraneous cognitive load and can decrease content specific learning for new players [24] [25]. However, as people play a game over time, they become more comfortable with game mechanics [22], allowing them to decrease the cognitive load of processing the game mechanics and redirect cognitive load toward learning content. Serge et al. [16] discovered that players improved performance significantly after their initial playing session if they had been presented with specific feedback acting as a "refresher" of training material. Longer exposure and repetition may improve memory of the content, but it may also lead to mental fatigue [26], which may increase reliance on heuristic processing to reduce cognitive load, which then increase the likelihood of making biased judgments. In a previous study testing the effects of the MACBETH game using either implicit or explicit instruction, we found that repeated play and longer duration of play were more effective than shorter or non-repeated gameplay (author citation removed for blind review). In light of these findings, we replicate the previous study and offer the following hypotheses:

H2: Longer exposure to MACBETH through a) repeated play or b) longer duration of play will be more effective at mitigating CB and FAE.

Finally, the funding agency that sponsored the game was also interested in testing whether the game would be more successful at mitigating cognitive bias compared to a more traditional learning video. They prepared a 30-minute instructional video that featured an instructor in a lab coat discussing the biases and vignettes demonstrating the bias through everyday interactions. We argue that playing the serious game would be more effective in mitigating CB and FAE than the instructional video because the game allow players to practice making active decisions and revise their decision-making methods by considering the feedback. We propose the following hypothesis:

H3: The MACBETH game will be superior to the control video at mitigating CB and FAE

3   Method

In this experiment, the key variable was Player Type (single vs. multiplayer), and exposure (repeated play, duration). Participants played either a single-player version of the game or a multiplayer version, in which they played with either at least one human participant or an artificial intelligence (AI) when another human player was not available.

Participants ($N = 626$ valid cases) were recruited by mass emails and classroom announcements at two large universities ($n = 309$ and 317). In total, 236 participants played a single-player game and 334 played a multiplayer game. Of those who played the multiplayer version, 71 played with another human, 114 played with the AI, and 149 played at least part of their time with a human and part with the AI (a mix of human and AI partners). Of the 626 participants involved in the initial experiment, 421 (67%) completed an 8-week follow-up survey measuring for long-term effects.

Research assistants at both locations followed an identical experimental script. Following their initial survey, voluntary participants arranged appointments using an online scheduling service. They were compensated $20 for participation at each laboratory session.

Upon arriving at the lab, participants were directed to a computer. Participants then completed pretest measures using the Qualtrics online survey tool, received the experimental treatment (game or video), completed post-measures, and were debriefed. If they were assigned to return to the lab, they made an appointment to return in one week. Some participants were assigned to the take-home condition, and they were given instructions for logging in to the game from home.

3.1 Independent Variables

Three independent variables were tested in various treatments of the MACBETH game, resulting in ten experimental conditions including the control video. The game treatment variables manipulated are as follows:

3.1.1 Player Type (Single vs. Multiplayer)

Participants played either a single-player version of the game or a multiplayer-version in which they played with either another human participant or an artificial intelligence (AI), the AI provided feedback to players just as another human participant. Comparisons between the multiplayer version players who played with a human to those who played with the AI were not significant so they were combined into a single condition. Qualitative analyses also revealed that players were unaware that the AI players were not human.

There were several ways in which the source of feedback differed in game play between the multiplayer and single player versions of the game. The single-player game had two computer agent analysts but they were not trained to mimic human players. In the multiplayer version, the players also had two "fellow analyst," one analyst was a computer agent similar to the ones in the single player version. The other analyst was either a human player or a computer agent simulating a human player.

In the single-player version of the game, players could request to receive either confirming or disconfirming intelligence from computer agents. The player received pre-programmed feedback based on their choice. For the multiplayer version, the player could request assistance from another player. The player receiving the request then provided Intel to the player and could possibly receive points. Intel sent from a request appeared in the other player's dropbox, a messaging system used for communication between each player in the multiplayer version. A player fulfilling a request received feedback based on the type of Intel submitted.

Intel review differed in each version. In the single-player version, the player could either justify his/her own hypothesis or disconfirm the computer agent's hypothesis. For the multiplayer version, the player could justify his/her own hypothesis or disconfirm the other player's hypothesis. If the player chose to provide Intel to the other player, the Intel appeared in that player's dropbox. In this way, the players interacted with each other as alternative sources of Intel collection and disconfirming/confirming feedback.

Another difference between multiplayer and single-player was in the final hypothesis section. In the single-player version, when the player submitted a final hypothesis they gained points based on correct items. If the player had insufficient evidence to prove the hypothesis they received a penalty. For the multiplayer version, when a player submitted a final hypothesis, it had to be approved or rejected by the other player. To reject a hypothesis, a player had to submit disconfirming Intel, which then appeared in the other player's dropbox. If a hypothesis was approved, the submitting player received a bonus. If a hypothesis was rejected, the rejecting player received points and the submitting player received a penalty. Both players shared the final approved hypothesis and gained points based on correct items.

3.1.2 Duration and Repetition

Players were randomly assigned to the 30- or 60-minute duration condition. The players were also randomly assigned to either a single play in the laboratory, repeated play in the laboratory, or the take-home condition. Participants in the take-home condition were given 60 minutes of gameplay in the lab and then sent home with instructions for how to play at home. 68 players elected to play at home, they spent an average of almost 3 hours playing the game ($M = 2:51:32$, $SD = 2:15:52$).

3.2 Bias Mitigation Measures

We designed and tested a new CB scale loosely modeled after Rassin's (2010) Test Strategy Scale. Six new CB measures were developed to make up two scales labeled "NewCB" scales (see Appendix A). Each of the two 3-item scales were used every other time period (pretest, posttests after in-lab play, and 8-week follow up) across the four time periods. The Cronbach's α reliability for NewCB was .68 for the pretest, .87 for Posttest 1, .91 for Posttest 2, and .90 for the 8-week follow-up test.

In order to measure susceptibility to FAE, we began with *Ron's Bad Day* from Riggio and Garcia [27] and created additional scenarios (including items depicting both positive and negative events) to measure the degree to which individuals rely on situational versus dispositional attributes. Participants saw two scenarios, one positive (e.g., Alex's successful day) and one negative (e.g., Ron's bad day) and were asked to explain the cause of the scenario. An example of the questions looked like this:

Ron was a bit late to work on Monday morning because there was a bad traffic jam. When he arrived at work he didn't feel very well and got a slow start on his work for the day. He made it to his 10:00 a.m. staff meeting, but because that meeting ran 10 minutes late, he arrived late at his 11:30 a.m. sales team meeting. At

that meeting Ron and three of his coworkers were supposed to present a new pro-
duction line to the Director, but the presentation wasn't finished and the laptop
projector wasn't functioning properly. At 2:30 p.m. when Ron was back at his
desk, three clients called and canceled their long-standing monthly supply con-
tracts with Ron's firm. At 4:00 p.m. Ron was called in to the Director's office and
fired. Using the scale below, please indicate the extent to which you believe these
factors contributed to Ron's day.
_____ *His skills*_____ *His personality*_____ *His abilities*_____ *His*
*workplace environment*_____ *His coworkers*_____ *His staff*_____ *His*
*clients*_____*His director*_____ *The traffic jam*_____ *His work technology*

The goal is to avoid dispositions and provide more situational cues. To calculate
their susceptibility to FAE, we summed their dispositional score based on ratings of
the 5 dispositional items (e.g. personality, skills, abilities) and also calculated an average situational score for the other 5 items related to the scenario (e.g. the weather).
When subjects are trained, they should have a lower dispositional score relative
to their situational score. The Cronbach's α reliabilities for the dispositional scores
were .85, .93, .90, and .89 for the four test periods and were .77, .88, .83, and .85 for
situational scores.

3.3   Personality Variables

Because the two Universities differed from one another in their cultural diversity, we
measured and controlled for cultural orientation using the items developed by Singe-
lis, Triandis, Bhawuk, and Gelfand (1995). Cronbach's α ranged from .65 to76. We
measured the Big Five personality traits (extroversion, agreeableness, conscientiousness, emotional stability and openness) which had α ranging from .75 to .88. We also
measured computer comfort, gaming experience, and other covariate measures but
they are not reported here due to space limitations.

4   Results

For all analyses reported below, we conducted a repeated-measures ANCOVA. The
analysis included Duration (30 vs. 60-min.), Repetition (one-shot, repeat-play, take-
home) and Player Type (multiplayer vs. single-player) as between-subject factors. To
maintain comparability across conditions, the within-subjects factor (test period) had
three levels: pretest, latest posttest (posttest 2 for the repeat players, posttest 1 for one-
shot and video players), and 8-week Posttest. Initial models included all covariates.
Non-significant covariates were pruned from the final analysis. Gender and Location
were also included as factors but were removed if they were not significant.

4.1   Confirmation Bias Mitigation Results

To test CB mitigation, we first conducted a repeated-measures ANCOVA on
the NewCB measure. Only one covariate, Agreeableness, was significant, thus, the

non-significant covariates were removed. Examination of the within subjects effects on the reduced model revealed a significant Test Period × Player Type, $F(2, 806) = 10.48$, $p < .001$, $\eta_p^2 = .025$, indicating, contrary to H1, that the single-player game was clearly more effective at mitigating confirmation bias than the multiplayer game, which in turn outperformed the control video (see Figure 1). A near-significant Test Period × Repetition interaction, $F(4, 806) = 2.22$, $p = .065$, $\eta_p^2 = .01$, showed the in-lab-repeat game tended to produce more bias mitigation than the one-shot and take-home conditions, which in turn outperformed the control video. The mitigation effect of the single player repeat condition was still significant at the 8-week Posttest.

The ANCOVA also revealed a significant 3-way Test Period × Repetition × Duration interaction, $F(2, 806) = 3.71$, $p = .025$, $\eta_p^2 = .01$, indicating the 60-minute, in-lab repeat game condition was more effective than the other two game conditions, which in turn were more effective than the control video. Again the mitigation effect of the 60 minutes single player repeat condition was significant after 8 weeks.

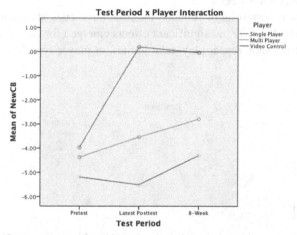

Covariates appearing in the model are evaluated at the following values: agreeableness = 5.4178

Fig. 1. Test Period x Player Interaction on NewCB (higher scores indicate less bias)

An independent samples t-test comparing the best performing game (60-minute, in-lab repeat, single-player) to the control video for NewCB indicated significantly less confirmation bias following the 8-week Posttest ($M = 0.55$, $SE = 1.29$) relative to the control video ($M = -4.58$, $SE = 0.78$), $t(78) = 3.40$, $p = .001$, $d = .77$, $r = .36$. Note, this large effect is due to the best game condition producing 100% mitigation with a mean above zero for NewCB at the 8-week Posttest, whereas the control video mean is well below zero and does not differ significantly from the control video pretest mean.

4.2   FAE Scenario Mitigation Results

Multivariate results indicated that Vertical Individualism, $F(2, 396) = 8.34$, $p < .001$, $\eta^2 = .041$ was the only significant covariate in the model. Omnibus results for reliance on dispositional cues revealed a significant effect for Repetition (one-shot, repeat-play, take-home), Wilk's $\lambda = .971$, $F(4, 790) = 2.94$, $p =.02$, $\eta^2 = .015$ and Duration (30 vs. 60-min.), Wilk's $\lambda = .983$, $F(2, 396) = 3.37$, $p =.035$, $\eta^2 = .02$. Player (single-player vs. multiplayer) failed to achieve significance.

Contrast effects showed a significant linear effect for Repetition (one-shot, repeat-play, take-home), $F(2, 397) = 5.23$, $p =.006$, $\eta^2 = .03$, with the players in the take-home condition achieving the lowest reliance on dispositional cues (Figure 2).

A significant quadratic contrast effect for Duration (30 vs. 60-min.), $F(1, 397) = 6.67$, $p =.01$, $\eta^2 = .02$, indicated that players in the 60-minute condition performed best at mitigating their reliance on dispositional cues, whereas participants in the 30-minute and video conditions showed a slight decay in their ability to mitigate the FAE. Here again, lower scores represent evidence of more effective mitigation of the FAE. Several of the game conditions significantly mitigated FAE but the control video only showed evidence of bias mitigation immediately after play but did not retain the mitigation after 8 weeks.

Omnibus results for analysis of reliance on situational cues shows no significant covariates emerged. Moreover, no significant effects emerged for Duration (30 vs. 60-min.), Repetition (one-shot, repeat-play, take-home), or player type (single-player vs. multiplayer).

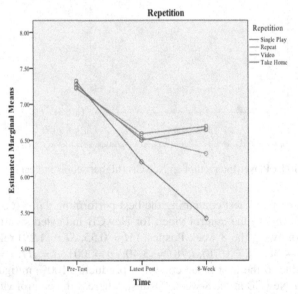

Fig. 2. Means for FAE Scenario - Dispositional Cues: Significant linear effect for Repetition (higher scores indicate more bias)

5   Discussion

Hypothesis 1 posited that the multiplayer game would outperform the single player game. It was not supported. In fact, the result showed that players in single player games performed better in bias mitigation, especially for confirmation bias. One possible explanation for this finding is that single players experienced less time waiting for their partners to react and had more engagement with the training materials. If multiplayer games force a trade-off between time learning skills and time interacting with partners, then the single-player version might be more successful at teaching mitigation strategies overall.

Hypothesis 2, that increased exposure to the game would enhance training, was supported. The longer game generally outperformed the shorter game and the repeated play conditions were superior to the single game play experience. The MACBETH game was a complex strategy game and had a steep learning curve. The players in the shorter conditions were just figuring out how to play when their sessions ended, so the additional sessions were especially beneficial for this game.

Hypothesis 3 predicted that the game would outperform the instructional video provided by the funding agency. One of the natural advantages of a game over a traditional lecture or video is the repeatability feature. You can play a game over and over and obtain more training with each session, whereas learners are unlikely to hear a lecture or watch a video more than once. However, even comparing the 30-minute game without repetition to the 30-minute control video, the means show that the game was superior at mitigating CB (although not FAE).

MACBETH significantly reduced bias from the pretests to the posttests for all the biases in most of the game conditions, producing similar mitigation results to those of the instructional video for FAE. However, the game produced a robust mitigation effect for CB, which significantly surpassed the video with an impressively large effect. For repeated play, the in-lab repeat-play and the take-home versions both substantially decreased bias and were generally equivalent. For FAE, the take-home proved the superior but the effect was small whereas for CB, the take-home and the in-lab repeat both were equally effective, demonstrating a large effect size for both.

6   Conclusions

Lave and Wenger [28] state that "knowledge is entwined with practice." We argue that serious games are more effective than training videos in cognitive bias training because it offers interactive decision-making practices and repeatable lessons. Cognitive biases are caused by over-relying on heuristics, which are difficult to tackle because they are so natural and require little cognitive effort. While the video can teach users about the biases, its ability to improve user "awareness" of their heuristics is limited because heuristics are most commonly applied in situations that require fast decision making and not deep considerations. In comparison, serious games can not only teach players about the biases, they also offer opportunities for players to repeatedly practice and reflect on their decisions. The interactive practices help players to identify situations in which cognitive bias may arise, and allow players to reroute their decision-making processes. The results showed that players' ability improved more with longer duration and repeated play, and even the 30-minutes short gameplay was superior to the video at mitigating some cognitive biases.

Another distinction from training videos is that serious games provide player with both performance and formative feedback. The feedback allow players to understand whether their decisions are biased or not and to adjust their decisions to improve their performance. We had initially hypothesized that feedback from other players (in the multiplayer game) would improve bias mitigation more than feedback from the game itself because the interaction would facilitate cooperation and competition and deepen attention to the decision. To our surprise, players of the multiplayer game performed worse than the single-player game, perhaps because players in the multiplayer game experienced more waiting time and were exposed to less practice. Another explanation is that the single-player game offered "correct" answers immediately, which helped players reflect on their decision. Comparatively, the multiplayer game required players to wait for their partners to provide feedback, feedback that might or might not be biased.

In summary, this study showed that serious games can be effective learning systems that change behaviors through interactive practice and feedback. The speed between the decision and the feedback may also be a vital part of game design that affects learning and persuasion effects.

Acknowledgements. This study was conducted according to the human subject protection procedures reviewed and approved by the internal review board at University of Oklahoma and the Air Force Research Laboratory.

The authors thank the graduate students in the CMI program at the University of Arizona and the students of Drs. Dunbar, Jensen, Bessarabova, and Miller at the University of Oklahoma for their suggestions and guidance through the development of this project. The authors would also like to thank the talented game development team at the K20 Center at the University of Oklahoma.

This research was supported by the Intelligence Advanced Research Projects Activity (IARPA) via the Air Force Research Laboratory (AFRL). The views and conclusions contained herein are those of the authors and should not be interpreted as necessarily representing the official policies or endorsements, either expressed or implied, of IARPA, AFRL, or the U.S. Government.

References

1. Chaiken, S.: Heuristic versus systematic information processing and the use of source versus message cues in persuasion. Journal of Personality and Social Psychology 39(5), 752–766 (1980)
2. Todorov, A., Chaiken, S., Henderson, M.D.: The heuristic-systematic model of social information processing. In: The Persuasion Handbook: Developments in Theory and Practice, pp. 195–211 (2002)

3. Chen, S., Chaiken, S.: Dual-process theories in social psychology. In: Dual-Process Theories in Social Psychology, pp. 73–96 (1999)
4. Nickerson, R.S.: Confirmation bias: A ubiquitous phenomenon in many guises. Review of General Psychology 2(2), 175 (1998)
5. Harvey, J.H., Town, J.P., Yarkin, K.L.: How fundamental is" the fundamental attribution error"? Journal of Personality and Social Psychology 40(2), 346 (1981)
6. Frank, M.G., Feeley, T.H.: To catch a liar: Challenges for research in lie detection training. Journal of Applied Communication Research 31(1), 58–75 (2003)
7. Vrij, A.: The impact of information and setting on detection of deception by police detectives. Journal of Nonverbal Behavior 18(2), 117–136 (1994)
8. Mayer, R.E.: Should there be a three-strikes rule against pure discovery learning? American Psychologist 59(1), 14 (2004)
9. Delacruz, G.C.: Impact of Incentives On the Use Of Feedback in Educational Videogames: CRESST report 813. National Center for Research on Evaluation, Standards, and Student Testing, 1–18 (2012)
10. Hays, R.T.: The effectiveness of instructional games: A literature review and discussion. In: Book The Effectiveness of Instructional Games: A Literature Review and Discussion (DTIC Document) (2005)
11. Mayer, R.E., Johnson, C.I.: Adding instructional features that promote learning in a game-like environment. Journal of Educational Computing Research 42(3), 241–265 (2010)
12. Moreno, R.: Decreasing cognitive load for novice students: Effects of explanatory versus corrective feedback in discovery-based multimedia. Instructional Science 32(1-2), 99–113 (2004)
13. Bangert-Drowns, R.L., Kulik, C.-L.C., Kulik, J.A., Morgan, M.: The instructional effect of feedback in test-like events. Review of Educational Research 61(2), 213–238 (1991)
14. Hattie, J., Timperley, H.: The power of feedback. Review of Educational Research 77(1), 81–112 (2007)
15. Kluger, A.N., DeNisi, A.: The effects of feedback interventions on performance: A historical review, a meta-analysis, and a preliminary feedback intervention theory. Psychological Bulletin 119(2), 254–284 (1996)
16. Serge, S.R., Priest, H.A., Durlach, P.J., Johnson, C.I.: The effects of static and adaptive performance feedback in game-based training. Computers in Human Behavior 29(3), 1150–1158 (2013)
17. Billings, D.R.: Adaptive feedback in simulation-based training. Unpublished doctoral dissertation, University of Central Florida Orlando, Florida (2010)
18. Shute, V.J.: Focus on formative feedback. Review of Educational Research 78(1), 153–189 (2008)
19. Kerschreiter, R., Schulz-Hardt, S., Mojzisch, A., Frey, D.: Biased Information Search in Homogeneous Groups: Confidence as a Moderator for the Effect of Anticipated Task Requirements. Personality and Social Psychology Bulletin 34(5), 679–691 (2008)
20. Silverman, B.G.: Modeling and critiquing the confirmation bias in human reasoning. IEEE Transactions on Systems, Man and Cybernetics 22(5), 972–982 (1992)
21. Michael, D.R., Chen, S.L.: Serious games: Games that educate, train, and inform. Thomson Course Technology (2006)
22. Dickey, M.D.: World of Warcraft and the impact of game culture and play in an undergraduate game design course. Computers & Education 56(1), 200–209 (2011)
23. Johnson, D.W., Johnson, R.T., Smith, K.A.: Active Learning: Cooperation in the College Classroom (1998)

24. Rey, G.D., Buchwald, F.: The expertise reversal effect: Cognitive load and motivational explanations. Journal of Experimental Psychology: Applied 17(1), 33–48 (2011)
25. Sweller, J.: Cognitive load theory, learning difficulty, and instructional design. Learning and Instruction 4(4), 295–312 (1994)
26. Gonzalez, C., Best, B., Healy, A.F., Kole, J.A., Bourne, L.E.: A cognitive modeling account of simultaneous learning and fatigue effects. Cognitive Systems Research 12(1), 19–32 (2011)
27. Riggio, H.R., Garcia, A.L.: The Power of Situations: Jonestown and the Fundamental Attribution Error. Teaching of Psychology 36(2), 108–112 (2009)
28. Lave, J., Wenger, E.: Situated Learning: Legitimate peripheral participation. Cambridge University Press (1991)

Appendix A: New CB Scale

1. You walk out to your car one morning and you notice some damage to the rear bumper. You suspect one of your neighbors, whom you've seen leaving in a hurry several days this week, and who likes to park near where you were parked. If you wanted to test your suspicion, what question(s) would you ask others about this neighbor? You may ask one or multiple questions, however, your task is to choose as few as you need to adequately test your suspicion:

   o   Is there any reason to believe this neighbor did not crash into your car?
   o   Was this neighbor in a hurry to get to work again this morning
   o   Did anyone see this neighbor parked near where your car was?
   o   Is there proof this neighbor was not parked near where your car was?

2. You return to your work desk and notice your cell phone is missing. You suspect the person in the next cubicle because he frequently comes to your cubicle looking around to borrow one of your pens, and he may have been around while you were away. If you wanted to test your suspicion, what question(s) would you ask others about this person?   You may ask one or multiple questions, however, your task is to choose as few as you need to adequately test your suspicion:

   o   Is there any reason to believe this person did not steal your phone?
   o   Was this person recently in your cubicle looking around for a pen again?
   o   Did anyone see this person near your desk while you were away?
   o   Is there proof this person was not around your desk while you were away?

3. You find out someone borrowed your laptop last night without your permission and let the battery run all the way down. You think it's one of your brother's friends because he's always forgetting his own laptop, and he was probably around last night. If you wanted to test your suspicion, what question(s) would you ask others about this person?   You may ask one or multiple questions, however, your task is to choose as few as you need to adequately test your suspicion:

- o   Is there any reason to believe your brother's friend did not use your laptop?
- o   Did anyone notice if your brother's friend forgot his own laptop yesterday?
- o   Did anyone notice if your brother's friend was around last night?
- o   Is there proof your brother's friend was not around last night?

4. Someone took the six-pack you had chilling in the refrigerator before the party earlier in the evening. You suspect one of your roommate's friends took it because she's always asking to bum a drink, and she probably showed up early, like she usually does. If you wanted to test your suspicion, what question(s) would you ask others about this person?   You may ask one or multiple questions, however, your task is to choose as few as you need to adequately test your suspicion.

- o   Is there proof this friend was not around earlier before the party?
- o   Did anyone see this friend around before the party started?
- o   Is there any reason to believe this friend did not take the six-pack?
- o   Was this friend asking to bum a drink earlier in the evening?

5. You come home one evening and notice the lamp in your living room is broken. You suspect one of your roommates because you know he is a little clumsy when he drinks, and was probably around earlier that evening. If you wanted to test your suspicion, what question(s) would you ask others about this roommate?   You may ask one or multiple questions, however, your task is to choose as few as you need to adequately test your suspicion:

- o   Is there any reason to believe this roommate did not break the lamp?
- o   Had this roommate been drinking that day?
- o   Is there proof this roommate was not around earlier that evening?
- o   Did anyone see this roommate around earlier that evening?

6. Someone has stolen money from the locked cashbox at your workplace. You suspect one of your co-workers because you think she is desperately behind on her bills, and she once had a key to the cashbox. If you wanted to test your suspicion, what question(s) would you ask others about this co-worker? You may ask one or multiple questions, however, your task is to choose as few as you need to adequately test your suspicion:

- o   Is there proof this co-worker does not actually have a key?
- o   Is there any reason to think this co-worker did not steal the money?
- o   Did anyone see this co-worker with the key?
- o   Did this co-worker actually fall desperately behind on her bills?

Sentiment Variations in Text
for Persuasion Technology*

Lorenzo Gatti[1], Marco Guerini[1], Oliviero Stock[2], and Carlo Strapparava[2]

[1] Trento RISE, Trento, Italy
{l.gatti,marco.guerini}@trentorise.eu
[2] FBK-irst, Trento, Italy
{stock,strappa}@fbk.eu

Abstract. Accurate wording is essential in persuasive verbal communication. Through it speakers can provide an affective connotation to the text and reveal their disposition or induce a similar disposition on the recipient. All this is apparent in persuasion texts *par excellence*, such as political speech and advertisement. Automatic sentiment variations of existing linguistic expressions open the way to promising applications, yet it is a challenging problem. In this paper we describe a system which takes up this challenge, together with a framework for evaluating the persuasiveness of the newly produced expressions.

Keywords: Language-based persuasion, affective NLP, persuasiveness evaluation.

1 Introduction

The same information can be presented linguistically from various angles or in a biased way. For instance we can load the description of a specific situation with vivid, connotative words and figures of speech, without changing the basic content. Words can provide an affective connotation to the text and reveal the affective disposition of the speaker or induce an affective disposition on the recipient in a subtle way. Slanted wording together with rhetorical structure is a fundamental tool for persuasion and is sometimes necessary even to grab the attention of the audience. As a scenario for application of this work let us consider a restaurant that receives criticism on a popular website saying "Though the restaurant serves good dishes, it is extremely expensive". The restaurant website may have a message personalization program that automatically produces the counter-slogan "Though our restaurant is a bit expensive, it serves exquisite dishes". This message personalization program may also adapt the message prepared by the owner - suppose "our restaurant serves very good dishes" - to different targets: e.g. to the young "our *trendy* restaurant serves *fantastic* dishes", to more mature clients "our *well located* restaurant serves *delicious* dishes", taking into account the context and dynamically choosing the appropriate wording.

---

* This work respects professional code of conduct and does not qualify as coercion or deceit.

A. Spagnolli et al. (Eds.): PERSUASIVE 2014, LNCS 8462, pp. 106–117, 2014.
© Springer International Publishing Switzerland 2014

In essence, this paper is about Natural Language Generation (NLG) [36] of persuasive messages (either written or spoken) with a focus on *affective* NLG. Still, we are not concerned with generating messages from scratch, but with modifying the wording of existing texts, changing their overall sentiment and rendering them more positive or negative in view of the desired persuasive effect. Affective variations of pre-existing texts have been studied and implemented in various domains, see for example [19,27,20]. The effectiveness of affective variations has also been assessed; in particular, [41] shows that biased variations of a message work better than the neutral condition. With regard to output quality, [43] demonstrated that adding bigram frequencies for the insertion of valenced modifiers significantly improve the perceived quality of the resulting texts. For an annotated bibliography on affective NLG, see [33].

The paper is structured as follows. In section 2 we describe the role of emotions in persuasive systems and some systems exploiting them. In section 3 we focus on the task of sentiment variation and introduce VALENTINO, a tool for automatically modifying existing texts, that can be plugged into persuasive systems. In section 4 we describe some linguistic phenomena that this tool needs to consider to produce an effective output, together with the new architecture we developed. Finally, section 5 describes some methodologies to evaluate the persuasiveness of sentiment modification tools.

2   The Role of Emotions in Persuasive Systems

Emotional load can enhance or lower message effectiveness. Gmytrasiewicz and Lisetti [15] propose a useful framework on how the emotions *felt* by an agent can change his or her own behavior. Still, for persuasive purposes, we shall focus on four dimensions about emotional elements that can increase or diminish the persuasiveness of a message: (i) the current emotional state of the persuadee, (ii) the current emotional state of the persuader, (iii) the emotional state expressed by the persuader and (iv) the emotional state possibly produced in the persuadee. In this paper we will focus on the third point, i.e. "the emotional state expressed by the persuader" in the delivered verbal message. This includes the chosen wording and word order of the message.

Since emotional reasoning is usually performed in order to modify/increase the impact of the message, affective NLG is strictly connected to persuasive NLG. There are also many computational models of emotion dynamics based on cognitive theories like the one proposed by Ortony *et al.* [29]. Yet, their focus is on *believability*, for a natural communication with the user or for simulation purposes, rather than on emotions use for an *effective* communication.

Some works, worth mentioning, follow. Elliott [11] presents a multi-agent platform for simulating simple emotional "reactions" among groups of agents, depending on personality traits. However, this system does not address persuasion directly, since it focuses on emotions dynamics in complex social environments rather than emotions induction for persuasive interactions. Carofiglio and de Rosis [6] focus on emotions as a core element for affective message generation. The

implemented model is more complex and more "persuasion oriented" than Elliott's. They use a dynamic belief network for modeling activations of emotional
states during dialogues. De Rosis and Grasso [9] also focus on affective language
generation. Their model uses plan operators - for text structuring - enriched
with applicability conditions depending on the user's emotional traits. In [35]
the focus is on the use of emotional display for communicative situations such
as social lies and deception. In their work, the authors try to understand how
users will react if the information conveyed nonverbally exhibits clues that are
not consistent with the verbal part of an agent's action. Persuasive system that
adapt messages to users' profiles were recently studied, in particular by Kaptein
and colleagues [23,24]. In general, one of the most recent subjects of interest in
this trend of research concerns widening the persuasion modes from considering
'rational' or 'cognitive' arguments to appealing to values and emotional states
[38,16,34].

3   Persuasion and Sentiment-Based Text Variations

Sentiment is one of the dimensions of emotions, together with arousal, and is
concerned with the polarity of an emotion (either positive or negative, while
arousal can be either high or low). For example, *sadness* and *anger* have both a
negative polarity but a different arousal (*low* for the former, *high* for the latter).
In the example below two sentiment variations (one positive and one negative)
of a sentence are expressed:

"You should try our dishes"
"You should try our delicious dishes" (+)
"You should try our tasteless dishes" (−)

VALENTINO is a tool for modifying existing textual expressions towards more
positively or negatively valenced versions as an element of a persuasive system.
For instance, a strategic planner may decide to intervene on a draft text with the
goal of "colouring" it emotionally. When applied to a text, the changes invoked
may be uniformly negative or positive; they can smooth all emotional peaks; or
they can be used in combination with deep rhetorical structure analysis, resulting
in different types of changes for key parts of the texts. Automatic variation of
the sentiment of a text is important for several applied scenarios. In general, any
system that wants to persuade the audience to change beliefs or attitudes may
benefit from this aspect [13,27,40,43].

Yet, the generation or variation of vivid textual material is not limited to sentences, but it can also involve *slogans* (short, not necessarily grammatical) and
brand names. Regarding automatic generation of slogans, [31] presents an exten-
sible framework for the generation of creative sentences in which users are able
to force words to appear in the sentence and to control the generation process
across several semantic dimensions, namely emotions, colors, domain relatedness
and phonetic properties. Regarding branding, [30] proposes a computational approach to the automation of creative naming for new products. The approach

allows generating neologisms based on homophonic puns and metaphors with reference to the service category to be named and the properties to be evoked.

4   An Architecture for Sentiment Text Variations

Even if approaches relying on simple strategies (e.g. adding or subtracting sentiment bearing adjectives to the text here and there [40]) can sometimes be effective, automatically modifying text sentiment with persuasive intents is indeed a complex task. One of the key aspects is that from an aesthetic point of view a given variation is more appreciated if the change is limited so that the original expression is still "present", as suggested by the optimal innovation theory [14]. The task of sentiment variation can then be defined as:

modifying existing textual expressions towards more positively or negatively valenced versions, while keeping the original meaning unchanged as much as possible and the original form still vivid.

This optimal innovation principle is then instantiated by a set of specific rules (both high level and low level). High level rules can decide which parts of the text should be modified (including relocation in another part of the sentence), which other parts should not be touched or somehow constrained in their modification (these last two points are in particular fundamental to maintain a proper semantic coherence). Low level rules, instead, take care of the single parts of the message, and in accordance with high level rule indications, they can modify, insert or delete sentiment bearing words.

VALENTINO in particular can modify existing textual expressions producing more positively or negatively *graded* variations. These graded variations are of paramount importance when contextual or demographic information about the receiver is provided (e.g. strong variations, up to hyperbole, are more effective with the young, while softer ones with adults). For example in the field of on-line advertising, where lot of small businesses want to reach their potential customers without the budget for copywriting their ads, and with the need of having geo-localized and personalized communication, VALENTINO is a useful tool for their needs. In the example below we provide a numeric coefficient that represents the desired valence for the final ad (for a restaurant) and some produced outputs to be used in different context with different audiences:

"You should try our [good dishes]"
"You should try our [very good dishes]" (+0.5)
"You should try our [delicious dishes]" (+0.7)
"You should try our [exquisite dishes]" (+1)

The new architecture of VALENTINO is built to work in an open domain and without lexical restrictions, its resources are automatically built from large scale corpora and English lexical repositories (e.g., Google Web n-grams and WordNet [12,5]). The slanting process is divided in two main steps: analysis of the original message and modification.

In the first step, the input text is analyzed and enriched with information like PoS, morphology, syntax, rhetoric and affective weight. The second step uses this enriched representation as an input, and applies a series of high and low level rules. High-level rules decide which parts of the sentence need to be modified given their current affective score and rhetorical structure. E.g. we could make the sentence "although the restaurant is expensive, the dishes are very good" slightly more positive by lowering the effect of the first negative part without touching the second: "although the restaurant is **a bit** expensive, the dishes are very good". Low-level rules control the actual word substitution, insertion and deletion. They first extract possible candidates using WordNet relations, and then filter them by the target valence score and a language model.

4.1 Analysis

Constituents and Dependencies. Text dependencies must be taken into account, so that the language models can be properly queried. To this end, the text is POS tagged, morphologically analyzed and divided into sentence constituents using the TextPro package [32]. Then its dependencies and coreference relations are reconstructed using the Stanford CoreNLP suite [8,25].

Constituents are informative for short distance dependencies where we need to choose the proper context for querying the language model. In the following example we need to know where 'good' should be attached (i.e. either to the article or to the noun) for a pertinent query. We need to look for a meaningful 'good dish', not for something like 'our good'.

You should try [our **good** dishes]$_{NP}$

Parsing is instead fundamental for non adjacent phrases, where we need to know – for example – what is the argument of an adjectival constituent:

[The **dishes**]$_{np}$ we prepare fresh every day are [very **good**]$_{adjp}$.

In this case we need to query 'very good dish' since 'very good' alone is not enough to rule out adjectives similar to 'good' that are not related to 'dishes'.

Anaphora resolution is also needed in many cases, for example to project the proper NP to its ADJP trough pronouns:

We serve many [**dishes**]$_{np}$. Everybody says [they] are [very **good**]$_{adjp}$.

Semantic Reasoning. It is necessary to distinguish modifiers that have a similar form but a different semantic function. We are currently working on the analysis of semantic roles using the Semafor parser [7] to deal with cases:

SOURCE: We ate [the dish]$_{patient}$ [with the fork]$_{mean}$
OK: We ate [the **pleasant** dish]$_{patient}$ [with the fork]$_{mean}$
SOURCE: We ate [the dish]$_{patient}$ [with pleasure]$_{manner}$
OK: We ate [the dish]$_{patient}$ [with **great** pleasure]$_{manner}$

Rhetorical Analysis. The rhetorical structure of the sentence is important too, since it can impose constraints in the modification phase or it can be exploited to achieve subtle variations. We analyse it using the Hilda rhetorical parser [22], which returns relations like the following:

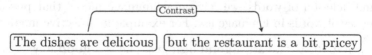

4.2   Modification

High Level Rules. Once the analysis has been completed, a set of high-level rules decide which part of the text should be modified. At present, we are including high-level rules of these 3 types:

- Rules that block the modification of a part of the sentence. For example, in statements of the form X_{NP} <be> Y_{ADJP} we want to modify chunk Y and leave X untouched, so that "Our dishes are very good" can become "Our dishes are delicious" but not "Our delicious dishes are delicious".
- Rules that move text spans in the same sentence. For example, since we know that when there is a `contrast` relation the second conjunct has a great recency effect, the system can swap the elements to have the positive one at the end to make the sentence more positive (i.e. "the dishes are delicious, but the place is a bit pricey" becomes "the place is a bit pricey, but the dishes are delicious").
- Rules that constraint the score of a constituent or of a phrase. For example, if we want to make the sentence "The restaurant is too expensive, but the dishes are delicious" more positive we cannot change "expensive" with a positive word like "affordable"; we can only mitigate valence by replacing it with "a bit pricey", otherwise the sentence would become nonsensical ("The restaurant is too affordable, but the dishes are delicious").

Low Level Rules. As can be seen from the above examples, most of the reasoning in VALENTINO is done on constituents and their relations (both inter-constituents and intra-constituents), and in general it follows these rules:

- Constituents are slanted as much as needed, but the target score should not be exceeded, limiting the variation to the minimum needed. E.g., it is not the case of saying "delicious dish" if "good dish" meets the target score.
- A constituent is modified considering first the dependents (from left to right) and then possibly the head (so for example, "very good dish" should be varied into "somewhat good dish" before than into "decent dish").

The rationale is that in a constituent as we move from the head outward the variation is less prominent. This way in general, if the valence sign is kept the same - positive or negative - at the same time we can minimize the meaning variation and let the user recognize the familiar initial sentence in the novel expression, creating a pleasing experience [14].

Both high and low level rules have been implemented in GBBopen[1], an open source blackboard system, that schedules which rules need to be applied first.

Language Models and Resources. To perform the actual substitution, insertion and deletion of words, we rely on a language model that provides the co-occurences of words in language use. For example in adjective modification:

SOURCE: "we ate a **good** dish" vs. "he is a **good** guy"
OK: "we ate a **delicious** dish" vs. "he is a **well-behaved** guy'
NO: "we ate a **well-behaved** dish"

Words relations (e.g. similar_to from WordNet or semantic similarity from LSA [10] are needed as well: in the above example they have been used to select the adjectives that are semantically similar to 'good'. The language model then tells us that 'delicious dish' is a viable option while 'well-behaved dish' is not, ensuring high quality output as experiments showed [43].

Metrics and Language Models. Given a language model different metrics can be used to choose among the best candidates for the shifting of the original expression. Metrics can be roughly divided into three groups:

- *Linguistic use* of a word/multiword expression, like n-gram frequency or Pointwise Mutual Information (PMI) [39]. The former is a measure that gives more relevance to very common terms/modifiers, while the latter favors words/modifiers that are specific to the term of interest ('dish' in the following case): '**exquisite** dish' has a low bigram frequency but a high PMI, the opposite is true for '**good** dish'.
- *Valence* of a word/multiword expression, so that we can state that 'fine' is less positive than 'good', which in turn is less positive than 'exquisite'.
- *Persuasiveness* of a word/multiword expression [17]: 'exquisite' and 'delicious' are synonyms (this implies that they have the same valence score) and have also a similar frequency/PMI. They are both good candidates for replacing 'good' in 'good dish', but if we consider their persuasive score 'delicious' is more "persuasive" than 'exquisite'.

To deal with the sentiment modification tasks described, we relied on an extended version of NgramQuery [1], a query-based engine that integrates WordNet with Google Web 1T 5-grams [5], which adds SentiWordNet [3] information. This tool allows to create a set of substitutes that match the target score and fit in the context. For example, the query for a strong positive substitute of 'good dish' is:

---

[1] http://gbbopen.org/

$$(\; similar\_to \; (\; adj \; good \;) \; \wedge \; affective\_score \; > 0.8 \;) + (\; noun \; dish \;)$$

The system will get all the adjectives similar to "good" from WordNet (finding, for example, "well-behaved", "delicious", "acceptable", "skilled", "exquisite"), then filter them according to the specified SentiWordNet affective score[2] 0.8 (so "acceptable" is removed because it is too weak). Then inappropriate adjectives ("well-behaved", "skilled") are ruled out because they are not co-occurring with "dish" in the language model. The remaining chunks can then be ranked by frequency or PMI between words, depending on the type of output we want to obtain. In addition specific n-gram patterns – see for example [42] – for extracting semantically exaggerated variations are used.

5 Evaluation Challenges

The evaluation of a linguistic persuasive system, which deals with many aspects of the produced text, involves many issues. The first step, especially at the prototyping stage, includes *output quality* (grammaticality and awkwardness) [43]. Another aspect fundamental at early stages of development is *output consistency*. This implies checking if the target score is effectively met in the final output, e.g. is "delicious dish" more positive than "good dish"? Is "decent dish" less positive? etc. Still, the paramount aspect of evaluation concerns *output effectiveness*: i.e. if the modified sentence has an actual effect on recipients behaviour. [21,40] The point is that the evaluation of the effectiveness of persuasive systems is very expensive and time consuming (as the STOP experience showed [37]): designing the experiment, recruiting subjects, making them take part in the experiment, dispensing questionnaires, gathering and analyzing data.

Existing methodologies for evaluating persuasion are usually split in two main sets, depending on the setup and domain: (i) long-term, in the field evaluation of behavioral change (as the STOP example mentioned before), and (ii) lab settings for evaluating short-term effects, as in [2]. While in the first approach it is difficult to take into account the role of external events that can occur over long time spans, in the second there are still problems of recruiting subjects and of time consuming activities such as questionnaire gathering and processing.

In addition, sometimes carefully designed experiments can fail because: (i) effects are too subtle to be measured with a limited number of subjects or (ii) participants are not engaged enough by the task to provoke usable reactions, see for example what reported in [40]. Especially the second point is critical: in fact, subjects can actually be convinced by the message to which they are exposed, but if they feel they do not care, they may not "react" at all, which is the case in many artificial settings.

---

[2] Since different senses of the same word can have different affective scores in SentiWordNet, and given that the Google corpus is not sense-disambiguated, we consider only prior polarity scores [18].

Partial Solution - Mechanical Turk. An emerging trend for behavioral studies is the use of Mechanical Turk [26] or similar tools to overcome a part of these limitations - such as subject recruitment. Still we believe that this poses other problems in assessing behavioral changes, and, more generally, persuasion effects. In fact: (i) studies must be as ecological as possible, i.e. conducted in real, even if controlled, scenarios; (ii) subjects should be neither aware of being observed, nor biased by external rewards.

In the case of Mechanical Turk for example, subjects are willingly undergoing a process of being 'tested' on their skills (e.g. by performing annotation tasks). Cover stories can be used to soften this awareness effect, nonetheless the fact that subjects are being paid for performing the task renders the approach unfeasible for behavioral change studies. It is necessary that the only reason for behavior induction taking place during the experiment (filling a form, responding to a questionnaire, clicking on an item, etc.) is the exposure to the experimental stimuli, not the external reward. Moreover, Mechanical Turk is based on the notion of a "gold standard" to assess contributors reliability, but for studies concerned with persuasion it is almost impossible to define such a reference: there is no "right" action the contributor can perform, so there is no way to assess whether the subject is performing the action because induced to do so by the persuasive strategy, or just in order to receive money. On the aspect of how to handle subject reliability in coding tasks, see the method proposed in [28].

Advanced Solution - Targeted Ads on the Web. Ecological studies (e.g. using tools for advertising on the web like Google AdWords[3]) offer a possible solution to the following challenges:

1. Time: apart from experimental design and setup, all the rest is automatically performed by the system. Experiments can yield results in a few hours as compared to several days/weeks.
2. Subject recruitment: the potential pool of subjects is the entire population of the web.
3. Subject motivation: ads can be targeted exactly to those who are most interested in the topic of the experiment in that precise moment throughout the world, and so potentially most prone to react.
4. Subject unawareness of test: subjects are totally unaware of being tested, testing is performed during their "natural" activity on the web.

We have developed a methodology using AdWords for the evaluation of short promotion expressions, suited for work in combination with VALENTINO. The basic idea of this approach is to test how different wording of an ad impact on (possibly different) audiences in an A/B test setting. One ad represent the control condition (i.e. the original message containing 'very good dish') while the experimental condition include the message modified with the VALENTINO tool (containing 'delicious dish'). Using metrics like Click-trough Rate (i.e. how many people exposed to the ad actually clicked on it) it is possible to understand if

---

[3] http://adwords.google.com/

the experimental condition has a statistically significant impact on the audience. Similar ecological approaches are beginning to be investigated also in other fields: for example in [4] an approach to assessing the social effects of content features on an on-line community is presented.

6 Conclusions

Language has been studied for a long time in connection with persuasion, mostly focusing on argumentation and rhetorics. Instead we focus on subtle sentiment variations of given short expressions. Expressing sentiment is in fact very effective factor in influencing people, and slanted wording is often adopted, for instance in advertisements, political speech or biased newspaper headlines. Minimal variation of a given expression is an important feature for aesthetic reasons, and it also consents to leave the original wording recognizable thus stressing the novel sentiment accent. Our goal was to develop technology for automatizing this task without domain restrictions. We have described our approach and the characteristics of the developed technology, integrated in a demonstrable system called VALENTINO. As for evaluation, we have briefly described the methodology we developed as an appropriate match for VALENTINO. It is suitable for a final user, who may want to check the persuasiveness of the expressions produced by the system. As far as future developments are concerned: we will include more variation rules (especially further rhetorical aspects in combination with lexical choice), we will consider languages other than English and introduce target profile as a parameter so that output is adapted accordingly.

Potential is great for taking into account the context of the message, including, a dynamic model of the recipients, their background and current affective and social state. News and other updates about the world may also be taken into account, even if only at a shallow level: for instance words with a high level of semantic similiarity with "president" may be particularly useful with positive valence in the period of the American elections. We shall work on the inclusion of several of these aspects and experiment the persuasive effect of various facets of this flexible technology.

In addition we shall study in detail some promising applied settings. The idea is to provide specific solutions for a selected class of potential users of language-based persuasive technology.

Acknowledgments. This work is part of the PerTe project, supported by Trento RISE.

References

1. Aleksandrov, M., Strapparava, C.: NgramQuery - smart information extraction from Google N-gram using external resources. In: Proceedings of LREC 2012, Istanbul, Turkey, pp. 563–568 (2012)

2. Andrews, P., Manandhar, S., De Boni, M.: Argumentative human computer dialogue for automated persuasion. In: Proceedings of SIGdial Workshop on Discourse and Dialogue, pp. 138–147. ACL (2008)
3. Baccianella, S., Esuli, A., Sebastiani, F.: SentiWordNet 3.0: An enhanced lexical resource for sentiment analysis and opinion mining. In: Proceedings of LREC 2010, Valletta, Malta, pp. 2200–2204 (2010)
4. Aral, S., Walker, D.: Creating social contagion through viral product design: A randomized trial of peer influence in networks. In: Proceedings of ICIS 2010 (2010)
5. Brants, T., Franz, A.: Web 1T 5-gram version 1. Linguistic Data Consortium (2006)
6. Carofiglio, V., de Rosis, F.: Combining logical with emotional reasoning in natural argumentation. In: Proceedings of the UM 2003 Workshop on Affect (2003)
7. Das, D., Schneider, N., Chen, D., Smith, N.A.: Probabilistic frame-semantic parsing. In: Proceedings of NAACL-HLT 2010, Los Angeles, USA, pp. 948–956 (2010)
8. De Marneffe, M.C., MacCartney, B., Manning, C.D.: Generating typed dependency parses from phrase structure parses. In: Proceedings of LREC 2006 (2006)
9. de Rosis, F., Grasso, F.: Affective natural language generation. In: Paiva, A.C.R. (ed.) IWAI 1999. LNCS (LNAI), vol. 1814, pp. 204–218. Springer, Heidelberg (2000)
10. Dumais, S.T.: Latent semantic analysis. Annual Review of Information Science and Technology 38(1), 188–230 (2004)
11. Elliott, C.: Multi-media communication with emotion driven 'believable agents'. In: AAAI Technical Report for the Spring Symposium on Believeable Agents, pp. 16–20. Stanford University (1994)
12. Fellbaum, C.: Wordnet: An electronic database (1998)
13. Gardiner, M., Dras, M.: Valence shifting: Is it a valid task? In: Australasian Language Technology Association Workshop 2012, p. 42 (2012)
14. Giora, R., Fein, O., Kronrod, A., Elnatan, I., Shuval, N., Zur, A.: Weapons of mass distraction: Optimal innovation and pleasure ratings. Metaphor and Symbol 19(2), 115–141 (2004)
15. Gmytrasiewicz, P.J., Lisetti, C.L.: Emotions and personality in agent design and modeling. In: Bauer, M., Gmytrasiewicz, P.J., Vassileva, J. (eds.) UM 2001. LNCS (LNAI), vol. 2109, p. 237. Springer, Heidelberg (2001)
16. Grasso, F., Cawsey, A., Jones, R.: Dialectical argumentation to solve conflicts in advice giving: a case study in the promotion of healthy nutrition. International Journal of Human-Computer Studies 53(6), 1077–1115 (2000)
17. Guerini, M., Strapparava, C., Stock, O.: CORPS: A corpus of tagged political speeches for persuasive communication processing. Journal of Information Technology & Politics 5(1), 19–32 (2008)
18. Guerini, M., Gatti, L., Turchi, M.: Sentiment analysis: How to derive prior polarities from SentiWordNet. In: Proceedings of EMNLP 2013 (2013)
19. Guerini, M., Stock, O., Strapparava, C.: Valentino: A tool for valence shifting of natural language texts. In: Proceedings of LREC 2008, pp. 243–246 (2008)
20. Guerini, M., Strapparava, C., Stock, O.: Slanting existing text with valentino. In: Proceedings of IUI 2011, Palo Alto, USA, pp. 439–440 (2011)
21. Guerini, M., Strapparava, C., Stock, O.: Ecological evaluation of persuasive messages using google adwords. In: Proceedings of ACL 2012, pp. 988–996 (2012)
22. Hernault, H., Prendinger, H., Ishizuka, M., et al.: HILDA: a discourse parser using support vector machine classification. Dialogue & Discourse 1(3), 1–33 (2010)
23. Kaptein, M., De Ruyter, B., Markopoulos, P., Aarts, E.: Adaptive persuasive systems: A study of tailored persuasive text messages to reduce snacking. ACM Transactions on Interactive Intelligent Systems 2(2), 10:1–10:25 (2012)

24. Kaptein, M., Halteren, A.: Adaptive persuasive messaging to increase service retention: using persuasion profiles to increase the effectiveness of email reminders. Personal and Ubiquitous Computing 17(6), 1173–1185 (2013)
25. Lee, H., Chang, A., Peirsman, Y., Chambers, N., Surdeanu, M., Jurafsky, D.: Deterministic coreference resolution based on entity-centric, precision-ranked rules. Computational Linguistics 39(4), 1–54 (2013)
26. Mason, W., Suri, S.: Conducting behavioral research on amazon's mechanical turk. Behavior Research Methods, 1–23 (2010)
27. Mateas, M., Vanouse, P., Domike, S.: Generation of ideologically-biased historical documentaries. In: Proceedings of AAAI 2000, Austin, USA, pp. 236–242 (2000)
28. Negri, M., Bentivogli, L., Mehdad, Y., Giampiccolo, D., Marchetti, A.: Divide and conquer: Crowdsourcing the creation of cross-lingual textual entailment corpora. In: Proceedings of EMNLP 2011 (2011)
29. Ortony, A., Clore, G.L., Collins, A.: The cognitive structure of emotions. Cambridge University Press (1988)
30. Özbal, G., Strapparava, C.: A computational approach to automatize creative naming. In: Proceedings of ACL 2012, Jeju Island, Korea (2012)
31. Özbal, G., Pighin, D., Strapparava, C.: Brainsup: Brainstorming support for creative sentence generation. In: Proceedings of ACL 2013, Sofia, Bulgaria (2013)
32. Pianta, E., Girardi, C., Zanoli, R.: The TextPro tool suite. In: Proceedings of LREC 2008, pp. 2603–2607 (2008)
33. Piwek, P.: An annotated bibliography of affective natural language generation. ITRI ITRI-02-02, University of Brighton (2002)
34. Poggi, I.: A goal and belief model of persuasion. Pragmatics and Cognition (2004)
35. Rehm, M., Andrè, E.: Catch me if you can – exploring lying agents in social settings. In: Proceedings of AAMAS 2005, pp. 937–944 (2005)
36. Reiter, E., Dale, R.: Building Natural Language Generation Systems. Cambridge University Press (2000)
37. Reiter, E., Robertson, R., Osman, L.: Lesson from a failure: Generating tailored smoking cessation letters. Artificial Intelligence 144, 41–58 (2003)
38. Sillince, J.A.A., Minors, R.H.: What makes a strong argument? emotions, highly-placed values and role playing. Communication and Cognition 24, 281–298 (1991)
39. Turney, P.D.: Mining the Web for synonyms: PMI-IR versus LSA on TOEFL. In: Proceedings of EMCL 2001, Freiburg, Germany, pp. 491–502 (2001)
40. van der Sluis, I., Mellish, C.: Towards empirical evaluation of affective tactical NLG. In: Krahmer, E., Theune, M. (eds.) Empirical Methods in NLG. LNCS (LNAI), vol. 5790, pp. 242–263. Springer, Heidelberg (2010)
41. Van Der Sluis, I., Mellish, C.: Towards empirical evaluation of affective tactical NLG. In: Proceedings of ENLG 2009, Athens, Greece, pp. 146–153 (2009)
42. Veale, T.: Creative language retrieval: A robust hybrid of information retrieval and linguistic creativity. In: Proceedings of HLT 2011, Portland, USA, pp. 278–287 (2011)
43. Whitehead, S., Cavedon, L.: Generating shifting sentiment for a conversational agent. In: Proceedings of NAACL-HLT 2010 Workshop on Computational Approaches to Analysis and Generation of Emotion in Text, pp. 89–97 (2010)

Do Persuasive Technologies Persuade?
- A Review of Empirical Studies

Juho Hamari[1,2], Jonna Koivisto[1], and Tuomas Pakkanen[2]

[1] Game Research Lab, University of Tampere, Tampere, Finland
{juho.hamari,jonna.koivisto}@uta.fi
[2] Aalto University, Helsinki, Finland
tuomas.pakkanen@aalto.fi

Abstract. This paper reviews the current body of empirical research on persuasive technologies (95 studies). In recent years, technology has been increasingly harnessed to persuade and motivate people to engage in various behaviors. This phenomenon has also attracted substantial scholarly interest over the last decade. This review examines the results, methods, measured behavioral and psychological outcomes, affordances in implemented persuasive systems, and domains of the studies in the current body of research on persuasive technologies. The reviewed studies have investigated diverse persuasive systems/designs, psychological factors, and behavioral outcomes. The results of the reviewed studies were categorized into fully positive, partially positive, and negative and/or no effects. This review provides an overview of the state of empirical research regarding persuasive technologies. The paper functions as a reference in positioning future research within the research stream of persuasive technologies in terms of the domain, the persuasive stimuli and the psychological and behavioral outcomes.

Keywords: persuasive technology, motivational affordance, gamification, persuasive computing, captology, game-based learning, behavioral change support system, sustainability, health technology.

1 Introduction

In recent years, technology has been increasingly harnessed in pursuit of persuading people and motivating them toward various individually and collectively beneficial behaviors. There are two dominant conceptual approaches: the longer-established persuasive technology[1] [1,2,3] and the more recent but increasingly popular gamification [4,5,6]. As Figure 1 shows, the number of gamification-related studies has rapidly increased; however, it seems that in the body of literature on persuasive technologies in particular, a relatively larger proportion of empirical studies exist [7]. Despite these differing titles, the conceptual core of both veins of development incorporates 1) the use of technology that 2) is aimed at affecting people's/users'

---

[1] Also referred to as "captology."

A. Spagnolli et al. (Eds.): PERSUASIVE 2014, LNCS 8462, pp. 118–136, 2014.
© Springer International Publishing Switzerland 2014

psychological attributes, such as attitudes or motivations, which are further presumed to 3) affect behavior. While the behaviors that are supported by these technologies may be similar, there are differences, which seem to stem mainly from the emphases in the articulation of the persuasive stimuli and the psychological mediators; whereas persuasive technology focuses more on social and communicative persuasion and attitude change, gamification centers more around invoking users' (intrinsic) motivations (through gameful experiences and affordances) (see e.g. [8]). The present paper contributes to research in this area by reviewing empirical studies of the persuasive technology field in particular.

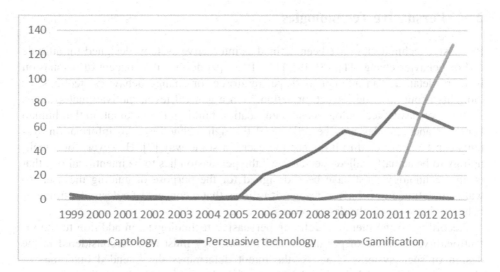

Fig. 1. Number of search hits, by year, for the main keywords associated with the relevant streams of research from paper titles, keywords, and abstracts in the Scopus database

The study of persuasive technologies first emerged in the academic environment in the late 1990s [9]. However, scholarly writing on them only truly began to proliferate in 2005. Since then, the amount of writing on the topic has been increasing steadily (see Figure 1). By 2013, research into persuasive technologies is abundant, with most of the studies being conducted in the field of human–computer interaction. A previous literature review [10] mapped research into persuasive technologies by looking at papers presented at the International Conferences on Persuasive Technology prior to 2009. The emphasis in its review of 51 studies (as compared to the 95 considered in the present work) was mainly on the design aspects presented in the studies.

Regardless of the conceptual framings and the steady increase in the quantity of related literature, it remains unclear what the actual empirical studies have investigated as persuasive stimuli, psychological mediators/outcomes, and behavioral outcomes. Consequently, there is still a dearth of coherent understanding of the field of persuasive technologies with respect to the research outcomes. This may be detrimental to future inquiries within these streams of research.

Therefore, this review systematically examines an extensive body of literature (95 studies) branding itself as addressing persuasive technologies. We investigate the system elements, the psychological mediators/outcomes, the behavioral outcomes, and the purposes for which persuasive technologies were harnessed in the reviewed studies. The results of the review provide insight into the field of persuasive technologies as a whole and enable comparison with parallel developments (such as gamification). Furthermore, the results outline the focus of the research so far and highlight which areas show a dearth of studies. For practitioners, this literature review provides a useful starting point for gaining an overview of the field of persuasive technologies.

2   Persuasive Technologies

Persuasive technologies have been defined as interactive systems designed for attitude and/or behavior change [1], [3], [9], [11]. Fogg [9] defines the concept of persuasion in more detail as "an attempt to shape, reinforce, or change behaviors, feelings, or thoughts about an issue, object, or action." On a general level, motivational systems such as persuasive technologies and gamification build on the assumption that human behavior and attitudes may be influenced through technology. All information systems can be considered to influence the users in some way [2]. However, for a technology to be actually called "persuasive," the persuasion has to be intentional [9]; that is, the technology must have been designed for the purpose of guiding the user towards an attitude or behavior change. It follows that a concept of a desired attitude or behavior has to guide the design process.

According to the literature defining persuasive technologies, in addition to the intentionality, the event of persuasion and the strategy must also be considered in the design of such systems [2,3]. As the intent determines the intended outcomes or changes in attitude or behavior, the event refers to the usage and user of the persuasive technology, and the strategy to the message and how it is delivered [2]. Previous discussion of the topic has emphasized the importance of contextual factors of persuasion and the interactions among persuader, user, and technology [3]. It has been suggested [2] that, for better discernment of the outcomes of persuasive technologies, these technologies could be categorized in terms of whether they are intended to 1) form, 2) alter, or 3) reinforce one of the following: 1) attitudes, 2) behaviors, or 3) an act of complying.

On the level of design, persuasive technologies have been considered to consist of 1) primary task support (i.e., features supporting the core activity or behavior), 2) computer–human dialogue support (i.e., feedback from the system), 3) perceived system credibility (i.e., features making the system seem credible and trustworthy), and 4) social influence (i.e., features inducing motivation through social influence) [2,3]. Design guidelines and principles for these elements have been presented [3].

Whether the actual empirical works on persuasive technologies implement these persuasive designs is as of yet unclear. Furthermore, regarding the aims of persuasive technology, the technologies seek to induce attitude change in addition to changing behaviors. However, attitude as such is rarely studied as a psychological outcome in studies of persuasive technology (see Table 4). Therefore, mapping of the actual empirical works is required.

To connect the conceptualizations of persuasive technologies to a wider framework, we integrate the definition of persuasive technologies with the concept of motivational affordances and its relationship to psychological and behavioral outcomes [12], [4], [13] in information technology (see Figure 2). This conceptual framing is suitable for a literature review because of its level of abstraction, which enables identification of the aforementioned aspects in all of the empirical studies reviewed.

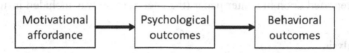

Fig. 2. The conceptual framing

3   The Review Process

3.1   The Literature Search and Criteria for Relevance

The review process began with selection of the sources to be used for the literature searches. We chose the Scopus database, the largest database of scholarly works, since it covers all the relevant publication venues for persuasion-related research. The search terms "persuasive technology" and "captology" were searched for in titles, abstracts, and keywords. The search produced 444 hits. For comparison, the IEEE database and ACM Digital Library yielded only 43 and 123 papers, respectively. However, the contents of both of these libraries are listed in the Scopus database.

For all hits in the search, the name and abstract were scanned, as was the information on whether the item was a full research paper rather than an abstract. All full research papers that potentially contained an empirical study entered a second round of review, in which the papers' content was scanned for the inclusion of an empirical study, to rule out ambiguous cases. This procedure was carried out by two researchers individually. The two resulting sets of papers by the researchers were largely the same, and the few divergences were further discussed in a team that assessed their meeting of the selection criteria. As a result, 95 studies (in 89 papers) were selected for review (see Appendix). The following criteria were applied for inclusion of papers:

1. The paper included an empirical study.
2. The research methods were explicated.
3. The paper described the persuasive stimuli/technology.
4. The paper investigated relationships between persuasive stimuli, psychological mediators/outcomes, and behavioral outcomes in some combination.

The papers excluded from the review belonged to at least one of the following categories:

1. Conceptual articles and frameworks.
2. Descriptions of the development of a system/application but without evaluation of the system.
3. Papers that mentioned persuasive technologies but did not actually study a topic connected with such technologies.
4. Limited research reports (pilot studies reported in sufficient detail were included).
5. Abstracts (including extended abstracts) and posters.
6. Studies reported upon in a later paper (the later version was included instead).

3.2   Analysis

Analysis of the selected studies was a two-stage process following the guidelines of the well-regarded MISQ article by Webster and Watson [14]. The first step features an author-centric analysis wherein studies are listed in a table, one per row. Selected details from the papers are entered in the various columns. For this review, the details included 1) the reference, 2) the domain to which the persuasive technology was related, 3) the psychological mediators/outcomes, 4) the behavioral outcomes, 5) the results, and – related to methodology – 6) the sample size and 7) methods used (including the data source). The second stage with the literature review framework is concept-centric. In this step, the author-centric analysis was pivoted and coded (with some abstraction to connect related papers under a given category) into concept-centric frequency tables. These tables are reported as the results of this review in the next section of the paper.

4   Results

4.1   Reported Results

Table 1 summarizes the reported results for the reviewed studies. In all, 52 studies reported positive results for the persuasive technology examined. These account for 54.7% of the reviewed studies. Partially positive results refer to situations wherein some but not all of the studied elements showed positive results. Partially positive results were reported in 36 studies (37.9%). The category "negative and other" covers papers with fully negative results, no negative or positive results, or no results at all. As is evident from Table 1, fully negative results were reported in very few papers (as is to be expected).

4.2   Types of Studies

Table 2 reports the types of the studies – that is, the methodology used. Papers employing quantitative methods were in the majority. These included both inferential as well as descriptive research. Of all reviewed studies, 54.7% were fully quantitative.

Table 1. Reported results (codes refer to the full list of studies, in the appendix)

Result	Study	Total	% of all
Positive	A02, A04, A05, A06, A07, A08, A09, A10, A11, A13, A14, A15, A16, A18, A19, A21, A23, A25, A26, A27, A28, A29, A31, A32, A34, A37, A41, A43, A48, A49, A51, A52b, A52c, A54, A55, A56, A61, A63, A64b, A66, A68, A69, A70, A71, A73, A74, A75, A76, A78, A83, A85, A88	52	54.7
Partially positive	A01, A03, A12, A17, A20, A22, A24, A30, A33, A35, A38, A39, A40a, A42, A44, A45, A46, A47, A50, A52a, A53, A57, A58, A59, A62, A64d, A67, A72, A77, A79, A80, A81, A82, A84, A86, A87	36	37.9
Negative or other	A36, A40b, A60, A64a, A64c, A65, A89	7	7.4

Table 2. Types of studies (codes refer to the full list of studies, in the appendix)

Type	Studies with positive results	Studies with partially positive results	Studies with negative results	Total	% of all
Quantitative	A05, A06, A08, A10, A11, A13, A16, A23, A26, A27, A29, A31, A32, A34, A37, A41, A51, A52b, A52c, A54, A55, A61, A66, A69, A73, A75, A76, A78, A85	A03, A12, A17, A20, A33, A35, A38, A40a, A42, A44, A52a, A53, A57, A58, A59, A67, A77, A80, A84, A87	A36, A40b, A65	52	54.7
Qualitative	A02, A04, A07, A09, A15, A18, A49, A56, A68, A71, A74	A62, A79, A81	A60	15	15.8
Mixed methods	A14, A19, A21, A25, A28, A43, A48, A63, A64b, A70, A83, A88	A01, A22, A24, A30, A39, A45, A46, A47, A50, A64d, A72, A82, A86	A64a, A64c, A89	28	29.5

Studies using mixed methods formed another large category, accounting for nearly a third of all studies (29.5%). Fully qualitative studies were in the minority (15.8%).

The most frequently used quantitative methods were surveys, manual or automatic data logs, and statistical analyses. The main qualitative methods were user interviews, focus-group discussions, and observations from persuasive technology use.

The sample sizes in the reviewed studies varied greatly, from 2 to 1,704. Furthermore, not all studies reported a sample size, and in some cases, the study process was composed of several phases, with different methods and differing sample sizes. The sample size was clearly reported in 87 of the studies, for which the mean size was 102 and the median 26.

In light of the literature review, the typical methods of a study of persuasive technology could be described in the following manner. The studies usually describe an implementation of a persuasive technology, often designed by the authors. A typical quantitative study included a survey or questionnaire for users of the implementation / test subjects and/or included tracking of use data. The qualitative studies mainly consisted of questionnaires or interviews carried out with users of the implementation. Typical mixed-method studies of persuasive technologies featured methods similar to those of the typical quantitative and qualitative studies.

4.3   Motivational Affordances

Table 3 reports the most prevalent motivational affordances in the reviewed studies. Some studies evaluated existing persuasive technologies, while in other papers the studied technology was a prototype or an application developed for purposes of the research.

Table 3. Motivational affordances (codes refer to the full list of studies, in the appendix)

Motivational affordance	Study	Total
Visual or audio feedback	A01, A09, A10, A11, A12, A13, A15, A21, A25, A34, A47, A48, A49, A50, A51, A54, A56, A59, A64b, A66, A70, A71, A72, A80, A83	25
Social support, comparisons, feedback, interaction, sharing	A13, A18, A25, A26, A28, A35, A36, A44, A46, A49, A58, A59, A64d, A66, A79, A81, A82, A83, A86, A88, A87, A89	22
Progress	A04, A10, A15, A18, A19, A39, A42, A45, A49, A54, A62, A68, A69, A79, A88, A89	16
Persuasive messages and reminders	A02, A04, A06, A13, A29, A42, A49, A53, A61, A62, A63, A65, A74, A77, A82, A86	16
Objectives and goals	A01, A04, A14, A15, A18, A27, A28, A39, A42, A49, A62, A63, A73, A75, A84	15
Rewards, credits, points, achievements	A04, A05, A08, A09, A10, A27, A36, A44, A49, A53, A60, A62, A64d, A70, A71, A80, A81	15
Ambient or public displays (displays embedded into the environment)	A18, A32, A37, A47, A48, A50, A64a, A64b, A64c, A64d, A70, A72, A83	13
Social agents (non-human, computerized assistants)	A02, A03, A31, A33, A34, A38, A55, A57, A58, A67, A73, A74	12
Competition, leaderboards, ranking	A04, A08, A09, A18, A25, A26, A27, A31, A36, A49, A81, A89	12
Emoticons and expressions	A03, A06, A34, A37, A53, A64a, A69, A74	8
Suggestions, advice	A27, A30, A49, A53, A69, A79	6
Tracking	A51, A80, A84	3
Video-based persuasion	A61, A76, A85	3
Positive reinforcement	A10, A68	2
Subliminal persuasion	A75	1
Not specified	A16, A17, A20, A23, A40a, A40b, A52a, A52b, A52c	9

The variety of motivational elements in the studies was wide. The affordances implemented most often were visual and audio feedback, social features, progress and persuasive messages, and reminders. In addition, many of the studied technologies featured also objectives and goals, rewards, and competition. Social agents and ambient displays were also found to be among the popular implementations.

4.4   Psychological Outcomes

Table 4 reports the studied psychological mediators/outcomes. As indicated by Table 4, most of the persuasive technologies studied in the reviewed papers featured design aimed at increasing engagement and encouragement, along with motivation through persuasion. Additionally, persuasive technologies increasing users' awareness pertaining to, for example, health and ecologically sound consumption were studied.

It should be noted that not all of the studies actually measured psychological elements; rather, they are discussed as intended consequences of persuasion in the given implementation.

Table 4. Psychological outcomes (codes refer to the full list of studies, in the appendix)

Psychological mediators/outcomes	Study	Total
Engagement, encouragement	A01, A02, A05, A09, A14, A15, A18, A19, A21, A25, A26, A28, A29, A30, A36, A42, A47, A49, A55, A60, A62, A63, A66, A67, A69, A76, A81, A86	28
Motivation	A01, A02, A05, A08, A10, A15, A18, A26, A27, A28, A31, A36, A42, A44, A45, A51, A56, A62, A63, A67, A69, A80, A81, A85	24
Awareness	A08, A11, A12, A21, A24, A25, A27, A28, A43, A47, A48, A50, A61, A64, A70, A74, A76, A80, A81, A83, A88	21
Enjoyment, "fun"	A01, A04, A05, A08, A09, A10, A19, A25, A36, A45, A49, A72, A80, A89	14
Negative attributes	A01, A03, A12, A64, A66, A73, A78, A79, A81, A82, A89	11
Attitude	A04, A22, A33, A44, A49, A54, A67, A76	8
Self-efficacy	A10, A11, A39, A49, A51, A67, A85	7
Trust, credibility	A16, A17, A23	3
Commitment	A28, A85	2
Sense of community	A22	1
Adherence	A85	1

Some of the studies were also concerned with negative attributes of the persuasive technologies. Among these were frustration (A01), cognitive overload (A03), anxiety (A12), perceived amateurness (A23), peer pressure (A66), threat to personal autonomy (A73), and feelings of guilt from neglecting the behavior one is being persuaded to perform (A81).

4.5   Target Behaviors of Persuasive Technologies

Table 5 reports the domains of the target behaviors of the persuasive technologies in the reviewed studies. In all, 47.4% of the studies examined persuasive technologies in a health and/or exercise context. The second most frequently studied implementation domain was ecological consumption (21.1%); this included, for example, technologies aimed at conserving energy. In addition, persuasive implementations in the domain of education and learning were common among the studies reviewed.

Table 5. Domains of target behaviors (codes refer to the full list of studies, in the appendix)

Context	Studies with positive results	Studies with partially positive results	Studies with negative results	Total	% of all
Health, exercise	A02, A05, A07, A13, A14, A15, A18, A19, A26, A28, A31, A43, A49, A51, A52b, A52c, A54, A55, A63, A64b, A66, A68, A78, A85, A88	A01, A30, A35, A39, A42, A44, A45, A46, A52a, A53, A57, A62, A72, A77, A79, A82, A86	A36, A64a, A89	45	47.4
Ecological consumption and/or behavior	A08, A21, A25, A27, A32, A37, A48, A73, A74, A75, A83	A47, A50, A58, A59, A64d, A80, A81, A84	A64c	20	21.1
Education, learning	A06, A10, A29, A56, A70	A03, A22, A33, A67	A60	10	10.5
Economic, commercial, marketing	A16, A76	A17, A20, A38	A65	6	6.3
Security, safety	A04, A11, A34, A61	A12, A24		6	6.3
Entertainment	A09, A71			2	2.1
No specific domain	A23, A41, A69	A40a, A87	A40b	6	6.3

5   Discussion

Addressing the title of this literature review, it can be concluded that, in the published literature, persuasive technologies indeed seem to persuade people into various behaviors. In the reviewed studies, a diverse array of psychological factors were discussed or measured as antecedents of the target behavior and/or as outcomes of the effects of persuasive technology. However, even though persuasive technologies are, by definition [1], aimed at changing attitudes in addition to behavior, only a few of the papers explicitly included general attitude as a variable [15].

Expectedly, but interestingly, it seems that persuasive technologies are implemented especially in contexts wherein people would be willing to undertake the target activities but find it difficult to start or continue working toward them. Among these activities are healthy habits, learning, and ecological behavior. This notion lends support to the idea that an important aspect with persuasive technologies and gamification is whether the encouraged activity is something the user is trying to accomplish regardless of the system or the user is instead persuaded toward a behavior that is valuable only for the designer of the system.

5.1   General Pitfalls in the Literature

Several shortcomings could be identified during the literature review. 1) The sample sizes were often rather small (median $N = 26$). 2) While many papers did measure experiences and attitudes with validated scales, many did not. 3) Some experiments lacked control groups and relied solely on user evaluation. 4) The persuasive system was often investigated as a whole instead of distinguishing between effects of individual affordances. 5) Many studies presented only descriptive statistics even though they could have easily made inferences about relationships among constructs. 6) Experiment timeframes were very short in most cases (novelty may have significantly skewed the test subjects' experiences). Finally, 7) there was lack of clarity in reporting the results. Further work should attempt in particular to avoid these pitfalls in order to refine research on persuasive technologies.

5.2   Limitations and Directions for Further Research

The literature search for this review included hits only for the keywords "persuasive technology" and "captology." This might have limited the body of literature with a few papers. In addition, similar technologies may have been investigated outside technology-oriented fields. In fact, we found two related meta-analyses conducted in the field of medical sciences. However, no noteworthy overlap with the present study was detected with regard to the reviewed papers (see [16,17]).

Another limitation of the research at this stage is that the present paper does not yet comprehensively report and distinguish which specific affordances affect which psychological or behavioral outcomes. Therefore, this work must be regarded as an exploratory overview of the field. Further research should break down the results stemming from persuasive technology implementations in more detail in order to further the mapping of the field.

Furthermore, many of the reviewed papers do not properly measure psychological factors; rather, they hypothesize and discuss them as psychological outcomes of the given persuasive technology implementations. Therefore, further research should distinguish between studies in a more comprehensive manner regarding the employed research models while also reporting more accurately which aspects have been properly measured.

Since the reviewed studies vary in their methods and in the details of the research questions, they might not all be directly comparable. For example, although many studies might be categorized as having positive results, finer details would be needed to be able to assign studies into more comparable, commensurate groups. Therefore, further studies should seek to establish more refined and detailed comparison regarding these issues.

One possible avenue for advancing the mapping of the field of persuasive technologies and related areas would be to conduct bibliometric analyses containing author, publication venue, year, keyword, and network analyses (see e.g. [19]). Bibliometric analyses facilitate distinguishing among sub-streams of research within and between disciplines / conceptual areas. They also support the consolidation of findings.

Although Scopus evidently features the most comprehensive collection of research papers related to persuasive technology, a meta-study could explore more database options, to guarantee the inclusion of all relevant research. We estimate that the searches of only Scopus captured most of the relevant studies.

Furthermore, one limitation of the paper is that, as in literature reviews in general, the possibility of publication bias must be considered. This bias, a tendency for papers with statistically significant or positive results to be more readily submitted and also accepted for publication, has been shown to exist (see e.g. [18]). For example, one analysis, looking mainly at studies in the medical field [18], has indicated that publication and outcome reporting biases are prevalent and affect the published research. According to that analysis, studies with positive findings were more likely to be published than were those with negative or null results. Even though the existence of publication bias among the studies included in this literature review is hard to ascertain, its potential effects on the findings should be kept in mind when considering the results of the review.

Ethics Statement. This work respects professional code of conduct and does not qualify as coercion or deceit.

Acknowledgements. This research has been supported by individual study grants from the Finnish Cultural Foundation as well as carried out as part of research projects (40311/12, 40134/13) funded by the Finnish Funding Agency for Technology and Innovation (TEKES).

References

1. Fogg, B.J.: Persuasive Technology: Using Computers to Change What We Think and Do. Morgan Kaufmann, San Francisco (2002)
2. Oinas-Kukkonen, H.: A Foundation for the Study of Behavior Change Support Systems. Personal and Ubiquitous Computing 17(6), 1223–1235 (2013)
3. Oinas-Kukkonen, H., Harjumaa, M.: Persuasive Systems Design: Key Issues, Process Model, and System Features. Communications of the Association for Information Systems 24(1), 485–500 (2009)
4. Huotari, K., Hamari, J.: Defining Gamification: A Service Marketing Perspective. In: MindTrek 2012 Proceedings of the 16th International Academic MindTrek Conference, pp. 17–22. ACM, New York (2012)
5. Deterding, S., Dixon, D., Khaled, R., Nacke, L.: From Game Design Elements to Gamefulness: Defining Gamification. In: MindTrek 2010 Proceedings of the 15th International Academic MindTrek Conference, pp. 9–15. ACM, New York (2011)

6. Hamari, J., Lehdonvirta, V.: Game Design as Marketing: How Game Mechanics Create Demand for Virtual Goods. International Journal of Business Science & Applied Management 5(1), 14–29 (2010)
7. Hamari, J., Koivisto, J., Sarsa, H.: Does Gamification Work? – A Literature Review of Empirical Studies on Gamification. In: HICSS 2014 Proceedings of the 47th Hawaii International Conference on System Sciences (2014)
8. Hamari, J., Koivisto, J.: Social Motivations to use Gamification: An Empirical Study of Gamifying Exercise. In: ECIS 2013 Proceedings of the 21st European Conference on Information Systems (2013)
9. Fogg, B.J.: Persuasive Computers: Perspectives and Research Directions. In: Karat, C.-M., Lund, A., Coutaz, J., Karat, J. (eds.) CHI 1998 Proceedings of the SIGCHI Conference on Human Factors in Computing Systems, pp. 225–232. ACM, New York (1998)
10. Torning, K., Oinas-Kukkonen, H.: Persuasive System Design: State of the Art and Future Directions. In: Persuasive 2009 Proceedings of the 4th International Conference on Persuasive Technology. ACM, New York (2009)
11. Oinas-Kukkonen, H., Harjumaa, M.: Towards Deeper Understanding of Persuasion in Software and Information Systems. In: Proceedings of the 1st International Conference on Advances in Computer-Human Interaction, pp. 200–205. IEEE Press (2008)
12. Zhang, P.: Motivational affordances: Reasons for ICT design and use. Communications of the ACM 51(11), 145–147 (2008)
13. Hamari, J.: Transforming Homo Economicus into Homo Ludens: A Field Experiment on Gamification in a Utilitarian Peer-To-Peer Trading Service. Electronic Commerce Research and Applications 12(4), 236–245 (2013)
14. Webster, J., Watson, R.T.: Analyzing the Past to Prepare for the Future: Writing a Literature Review. MIS Quarterly 26(2), xiii–xxiii (2002)
15. Ajzen, I.: The Theory of Planned Behavior. Organizational Behavior and Human Decision Processes 50(2), 179–211 (1991)
16. Cugelman, B., Thelwall, M., Dawes, P.: Online Interventions for Social Marketing Health Behavior Change Campaigns: A Meta-Analysis of Psychological Architectures and Adherence Factors. Journal of Medical Internet Research 13(1) (2011)
17. Kelders, S.M., Kok, R.N., Ossebaard, H.C., van Gemert-Pijnen, J.E.: Persuasive System Design Does Matter: A Systematic Review of Adherence to Web-Based Interventions. Journal of Medical Internet Research 14(6) (2012)
18. Dwan, K., Altman, D.G., Arnaiz, J.A., Bloom, J., Chan, A.-W., et al.: Systematic Review of the Empirical Evidence of Study Publication Bias and Outcome Reporting Bias. PLoS ONE 3(8) (2008)
19. Bragge, J., Korhonen, P., Wallenius, H., Wallenius, J.: Bibliometric Analysis of Multiple Criteria Decision Making/Multiattribute Utility Theory. In: Ehrgott, M., Naujoks, B., Stewart, T.J., Wallenius, J. (eds.) Multiple Criteria Decision Making for Sustainable Energy and Transportation Systems. LNEMS, vol. 634, pp. 259–268. Springer, Heidelberg (2010)

Appendix

Appendix. Reviewed Studies

A1. Albaina, I.M., Visser, T., Van Der Mast, C.A.P.G., Vastenburg, M.H.: Flowie: A persuasive virtual coach to motivate elderly individuals to walk. In: 3rd International Conference on Per-vasive Computing Technologies for Healthcare, pp. 1–7 (2009)

A2. Arteaga, S.M., Kudeki, M., Woodworth, A., Kurniawan, S.: Mobile system to motivate teen-agers' physical activity. In: 9th International Conference on Interaction Design and Children, pp. 1–10. ACM, New York (2010)

A3. Baylor, A.L., Kim, S.: Designing nonverbal communication for pedagogical agents: When less is more. Computers in Human Behavior 25(2), 450–457 (2009)

A4. Bergmans, A., Shahid, S.: Reducing speeding behavior in young drivers using a persuasive mobile application. In: Kurosu, M. (ed.) HCII/HCI 2013, Part II. LNCS, vol. 8005, pp. 541–550. Springer, Heidelberg (2013)

A5. Berkovsky, S., Freyne, J., Coombe, M.: Physical activity motivating games: Be active and get your own reward. ACM Transactions on Computer-Human Interaction 19(4) (2012)

A6. Berque, D., Billingsley, A., Bonebright, T.L., Burgess, J., Johnson, S.K., Wethington, B.: De-sign and evaluation of persuasive technology to encourage healthier typing behaviors. In: Haugtvedt, C.P., Stibe, A. (eds.) PERSUASIVE 2011 Proceedings of the 6th International Con-ference on Persuasive Technology. ACM, New York (2011)

A7. Bhatnagar, N., Sinha, A., Samdaria, N., Gupta, A., Batra, S., Bhardwaj, M., Thies, W.: Biometric monitoring as a persuasive technology: Ensuring patients visit health centers in india's slums. In: Bang, M., Ragnemalm, E.L. (eds.) PERSUASIVE 2012. LNCS, vol. 7284, pp. 169–180. Springer, Heidelberg (2012)

A8. Centieiro, P., Romão, T., Dias, A.E.: A location-based multiplayer mobile game to encourage pro-environmental behaviours. In: Romão, T., Correia, N., Inami, M., Kato, H., Prada, R., Terada, T., Dias, E., Chambel, T. (eds.) ACE 2011 International Conference on Advances in Computer Entertainment Technology. ACM, New York (2011)

A9. Centieiro, P., Romão, T., Dias, A.E.: Applaud having fun: A mobile game to cheer your favourite sports team. In: Nijholt, A., Romão, T., Reidsma, D. (eds.) ACE 2012. LNCS, vol. 7624, pp. 1–16. Springer, Heidelberg (2012)

A10. Chang, Y.-C., Lo, J.-L., Huang, C.-J., Hsu, N.-Y., Chu, H.-H., Wang, H.-Y., Chi, P.-Y., Hsieh, Y.-L.: Playful Toothbrush: UbiComp technology for teaching tooth brushing to kindergarten children. In: Proceedings of the SIGCHI Conference on Human Factors in Computing Systems 2008, pp. 363–372. ACM, New York (2008)

A11. Chittaro, L.: Passengers' safety in aircraft evacuations: Employing serious games to educate and persuade. In: Bang, M., Ragnemalm, E.L. (eds.) PERSUASIVE 2012. LNCS, vol. 7284, pp. 215–226. Springer, Heidelberg (2012)

A12. Chittaro, L., Zangrando, N.: The persuasive power of virtual reality: Effects of simulated human distress on attitudes towards fire safety. In: Ploug, T., Hasle, P., Oinas-Kukkonen, H. (eds.) PERSUASIVE 2010. LNCS, vol. 6137, pp. 58–69. Springer, Heidelberg (2010)

A13. Chiu, M.-C., Chang, S.-P., Chang, Y.-C., Chu, H.-H., Chen, C.C.-H., Hsiao, F.-H., Ko, J.-C.: Playful bottle: A mobile social persuasion system to motivate healthy water intake. In: Ubicomp 2009: Proceedings of the 11th International Conference on Ubiquitous Computing, pp. 185–194. ACM, New York (2009)

A14. Consolvo, S., Klasnja, P., McDonald, D.W., Avrahami, D., Froehlich, J., Legrand, L., Libby, R., Mosher, K., Landay, J.A.: Flowers or a robot army?: Encouraging awareness & activity with personal, mobile displays. In: UbiComp 2008: Proceedings of the 10th International Conference on Ubiquitous Computing, pp. 54–63. ACM, New York (2008)

A15. Consolvo, S., McDonald, D.W., Toscos, T., Chen, M.Y., Froehlich, J., Harrison, B., Klasnja, P., LaMarea, A., LeGrand, L., Libby, R., Smith, I., Landay, J.A.: Activity sensing in the wild: A field trial of UbiFit Garden. In: CHI 2008 Proceedings of the SIGCHI Conference on Human Factors in Computing Systems, pp. 1797–1806. ACM, New York (2008)

A16. Cugelman, B., Thelwall, M., Dawes, P.: Website credibility, active trust and behavioural intent. In: Oinas-Kukkonen, H., Hasle, P., Harjumaa, M., Segerståhl, K., Øhrstrøm, P. (eds.) PERSUASIVE 2008. LNCS, vol. 5033, pp. 47–57. Springer, Heidelberg (2008)

A17. Cugelman, B., Thelwall, M., Dawes, P.: The Dimensions of Web Site Credibility and Their Relation to Active Trust and Behavioural Impact. Communications of the Association for Information Systems 24 (2009)

A18. Faber, J.P., Markopoulos, P., Dadlani, P., van Halteren, A.: AULURA: Engaging users with ambient persuasive technology. In: Keyson, D.V., Maher, M.L., Streitz, N., Cheok, A., Augusto, J.C., Wichert, R., Englebienne, G., Aghajan, H., Kröse, B.J.A. (eds.) AmI 2011. LNCS, vol. 7040, pp. 215–221. Springer, Heidelberg (2011)

A19. Fabri, M., Wall, A., Trevorrow, P.: Changing eating behaviors through a cooking-based website for the whole family. In: Marcus, A. (ed.) DUXU 2013, Part III. LNCS, vol. 8014, pp. 484–493. Springer, Heidelberg (2013)

A20. Felfernig, A., Friedrich, G., Gula, B., Hitz, M., Kruggel, T., Leitner, G., Melcher, R., Riepan, D., Strauss, S., Teppan, E., Vitouch, O.: Persuasive recommendation: Serial position effects in knowledge-based recommender systems. In: de Kort, Y.A.W., IJsselsteijn, W.A., Midden, C., Eggen, B., Fogg, B.J. (eds.) PERSUASIVE 2007. LNCS, vol. 4744, pp. 283–294. Springer, Heidelberg (2007)

A21. Filonik, D., Medland, R., Foth, M., Rittenbruch, M.: A customisable dashboard display for environmental performance visualisations. In: Berkovsky, S., Freyne, J. (eds.) PERSUASIVE 2013. LNCS, vol. 7822, pp. 51–62. Springer, Heidelberg (2013)

A22. Firpo, D., Kasemvilas, S., Ractham, P., Zhang, X.: Generating a sense of community in a graduate educational setting through persuasive technology. In: Proceedings of the 4th International Conference on Persuasive Technology. ACM, New York (2009)

A23. Fogg, B.J., Marshall, J., Laraki, O., Osipovich, A., Varma, C., Fang, N., Paul, J., Rangnekar, A., Shon, J., Swani, P., Treinen, M.: What makes Web sites credible?: a report on a large quantitative study. In: CHI 2001 Proceedings of the SIGCHI Conference on Human Factors in Computing Systems, pp. 61–68. ACM, New York (2001)

A24. Forget, A., Chiasson, S., van Oorschot, P.C., Biddle, R.: Improving text passwords through persuasion. In: SOUPS 2008 Proceedings of the 4th Symposium on Usable Privacy and Security, pp. 1–12. ACM, New York (2008)

A25. Foster, D., Lawson, S., Blythe, M., Cairns, P.: Wattsup?: Motivating reductions in domestic energy consumption using social networks. In: NordiCHI 2010: Proceedings of the 6th Nordic Conference on Human-Computer Interaction, pp. 178–187. ACM, New York (2010)

A26. Foster, D., Linehan, C., Kirman, B., Lawson, S., James, G.: Motivating physical activity at work: Using persuasive social media for competitive step counting. In: MindTrek 2010 Proceedings of the 14th International Academic MindTrek Conference, pp. 111–116. ACM, New York (2010)

A27. Gamberini, L., Spagnolli, A., Corradi, N., Jacucci, G., Tusa, G., Mikkola, T., Zamboni, L., Hoggan, E.: Tailoring feedback to users' actions in a persuasive game for household electricity conservation. In: Bang, M., Ragnemalm, E.L. (eds.) PERSUASIVE 2012. LNCS, vol. 7284, pp. 100–111. Springer, Heidelberg (2012)

A28. Gasca, E., Favela, J., Tentori, M.: Persuasive virtual communities to promote a healthy lifestyle among patients with chronic diseases. In: Briggs, R.O., Antunes, P., de Vreede, G.-J., Read, A.S. (eds.) CRIWG 2008. LNCS, vol. 5411, pp. 74–82. Springer, Heidelberg (2008)

A29. Goh, T.-T., Seet, B.-C., Chen, N.-S.: The impact of persuasive SMS on students' self-regulated learning. British Journal of Educational Technology 43(4), 624–640 (2012)

A30. Graham, C., Benda, P., Howard, S., Balmford, J., Bishop, N., Borland, R.: Heh - Keeps me off the smokes...: Probing technology support for personal change. In: Kjeldskov, J., Paay, J. (eds.) OZCHI 2006 Proceedings of the 18th Australia Conference on Computer-Human Interaction, pp. 221–228. ACM, New York (2006)

A31. Halan, S., Rossen, B., Cendan, J., Lok, B.: High score! - Motivation strategies for user participation in virtual human development. In: Allbeck, J., Badler, N., Bickmore, T., Pelachaud, C., Safonova, A. (eds.) IVA 2010. LNCS (LNAI), vol. 6356, pp. 482–488. Springer, Heidelberg (2010)

A32. Ham, J., Midden, C.: Ambient persuasive technology needs little cognitive effort: The differential effects of cognitive load on lighting feedback versus factual feedback. In: Ploug, T., Hasle, P., Oinas-Kukkonen, H. (eds.) PERSUASIVE 2010. LNCS, vol. 6137, pp. 132–142. Springer, Heidelberg (2010)

A33. Ham, J., Bokhorst, R., Cuijpers, R., van der Pol, D., Cabibihan, J.-J.: Making robots persuasive: The influence of combining persuasive strategies (Gazing and gestures) by a storytelling robot on its persuasive power. In: Mutlu, B., Bartneck, C., Ham, J., Evers, V., Kanda, T. (eds.) ICSR 2011. LNCS, vol. 7072, pp. 71–83. Springer, Heidelberg (2011)

A34. Hartwig, M., Windel, A.: Safety and health at work through persuasive assistance systems. In: Duffy, V.G. (ed.) DHM/HCII 2013, Part II. LNCS, vol. 8026, pp. 40–49. Springer, Heidelberg (2013)

A35. Jeen, Y., Han, J., Kim, H., Lee, K.W., Park, P.: Persuasive interaction strategy for self diet system: Exploring the relation of user attitude and intervention by computerized systematic methods. In: Jacko, J.A. (ed.) HCI 2007, Part IV. LNCS, vol. 4553, pp. 450–458. Springer, Heidelberg (2007)

A36. Johnston, H., Whitehead, A.: Pose presentation for a dance-based massively multiplayer online exergame. Entertainment Computing 2(2), 89–96 (2011)

A37. Kalnikaite, V., Rogers, Y., Bird, J., Villar, N., Bachour, K., Payne, S., Todd, P.M., Schöning, J., Krüger, A., Kreitmayer, S.: How to nudge in situ: Designing lambent devices to deliver salient information in supermarkets. In: UbiComp 2011: Proceedings of the 13th International Conference on Ubiquitous Computing. ACM, New York (2011)

A38. Kamei, K., Shinozawa, K., Ikeda, T., Utsumi, A., Miyashita, T., Hagita, N.: Recommendation from robots in a real-world retail shop. In: ICMI-MLMI 2010: International Conference on Multimodal Interfaces and the Workshop on Machine Learning for Multimodal Interaction. ACM, New York (2010)

A39. Kaplan, B., Farzanfar, R., Friedman, R.H.: Personal relationships with an intelligent interactive telephone health behavior advisor system: A multimethod study using surveys and ethnographic interviews. International Journal of Medical Informatics 71(1), 33–41 (2003)

A40. a) Kaptein, M., Duplinsky, S., Markopoulos, P.: Means based adaptive persuasive systems (study 1). In: CHI 2011 Proceedings of the SIGCHI Conference on Human Factors in Computing Systems, pp. 335–344. ACM, New York (2011)
b) Kaptein, M., Duplinsky, S., Markopoulos, P.: Means based adaptive persuasive systems (study 2). In: CHI 2011 Proceedings of the SIGCHI Conference on Human Factors in Computing Systems, pp. 335–344. ACM, New York (2011)

A41. Kaptein, M., Markopoulos, P., de Ruyter, B., Aarts, E.: Can you be persuaded? Individual differ-ences in susceptibility to persuasion. In: Gross, T., Gulliksen, J., Kotzé, P., Oestreicher, L., Palanque, P., Prates, R.O., Winckler, M. (eds.) INTERACT 2009. LNCS, vol. 5726, pp. 115–118. Springer, Heidelberg (2009)

A42. Kaptein, M., Van Halteren, A.: Adaptive persuasive messaging to increase service retention: Using persuasion profiles to increase the effectiveness of email reminders. Personal and Ubiquitous Computing 17(6), 1173–1185 (2013)

A43. Kehr, F., Hassenzahl, M., Laschke, M., Diefenbach, S.: A transformational product to improve self-control strength: The Chocolate Machine. In: CHI 2012 Proceedings of the SIGCHI Conference on Human Factors in Computing Systems, pp. 689–694. ACM, New York (2012)

A44. Khaled, R., Barr, P., Biddle, R., Fischer, R., Noble, J.: Game design strategies for collectivist persuasion. In: Spencer, S.N. (ed.) Sandbox 2009 Proceedings of the 2009 ACM SIGGRAPH Symposium on Video Games, pp. 31–38. ACM, New York (2009)

A45. Khalil, A., Abdallah, S.: Harnessing social dynamics through persuasive technology to promote healthier lifestyle. Computers in Human Behavior 29(6), 2674–2681 (2013)

A46. Kim, S., Kientz, J.A., Patel, S.N., Abowd, G.D.: Are you sleeping? Sharing portrayed sleeping status within a social network. In: CSCW 2008 Proceedings of the 2008 ACM Conference on Computer Supported Cooperative Work, pp. 619–628. ACM, New York (2008)

A47. Kim, S., Paulos, E.: inAir: Sharing indoor air quality measurements and visualizations. In: CHI 2010 Proceedings of the SIGCHI Conference on Human Factors in Computing Systems, pp. 1861–1870. ACM, New York (2010)

A48. Kim, T., Hong, H., Magerko, B.: Design requirements for ambient display that supports sustainable lifestyle. In: DIS 2010 Proceedings of the 8th ACM Conference on Designing Interactive Systems, pp. 103–112. ACM, New York (2010)

A49. Kroes, L., Shahid, S.: Empowering young adolescents to choose the healthy lifestyle: A persuasive intervention using mobile phones. In: Kurosu, M. (ed.) HCII/HCI 2013, Part II. LNCS, vol. 8005, pp. 117–126. Springer, Heidelberg (2013)

A50. Kuznetsov, S., Paulos, E.: UpStream: Motivating water conservation with low-cost water flow sensing and persuasive displays. In: CHI 2010 Proceedings of the SIGCHI Conference on Human Factors in Computing, pp. 1851–1860. ACM, New York (2010)

A51. Lacroix, J., Saini, P., Goris, A.: Understanding user cognitions to guide the tailoring of persuasive technology-based physical activity interventions. In: Proceedings of the 4th International Conference on Persuasive Technology. ACM, New York (2009)

A52. a) Lee, M.K., Kiesler, S., Forlizzi, J.: Mining behavioral economics to design persuasive tech-nology for healthy choices (study 1). In: CHI 2011 Proceedings of the SIGCHI Conference on Human Factors in Computing, pp. 325–334. ACM, New York (2011)
b) Lee, M.K., Kiesler, S., Forlizzi, J.: Mining behavioral economics to design persuasive technology for healthy choices (study 2). In: CHI 2011 Proceedings of the SIGCHI Conference on Human Factors in Computing, pp. 325–334. ACM, New York (2011)
c) Lee, M.K., Kiesler, S., Forlizzi, J.: Mining behavioral economics to design persuasive technology for healthy choices (study 3). In: CHI 2011 Proceedings of the SIGCHI Conference on Human Factors in Computing, pp. 325–334. ACM, New York (2011)

A53. Li, H., Chatterjee, S.: Designing effective persuasive systems utilizing the power of entanglement: Communication channel, strategy and affect. In: Ploug, T., Hasle, P., Oinas-Kukkonen, H. (eds.) PERSUASIVE 2010. LNCS, vol. 6137, pp. 274–285. Springer, Heidelberg (2010)

A54. Lim, B.Y., Shick, A., Harrison, C., Hudson, S.E.: Pediluma: motivating physical activity through contextual information and social influence. In: TEI 2011 Proceedings of the Fifth International Conference on Tangible, Embedded, and Embodied Interaction, pp. 173–180. ACM, New York (2010)

A55. Looije, R., Cnossen, F., Neerincx, M.A.: Incorporating guidelines for health assistance into a socially intelligent robot. In: ROMAN 2006 15th International Symposium on Robot and Human Interactive Communication, pp. 515–520. IEEE Press (2006)

A56. Lucero, A., Zuloaga, R., Mota, S., Muñoz, F.: Persuasive technologies in education: Improving motivation to read and write for children. In: IJsselsteijn, W.A., de Kort, Y.A.W., Midden, C., Eggen, B., van den Hoven, E. (eds.) PERSUASIVE 2006. LNCS, vol. 3962, pp. 142–153. Springer, Heidelberg (2006)

A57. McCalley, T., Mertens, A.: The pet plant: Developing an inanimate emotionally interactive tool for the elderly. In: de Kort, Y.A.W., IJsselsteijn, W.A., Midden, C., Eggen, B., Fogg, B.J. (eds.) PERSUASIVE 2007. LNCS, vol. 4744, pp. 68–79. Springer, Heidelberg (2007)

A58. Midden, C., Ham, J.: The illusion of agency: The influence of the agency of an artificial agent on its persuasive power. In: Bang, M., Ragnemalm, E.L. (eds.) PERSUASIVE 2012. LNCS, vol. 7284, pp. 90–99. Springer, Heidelberg (2012)

A59. Midden, C., Kimura, H., Ham, J., Nakajima, T., Kleppe, M.: Persuasive power in groups: The influence of group feedback and individual comparison feedback on energy consumption be-havior. In: Haugtvedt, C.P., Stibe, A. (eds.) PERSUASIVE 2011 Proceedings of the 6th International Conference on Persuasive Technology. ACM, New York (2011)

A60. Mintz, J., Branch, C., March, C., Lerman, S.: Key factors mediating the use of a mobile technology tool designed to develop social and life skills in children with Autistic Spectrum Disorders. Computers and Education 58(1), 53–62 (2012)

A61. Miranda, B., Jere, C., Alharbi, O., Lakshmi, S., Khouja, Y., Chatterjee, S.: Examining the efficacy of a persuasive technology package in reducing texting and driving behavior. In: Berkovsky, S., Freyne, J. (eds.) PERSUASIVE 2013. LNCS, vol. 7822, pp. 137–148. Springer, Heidelberg (2013)

A62. Munson, S.A., Consolvo, S.: Exploring goal-setting, rewards, self-monitoring, and sharing to motivate physical activity. In: PervasiveHealth 2012 6th International Conference on Pervasive Computing Technologies for Healthcare, pp. 25–32. IEEE Press (2012)

A63. Mutsuddi, A.U., Connelly, K.: Text messages for encouraging physical activity: Are they effective after the novelty effect wears off? In: PervasiveHealth 2012 6th International Conference on Pervasive Computing Technologies for Healthcare, pp. 33–40. IEEE Press (2012)

A64. a) Nakajima, T., Lehdonvirta, V.: Designing motivation using persuasive ambient mirrors (study 1). Personal and Ubiquitous Computing 17(1), 107–126 (2013)
b) Nakajima, T., Lehdonvirta, V.: Designing motivation using persuasive ambient mirrors (study 2). Personal and Ubiquitous Computing 17(1), 107–126 (2013)
c) Nakajima, T., Lehdonvirta, V.: Designing motivation using persuasive ambient mirrors (study 3). Personal and Ubiquitous Computing 17(1), 107–126 (2013)
d) Nakajima, T., Lehdonvirta, V.: Designing motivation using persuasive ambient mirrors (study 4). Personal and Ubiquitous Computing 17(1), 107–126 (2013)

A65. Orino, M., Kitamura, Y.: An approach to create persuasive web sites. In: Proceedings of 2010 International Conference on Web Intelligence and Intelligent Agent Technology, pp. 116–119. IEEE Press (2010)

A66. Parmar, V., Keyson, D.V., deBont, C.: Persuasive technology for shaping social beliefs of rural women in india: An approach based on the theory of planned behaviour. In: Oinas-Kukkonen, H., Hasle, P., Harjumaa, M., Segerståhl, K., Øhrstrøm, P. (eds.) PERSUASIVE 2008. LNCS, vol. 5033, pp. 104–115. Springer, Heidelberg (2008)

A67. Plant, E.A., Baylor, A.L., Doerr, C.E., Rosenberg-Kima, R.B.: Changing middle-school stu-dents' attitudes and performance regarding engineering with computer-based social models. Computers and Education 53(2), 209–215 (2009)

A68. Ploderer, B., Howard, S., Thomas, P., Reitberger, W.: "Hey world, take a look at me!": Appreciating the human body on social network sites. In: Oinas-Kukkonen, H., Hasle, P., Harjumaa, M., Segerståhl, K., Øhrstrøm, P. (eds.) PERSUASIVE 2008. LNCS, vol. 5033, pp. 245–248. Springer, Heidelberg (2008)

A69. Pribik, I., Felfernig, A.: Towards persuasive technology for software development environments: An empirical study. In: Bang, M., Ragnemalm, E.L. (eds.) PERSUASIVE 2012. LNCS, vol. 7284, pp. 227–238. Springer, Heidelberg (2012)

A70. Reis, S., Correia, N.: The perception of sound and its influence in the classroom. In: Campos, P., Graham, N., Jorge, J., Nunes, N., Palanque, P., Winckler, M. (eds.) INTERACT 2011, Part I. LNCS, vol. 6946, pp. 609–626. Springer, Heidelberg (2011)

A71. Reitberger, W., Güldenpfennig, F., Fitzpatrick, G.: Persuasive technology considered harmful? An exploration of design concerns through the TV companion. In: Bang, M., Ragnemalm, E.L. (eds.) PERSUASIVE 2012. LNCS, vol. 7284, pp. 239–250. Springer, Heidelberg (2012)

A72. Rogers, Y., Hazlewood, W.R., Marshall, P., Dalton, N., Hertrich, S.: Ambient influence: Can twinkly lights lure and abstract representations trigger behavioral change? In: Ubicomp 2010: Proceedings of the 12th International Conference on Ubiquitous Computing, pp. 261–270. ACM, New York (2010)

A73. Roubroeks, M.A.J., Ham, J.R.C., Midden, C.J.H.: The dominant robot: Threatening ro-bots cause psychological reactance, especially when they have incongruent goals. In: Ploug, T., Hasle, P., Oinas-Kukkonen, H. (eds.) PERSUASIVE 2010. LNCS, vol. 6137, pp. 174–184. Springer, Heidelberg (2010)

A74. Ruijten, P.A.M., de Kort, Y.A.W., Kosnar, P.: Bridging the gap between the home and the lab: A qualitative study of acceptance of an avatar feedback system. In: Bang, M., Ragnemalm, E.L. (eds.) PERSUASIVE 2012. LNCS, vol. 7284, pp. 251–255. Springer, Heidelberg (2012)

A75. Ruijten, P.A.M., Midden, C.J.H., Ham, J.: Unconscious persuasion needs goal-striving: The effect of goal activation on the persuasive power of subliminal feedback. In: Haugtvedt, C.P., Stibe, A. (eds.) PERSUASIVE 2011 Proceedings of the 6th International Conference on Persuasive Technology. ACM, New York (2011)

A76. Russell, M.G.: Benevolence and effectiveness: Persuasive technology's spillover effects in retail settings. In: Oinas-Kukkonen, H., Hasle, P., Harjumaa, M., Segerståhl, K., Øhrstrøm, P. (eds.) PERSUASIVE 2008. LNCS, vol. 5033, pp. 94–103. Springer, Heidelberg (2008)

A77. Sakai, R., Van Peteghem, S., van de Sande, L., Banach, P., Kaptein, M.: Personalized persuasion in ambient intelligence: The APStairs system. In: Keyson, D.V., Maher, M.L., Streitz, N., Cheok, A., Augusto, J.C., Wichert, R., Englebienne, G., Aghajan, H., Kröse, B.J.A. (eds.) AmI 2011. LNCS, vol. 7040, pp. 205–209. Springer, Heidelberg (2011)

A78. Salam, S.N.-A., Yahaya, W.A.J.-W., Ali, A.-M.: Using persuasive design principles in motivational feeling towards Children Dental Anxiety (CDA). In: Ploug, T., Hasle, P., Oinas-Kukkonen, H. (eds.) PERSUASIVE 2010. LNCS, vol. 6137, pp. 223–237. Springer, Heidelberg (2010)

A79. Segerståhl, K., Kotro, T., Väänänen-Vainio-Mattila, K.: Pitfalls in persuasion: How do users experience persuasive techniques in a web service? In: Ploug, T., Hasle, P., Oinas-Kukkonen, H. (eds.) PERSUASIVE 2010. LNCS, vol. 6137, pp. 211–222. Springer, Heidelberg (2010)

A80. Takayama, C., Lehdonvirta, V., Shiraishi, M., Washio, Y., Kimura, H., Nakajima, T.: ECOISLAND: A system for persuading users to reduce CO_2 emissions. In: STFSSD 2009 Proceedings of the 2009 Software Technologies for Future Dependable Distributed Systems, pp. 59–63. IEEE Press (2009)

A81. Thieme, A., Comber, R., Miebach, J., Weeden, J., Krämer, N., Lawson, S., Olivier, P.: "We've bin watching you" - Designing for reflection and social persuasion to promote sustainable life-styles. In: CHI 2012 Proceedings of the SIGCHI Conference on Human Factors in Computing Systems, pp. 2337–2346. ACM, New York (2012)

A82. Toscos, T., Faber, A., Connelly, K., Upoma, A.M.: Encouraging physical activity in teens can technology help reduce barriers to physical activity in adolescent girls? In: PervasiveHealth 2008 International Conference on Pervasive Computing Technologies for Healthcare, pp. 218–221. IEEE Press (2008)

A83. Valkanova, N., Jorda, S., Tomitsch, M., Vande Moere, A.: Reveal-it!: the impact of a social visualization projection on public awareness and discourse. In: CHI 2013 Proceedings of the SIGCHI Conference on Human Factors in Computing Systems, pp. 3461–3470. ACM, New York (2013)

A84. van Dam, S.S., Bakker, C.A., van Hal, J.D.M.: Home energy monitors: impact over the me-dium-term. Building Research & Information 38(5), 458–469 (2010)

A85. van Leer, E., Connor, N.P.: Use of portable digital media players increases patient motivation and practice in voice therapy. Journal of Voice 26(4), 447–453 (2012)

A86. VanDeMark, N.R., Burrell, N.R., LaMendola, W.F., Hoich, C.A., Berg, N.P., Medina, E.: An exploratory study of engagement in a technology-supported substance abuse intervention. Substance Abuse: Treatment, Prevention, and Policy 5(1) (2010)

A87. Waardenburg, T., Winkel, R., Lamers, M.H.: Normative social influence in persuasive technology: Intensity versus effectiveness. In: Bang, M., Ragnemalm, E.L. (eds.) PERSUASIVE 2012. LNCS, vol. 7284, pp. 145–156. Springer, Heidelberg (2012)

A88. Young, M.M.: Twitter me: Using micro-blogging to motivate teenagers to exercise. In: Winter, R., Zhao, J.L., Aier, S. (eds.) DESRIST 2010. LNCS, vol. 6105, pp. 439–448. Springer, Heidelberg (2010)

A89. Zwinderman, M.J., Shirzad, A., Ma, X., Bajracharya, P., Sandberg, H., Kaptein, M.C.: Phone row: A smartphone game designed to persuade people to engage in moderate-intensity physical activity. In: Bang, M., Ragnemalm, E.L. (eds.) PERSUASIVE 2012. LNCS, vol. 7284, pp. 55–66. Springer, Heidelberg (2012)

Wicked Persuasion: A Designerly Approach

Bran Knowles, Paul Coulton, Mark Lochrie, and Jon Whittle

Lancaster University, Lancaster, United Kingdom
{b.h.knowles,p.coulton,m.lochrie,j.n.whittle}@lancaster.ac.uk

Abstract. Persuasive computing has tended to be applied toward the promotion of minor behavior change in the direction of easily understood and uncontroversial goals. Such approaches may not make sense, however, when designing for so called 'wicked problems'. We argue that while wicked problems *can* be effectively addressed through persuasive technology, a 'designerly' (as opposed to engineering or experimental psychology) approach is required in their creation. We illustrate this approach through the design of our own persuasive system directed at the wicked problem of encouraging local spending, and we draw lessons for persuasive design more generally.

Keywords: persuasion, persuasive games, interaction design, wicked problems, rhetoric.

The common wisdom for persuasive computing is that success depends on choosing a 'simple behavior to target' [1]. For example, when trying to address the complex challenge of helping people lead healthier lives, a persuasive computing solution might focus on a reductionist approach of getting people to go to the gym more often.

We are using the word 'reductionist' in a descriptive, rather than derogatory, sense. There are instances where this approach to persuasive computing is appropriate, such as those for which there is an understood and uncontroversial behavioral solution, and for which there is a clear and short path for the target user to take from the undesired behavior to the desired behavior. However, there are instances where this approach is less than ideal, and for which new strategies need to be developed: for example, where there is no obvious or recognized behavioral solution; where there are multiple behavioral laws operating in conflict in a given situation, or behaviors are demonstrably unpredictable; or where the problem pertains not to a single behavior but to a set of interrelated behaviors, or a culturally intractable 'norm'. Such complexities are often termed 'wicked problems' [2], so named for their indeterminacy and for being inherently 'unsolvable' in the traditional sense. To date, persuasive computing has shied away from these wicked problems, and the purpose of this paper is to show how the community may effectively tackle such interesting challenges.

Designers commonly face wicked problems [3], and have developed a qualitatively different process for arriving at solutions, which are often cryptically referred to as a 'designerly approach' [4]. In this paper, we attempt to demystify

A. Spagnolli et al. (Eds.): PERSUASIVE 2014, LNCS 8462, pp. 137–142, 2014.

some of what this approach entails — specifically, how to embrace the 'messiness' [5] (cf. Practice Theory) with which we are faced. We describe a wicked problem for which we are currently designing a persuasive system (named BARTER), and present the design thinking involved in understanding and responding to this problem. We first provide the context for our chosen problem and our process of identifying and framing that problem. We then unpack the design complexities that emerge and how our awareness of these challenges affects the design of our system. We conclude with a discussion of more broadly generalizable lessons for persuasive solutions for wicked problems.

1   Problem

Verplank [6] developed a framework of concerns underpinning successful interaction designs, which we adopt as a way of organizing this paper. We begin by describing the *motivation* that underpins our design ambitions and the *meanings* that frame what we think we are doing — i.e. the metaphors that have influenced our understanding and which we seek to communicate to our users. The remaining two concerns — *modes* and *mappings* — are addressed in the System Design Considerations section.

1.1   Motivation

The backdrop of our project is the global recession, the academic and media response to the crisis, and the growing insecurity surrounding the future of modern capitalist society. Of particular concern, many of the UK's town centers are witnessing significant shop vacancy as consumers seek the bargains and convenience available from mega retail outlets and online stores [7]. While non-local spending appears to bring short-term individual economic wins, it comes at the expense of long-term community losses.

An increasingly common approach to interrupt this trend is the establishment of local currencies [8]. As these currencies are only recognized tender within the locale, they represent a pool of local wealth that cannot be siphoned away from the community. By taking away the option to spend non-locally, local currencies function as a kind of 'tunnelling' (one of Fogg's tools of persuasion [9]) by reducing the uncertainty of consumer spending and directing it locally.

Unfortunately, local currencies often fail [10], and we suggest that this is in part because they do not engage consumers in a discussion about the *reasons* for spending locally. No matter how outspoken proponents are about why they support the idea of local currency, the currency itself does not illustrate the benefits of spending locally or the negative impacts of not doing so. As a result, although individuals who are already convinced that local spending is important may enthusiastically embrace a local currency, those for whom the rationale is not fully understood or accepted are unlikely to be won over [8].

While we have come to believe that local spending is a far more desirable behavior than non-local spending, we accept that understanding why takes some persuasion. . . and that this is an *opinion*. Our aim, therefore, is to convince others of this position — to persuade in the rhetorical sense of the term — and to use technology to catalyze internally motivated behavior change.

1.2 Meanings

Metaphors were instrumental in developing a shared understanding of our chosen problem and revealing potential opportunities for intervention, and we describe these metaphors in the subsequent paragraphs.

The Leaky Bucket. We were inspired by the New Economics Foundation's use of the metaphor of a 'bucket' to describe local economies [11] and their assertion that the reason certain communities are struggling is because they have too many holes in their bucket. Specifically, the holes allow money coming in to leak out faster than it is able to grow, and thus the overall level of wealth is dropping. This suggests two initial objectives for address this wicked problem. 1) We could attempt to *plug these holes*, i.e. substituting non-local transactions with local transactions in instances where there is no *need* to buy from a non-local trader [11]. 2) We could attempt to increase the rate at which a community's wealth grows by seeking to *increase the number of transactions* through which profit is accummulated and added to the local economy.

Money as an Information System. Money is an information system that records information in a way that enables tradable value. Like all information systems, money both 'remembers' and 'forgets'. While money remembers an abstracted value, it does not remember where this value derives from. This provides insight into a specific *error* [6] that can be addressed, namely that people cannot recognize the impact of their spending behavior on their local community. To correct this, technological interventions could increase the 'transfer rate' of money, by providing a new or additional view of money that allows greater information about the social consequences of spending behavior to be communicated.

Flow. The health of any economy depends on a continuous flow of money between individuals. When money is hoarded, wealth not only fails to grow, but the value of the currency plummets as it loses its perceived value as a means of facilitating trade. Systems can be designed to support flow by creating incentives for spending over hoarding. A similar principle underpins an alternative to local currencies, namely local economic transfer systems (LETS) [8]. In these systems, the currency of exchange exists only in the trade itself (it *is* the trade).

By combining these different ideas, we have a sense of the means through which we might promote behavior change. Our strategy is to present a persuasive argument for the long-term community benefits of local spending, which is not currently obvious because certain information that would lead one to this conclusion is hidden. To this end, we propose to make it visible through an information layer that allows individuals to see the flow of money around their community over time. We will also reveal any potential 'leaks', which could signal opportunities for motivated individuals to identify alternative local traders, and may highlight gaps in the market for new local businesses to fill.

2   System Design Considerations

Verplank [6] described the three questions that interaction designers need to answer as: 1) 'How do you do?' — how does the person you are designing for affect the world? 2) 'How do you feel?' — what feedback do you want the person you are designing for to receive, and what emotions do you seek to elicit? 3) 'How do you know?' — what does the person you are designing for need to understand in order to carry out the desired action? We explore each of these in reverse order to develop the design features for our system. In so doing, we address the conceptual development of the *modes* (the models and tasks) and *mappings* (the displays and controls) our system might accommodate.

2.1   Know

There are two basic forms that knowledge might take. *Path knowledge* is step-by-step and specific to a particular context [6]. For example, when designing the interaction for an emergency exit it makes sense to give people a path for getting to safety without the need for the user to understand why that path is the best path. *Map knowledge* is required when the goal is to enable people to make their own determination of the appropriate thing to do [6]. Map knowledge enables individuals to make decisions in the future based on an understanding of how the system works.

If our goal were to get people to spend money at a particular shop, it may be appropriate to develop a simple path for users. But the desired behavior for BARTER is far less prescriptive, as we are trying to create a new *sensibility* whereby local spending becomes the norm. To enable this sensibility, we are primarily interested in conveying the general *rationale* for spending locally and believe that map knowledge is therefore required.

What better way to impart map knowledge about the dynamics of a local economy than to develop a system that displays a map of the flow of money? However, the key characteristics of any successful map are 1) accuracy and 2) legibility, and we recognize that the accuracy of our map will be highly dependent on a high percentage of the target community participating in having their transactions recorded. With regards to legibility, we are experimenting with visualizations of the transaction data recorded by the system in order to determine how best to help users navigate through and comprehend a local spending map.

The point we are making here is how different a challenge this is from most common persuasive technologies, in particular systems that seek to provide feedback to individuals to get them to change a specific behavior. In these systems, the path is obvious — it is short and easy to follow, and the user accepts the basic premise of the 'correctness' of the end behavior. Therefore there is no rhetorical persuasion, as behavior change is induced by getting the user to follow the path enough times that it becomes habitual. In our case, accepting the premise behind local spending requires a greater level of understanding by the user, which can only be facilitated by revealing the relevant dynamics.

2.2   Feel

Most persuasive technologies attempt to leverage people's self-interest, which in this case may be a self-interested economic argument for spending locally. But a central premise of our argument is that if everyone acted in their short-term economic self-interest the whole community will be worse off in the long-term, so it would be contradictory to design the system around extrinsic or self-interest motivations. Instead, the system must promote intrinsic rewards and community spirit, which we aim to achieve by displaying one's personal behaviors only in terms of the community impact these have, and to represent success in terms of the growing pool of wealth of the community.

Note that this premise also goes against the dominant economic narrative, which proposes that the economy functions precisely because each individual is pursuing their own personal self-interest. We recognize, therefore, that we are making a *political* argument about how a major societal structure (the global free market) is failing to support widespread wellbeing, and as such we adopt a similar approach to political videogames [12]. Our political rhetoric for the system is to reveal, in part, how the global free market model does not work, and to create a motivation for people to adopt more altruistic behavior.

2.3   Do

There are two metaphorical types of control we could design: the 'button' representing simple, discrete control, or the 'lever' which allows continuous control. It is likely that we will require a mix of the two. Interactions that are unrelated to the process of learning the map but integral to the working of the system should be as quick and simple as possible ('button'). However, when trying to engage people with the flow of money, we might be better evoking this engagement through continuous interaction ('lever'). This is reflected in the kind of feedback we ought to present — e.g. we do not provide instantaneous points or badges for pressing a button, but rather show how various button presses (or transactions) join the continuous flow of money and gratification will only be achieved through cooperation.

3   Conclusion

In this paper we have built a case for the need for a designerly approach to persuasion when faced with wicked problems, which is characterized by the embracing of complexity. This approach is illustrated through the development of our (evolving) system design and holistically addressing the *motivation, meanings, modes* and *mappings*.

Our experience thus far in developing the BARTER system has led to specific insights regarding the requirements of persuasive computing when applied to wicked problems. Firstly, we suggest that because the prescribed behavior change for wicked problems is not obvious to the target users, systems will need to foster map knowledge rather than path knowledge. Secondly, wicked problems are wicked in part because the target behavior(s) are often intertwined with social practices and cultural norms, and any persuasive system that aims to change these behaviors is, therefore, making a *political* argument. Thirdly, persuasive games seem well suited for fostering the engaged participation required for mastering map knowledge, and they are congruent with the rhetorical nature of the designerly approach, as they motivate behavior change by 'engaging users in a discourse about the behavior itself or the logics that would recommend such actions or beliefs' [12, p. 60–1]. They function to reveal underlying ideologies in a way that can provoke changes in *understanding* as a route to changing behavior, which is precisely what is required to address wicked problems.

Acknowledgements. This research is made possible by EPSRC grants EP/K012584/1 and EP/I033017/1. The project is in collaboration with Michael Hallam of the Ethical Small Traders Association.

References

[1] Fogg, B.: Creating persuasive technologies: an eight-step design process. In: Persuasive, p. 44 (2009)
[2] Buchanan, R.: Wicked problems in design thinking. Design Issues 8(2), 5–21 (1992)
[3] Stolterman, E.: The nature of design practice and implications for interaction design research. International Journal of Design 2(1), 55–65 (2008)
[4] Cross, N.: Designerly ways of knowing: design discipline versus design science. Design Issues 17(3), 49–55 (2001)
[5] Law, J.: After method: Mess in social science research. Routledge (2004)
[6] Verplank, B.: Interaction design sketchbook. Unpublished paper for CCRMA course Music 250a (2003)
[7] Portas, M., Britain, G.: The Portas Review: An independent review into the future of our high streets. Department for Business, Innovation and Skills (2011)
[8] Helleiner, E.: Think globally, transact locally: Green political economy and the local currency movement. Global Society 14(1), 35–51 (2000)
[9] Fogg, B.J.: Persuasive Technology: Using Computers to Change What We Think and Do. Morgan Kauffman, San Francisco (2003)
[10] Collom, E.: Community currency in the united states: the social environments in which it emerges and survives. Environment and Planning A 37(9), 1565 (2005)
[11] Ward, B., Lewis, J., Britain, G., Unit, N.R.: Plugging the Leaks: Making the most of every pound that enters your local economy. New Economics Foundation London (2002)
[12] Bogost, I.: Persuasive games: The expressive power of videogames. MIT Press (2007)

Credibility and Interactivity: Persuasive Components of Ideological Group Websites

Genevieve Johnson, William D. Taylor, Alisha M. Ness, Michael K. Ault,
Norah E. Dunbar, Matthew L. Jensen, and Shane Connelly

University of Oklahoma, Norman, OK, United States
{johnson.gen,wtaylor,alishaness,michael.ault-1,
ndunbar,mjensen,sconnelly}@ou.edu

Abstract. The quickly growing presence of ideological groups on the Internet has garnered interest into how these groups use technology to persuade others. This study extends current research on the influential effects of website credibility and interactivity to the context of ideological group websites. Results of this study indicated that credibility and interactivity had direct and interactive effects on outcomes of agreement with the ideology, negative affective responses, and strength of argument when responding to the website. A number of these results may be due to (in)consistency with previous beliefs or violations of expectations regarding ideological group websites. Limitations and future directions are also discussed.

Keywords: Ideological groups, websites, credibility, interactivity.

1   Introduction

The Internet and various forms of new media have allowed ideological groups to have a growing presence on the World Wide Web, prompting interest in how these groups use this technology to persuade others. Ideological groups hold clear, persistent values and beliefs and provide a structure or mental model to help their members interpret and navigate the world [31], [45]. As a result, ideological groups can fulfill a number of basic human needs, such as providing a sense of identity and strategies for acting upon one's environment [3], [46]. Group ideologies range from social movements to political or religious causes[1] [45], and the widespread nature of ideological groups underscores their ability to perpetuate shared beliefs and motivate action [45]. The Internet provides an outlet for meeting these goals, and research is needed to understand how these groups use websites to exert influence.

Traditionally, it has been difficult to study ideological group communications due to their limited accessibility [14]. However, the Internet has become critical to these groups and serves as a central way for group members to communicate, interact, and

---

[1] Examples include English Defense League (EDL), Sierra Club, People for the Ethical Treatment of Animals (PETA), and National Rifle Association (NRA).

A. Spagnolli et al. (Eds.): PERSUASIVE 2014, LNCS 8462, pp. 143–154, 2014.

build relationships [40]. An online presence enables recruitment of members who would be unwilling or unable to attend in-person functions or meetings [22]. In addition, the Internet provides an economical and less regulated way to reach individuals directly [4], [26] while fostering an international appeal and tightly controlling the group's image [12], [18]. There is sparse research on how aspects of website technology influence those who browse ideological group websites. One central goal of websites is to persuade its visitors to think and/or act in a particular way [11], but much of the website research to date has been done in marketing or political domains. Ideological group websites offer an important and rich extension to this literature, and we investigate two persuasive tools commonly seen on websites – credibility and interactivity. Specifically, we manipulate these website features to assess their impact on viewers' thoughts, feelings, and behavior.

1.1   Credibility

The level of credibility attributed to information is generally based on the overall believability of the information and/or its source [16], [11]. Trustworthiness and expertise of the message source are two traditional components of credibility [9], [17], [27], [35]. However, theory and research has expanded the construct to include other factors such as authority and character [28], experience [16], [35], goodwill [29], and external support [30].

Credibility is theorized to be one of the main ways in which a message can persuade [34], and sources high in credibility are generally found to be more persuasive than sources lacking credible properties [17], [27], [35]. Credible sources influence opinions, attitudes, and behavior [17], [41, [33]. Wilson and Sherrell's (1993) meta-analysis showed that a credible message from an expert source is a powerful source of attitude change. Furthermore, Pornpitakan (2004), citing Braunsberger (1996), points out that advertisement research has found that interacting with a more credible source results in more positive attitudes regarding a brand and its product. Presenting credible arguments on a website may therefore help ideological groups accomplish their goal of indoctrinating their members with their beliefs [3] and evoking attitudes consistent with their viewpoints. Furthermore, website features themselves, independent of the website sponsor, have been found to have an influence on credibility perceptions [10]. Therefore, we propose the following:

> *Hypothesis 1: Viewing high-credibility websites will lead to more agreement with the ideological position presented on the website than viewing low-credibility websites.*

1.2   Interactivity

Website interactivity refers to features of websites that allow participation by visitors such that they can actively control what information to access and and/or engage in two-way communication with the website host or other visitors [15], [23], [25]. Hyperlinks [8], website search capability, online bulletin boards [25], chatrooms, and drop-down menus [48] are some examples of interactive website components. Websites with these features are seen as more interactive than those without them.

The core function of website interactivity is to facilitate engagement with other users, members, and the website sponsor [15], [24], and the literature on interactivity oftentimes affirms interactivity's ability to create a highly involved and cognitively engaging website experience [20], [24], [36]. As a result, interactivity enhances attitudes and trust towards a website, the website sponsor, and its featured product [7], [19], [42], [43], [48]. Interactive websites have also been linked to favorable viewpoint adjustments [20] and greater acceptance of website information [5]. In addition, interactive websites increase satisfaction and reduce frustration by decreasing feelings of being ignored or manipulated [24] and are seen as more appealing than less interactive websites [13]. Such components are also important for ideological groups, as they aim to generate positive impressions of the group and their message. Accordingly, we suggest:

> *Hypothesis 2: Viewing websites low in interactivity will lead to a) less agreement with the ideological position presented on the website and b) more negative affective responses than viewing highly interactive websites.*

These components have not been considered in tandem, especially for the websites of ideological groups. Credibility and interactivity may interact to influence reactions to the website. For example, a credible, interactive website may appear more legitimate and therefore synergistically boost agreement and positive affective responses to the website. Another possibility may be that the legitimacy conferred by websites high in credibility and interactivity heightens awareness of the extreme nature of the ideology. This heightened salience could evoke negative responses in website viewers whose own beliefs and values run counter to the ideology, prompting more negative responses and less agreement with the ideological views. We therefore ask:

> *RQ1: How will credibility and interactivity interact to influence agreement with ideological views presented on the website and affective responses towards the ideological group?*

Attitudes and intentions are believed to be directly linked to behaviors [1, 2], and both credibility and interactivity has been linked to behavioral intentions and behavioral compliance [32], [35], [49]. Credibility and interactivity could have main effects or interactive ones on behavior. Similar to agreement and affect, credibility and interactivity may work together to foster a viewer's desire to express strong arguments in response to the ideological beliefs whether they are consistent with an individual's own beliefs or against them if they are perceived as a threat to an individual's beliefs. For example, seeing a website high in credibility and interactivity may motivate someone who is against the ideology to respond with a more thorough argument as they may feel that the views expressed are a real threat to his or her worldview. Alternatively, those same individuals may react to a highly credible and interactive website by withdrawing from engaging with this significant threat to their worldview, and consequently offer weak arguments in response to comments on the website.

Credibility and interactivity could also work together in other ways. For example, seeing a website high in credibility but low in interactivity may seem inconsistent, prompting someone who is in favor of the ideology to feel a need to provide a strong argument to make up for the weaknesses seen on the website. Alternatively, someone who is against the ideology could potentially react to such an inconsistency by seeing the group as illegitimate and not a threat, thereby not feeling the need to speak out strongly against the group. We therefore ask the following:

> *RQ2: How will credibility and interactivity function to influence strength of arguments (writing quality, persuasiveness, soundness of arguments) when responding to the group?*

2   Method

2.1   Participants and Design

Participants included 212 undergraduate students from a large university in the United States. All data were collected in a lab via online survey software. Mean age of the participants was 18.5 ($SD = 1.47$), and 24% were male ($n = 51$). A 2 x 2 x 2 between-subjects design was used (credibility, interactivity, and violence were each high or low), and participants were randomly assigned to one of the eight conditions. Due to space considerations, only the credibility and interactivity manipulations are examined in this paper. Their effects are considered across both violent and non-violent group websites, and violence did not have an effect in any analyses here.

2.2   Procedure

Upon arrival, participants read and signed informed consent forms which indicated they would be looking at a website and answering questions about it. Participants were led to believe the website was associated with an actual group rather than created for the purpose of this research. They were not informed that the website was fictitious[2] until the debriefing. Participants first completed a set of covariate measures. Following these measures, participants viewed the fictitious website then answered a series of questions about the website and the ideology as well as manipulation check questions and additional covariate surveys. The consenting, data collection, and debriefing processes were guided by the Institutional Review Board to ensure no coercion or undue stress or strain occurred.

2.3   Manipulations

To select an ideological view to represent on this website, we conducted a survey in an undergraduate psychology class that assessed their interest and viewpoints on a

---

[2] Website creation was assisted by a professional web developer. All versions of the website were only available by login codes. They were not accessible by the general public or indexed in search engines. Data were always collected with an experimenter present.

variety of topics (e.g., human rights, environmental issues, animal rights, etc.) on 7-point scales. We selected the topic of separation of church and state based on its importance to participants and variation with regards to agreement with the ideology (importance $M = 5.81$, $SD = 1.31$, agreement with issues $M = 4.73$, $SD = 1.86$). We then created a website for a group called "The Christian Liberty Foundation" that included content such as the history of the group, issues on which the group acts, and upcoming events. The generated content was based on typical ideological group websites, and each website contained interactivity and credibility manipulations. Manipulated facets of credibility included authority, character, expertise, goodwill, external support, experience, education, position and writing quality, and were all either high or low. For example, for external support, on the high credibility websites, studies at prominent universities were cited to support numerous claims that were made, while obscure sources were cited for those same claims on the low credibility websites. As another example, the description of the founders of the group differed across websites, with the high credibility websites indicating that one of the founders had received a Master's degree from a prominent university, while for the low credibility websites the description stated he had received a lower degree at an obscure college. Two judges with communication expertise and who were blind to the manipulations evaluated the credibility of each condition. Their ratings confirmed that the high credibility conditions included high credibility cues to a much greater extent than the low credibility conditions ($M = 4.44$ for high credibility websites vs. $M = 1.92$ for low credibility websites on an 18-item, 7-point scale).

We manipulated interactivity through altering the ease with which participants could communicate with and navigate the website and through the presence of external links. For example, the high interactive websites had drop-down menus and the ability to post comments, offer feedback, request information, and click on external links, while the low interactive websites did not. The interactivity manipulation check based on Liu's (2003) measure was successful such that a t-test demonstrated that those in the high interactivity conditions perceived the websites as more interactive ($M = 3.72$, $SD = .62$) than those in the low interactivity conditions ($M = 3.26$, $SD = .51$), $t(210) = -5.91$, $p \leq .001$.

2.4   Measures

Open-Ended Responses. After browsing the website, the participants responded to two comments they were told had been posted on the website in the past. The first comment was in favor of the integration of church and state (pro-ideology) while the second comment argued for the separation of church and state (anti-ideology). Trained raters coded the responses for numerous dimensions which were combined to create three scales: agreement with ideology ($\alpha = .85$), negative affective response ($\alpha = .76$), and argument strength ($\alpha = .85$). R^*_{wg} was calculated for each of the ratings variables and ranged from .67 to .85.

Covariates. Several covariates were included in the analyses. We assessed levels of intrinsic religiosity, or personal religious commitment, using a 3-item scale from the

Duke University Religion Index (DUREL; [21]). Participants responded using a 5-point Likert scale (Definitely NOT true to Definitely true) (α = .92). We measured conservatism using Ray's (1983) 22-item measure with a 7-point scale (1 = Strongly disagree, 5 = Strongly agree) (α = .76). We assessed intelligence using the Employee Aptitude Survey (EAS; [38]), a 5-minute timed measure of verbal reasoning. We measured the level to which the participants perceived themselves to be personally affected by the issue using a 1-item measure on a 7-point Likert scale (1 = Does not affect me at all, 7 = Affects me very much). Time spent on the website was also recorded. Covariates significant at the .05 level for a given analysis were retained.

3   Results

We tested hypotheses 1 and 2a, which predicted that credibility and interactivity would lead to higher levels of agreement, using one-way between group ANCOVAs. These hypotheses were unsupported. We also conducted a t-test to assess the perceived credibility of the websites as measured by 25 items based on the manipulated credibility facets (7-point Likert scale, strongly disagree to strongly agree, α = .96). There were no significant differences in perceived credibility in the high (M = 3.26, SD = 1.17) versus low credibility (M = 3.31, SD = 1.26) conditions, $t(210)$ = -.303, p = .76. However, for research question 1, there was a significant interactive effect for credibility and interactivity in the responses to the anti-ideological comment when controlling for intrinsic religiosity, conservatism, and total time on website, $F(1, 204)$ = 4.69, p = .032 , η_p^2 = .02. The lowest levels of agreement resulted after viewing websites low in credibility and high in interactivity (M = 1.55, SE = .08) while the highest levels resulted following browsing websites both low (M = 1.76, SE = .08) or high (M = 1.77, SE = .09) in interactivity and credibility (See Figure 1).

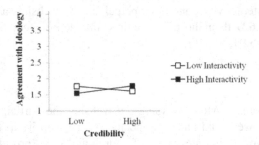

Fig. 1. Interactive effects for website credibility and interactivity on agreement

We also used between-subject ANCOVAs to test the hypothesis regarding negative affective responses. Controlling for intrinsic religiosity, hypothesis 2b was unsupported as the analyses resulted in a finding opposite as expected. Highly interactive websites actually resulted in higher levels of negative affective reactions (M = 2.83, SE = .07) than websites lower in interactivity (M = 2.59, SE = .07), $F(1, 207)$ = 5.55,

$p = .019$, $\eta_p^2 = .03$, when responding to the pro-ideology prompt. Follow-up analyses revealed that this was not due to differences in agreement with the ideological views across the high and low interactivity conditions ($t(210) = .259$, $p = .796$). An additional unexpected finding resulted for the credibility manipulation. Responses to the anti-ideological prompt for those who viewed websites higher in credibility had more expressions of negative affect ($M = 2.89$, $SE = .07$) than those who viewed websites lower in credibility ($M = 2.55$, $SE = .07$), $F(1, 207) = 11.79$, $p = .001$, $\eta_p^2 = .05$. Again, this was not due to levels of agreement with the ideology across credibility conditions, $t(209) = -.672$, $p = .502$. No interactive effects were found for negative affect.

Research question 2, which asked about the effects of the manipulations on argument strength, was also tested using a between-subjects ANCOVA, controlling for intelligence and the level to which they were personally affected by the issue. The interaction of credibility and interactivity was significant, $F(1, 206) = 4.13$, $p = .043$, $\eta_p^2 = .02$, when responding to the pro-ideological prompt. Viewing websites high in credibility and low in interactivity led to the strongest argument ($M = 3.64$, $SE = .08$) while viewing websites that were both high in credibility and interactivity (3.43, $SE = .08$) or low in credibility and interactivity ($M = 3.43$, $SE = .08$) resulted in the lowest levels of argument strength (See Figure 2).

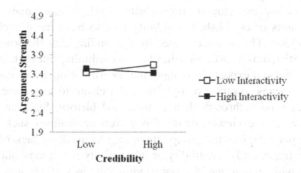

Fig. 2. Interactive effects for website credibility and interactivity on argument strength in a response to an ideologically-based prompt

4   Discussion

Persuasive technology is becoming more prominent with the rise of the Internet. This study supports the idea that website credibility and interactivity influence website visitors' perceptions of and responses to ideological views in ways that can either facilitate or impede ideological group goals. First-time visitors to an ideological website were impacted in different and sometimes opposite ways by the established credibility of the group (e.g, expertise, authority) and the ability to interact with the group's website compared to more traditional persuasive contexts (e.g., marketing messages). This may be largely due to the fact that ideologies are important for life meaning, reflecting part of peoples' identities. Participants' pre-existing beliefs on the separation of church and state may have prompted reactions to protect their identity, whether it was consistent with or threatened by the ideological group. For example, participants who may have desired more integration of church and state may have still reacted negatively to the extreme position taken up by the group such that they agreed with the issue but not the group's approach to it[3]. This is consistent with our finding that even the websites with high credibility cues were perceived as having low to moderate credibility. Use of a less extreme stance on this ideological view might have produced different findings and could be examined in future research. Such pre-existing beliefs connected to an individual's life meaning and identity are not likely to exist or be as strong for those products and topics that are researched in other credibility and interactivity literature, possibly leading to the discrepant findings.

Although strong main effects were not seen, their interactive effects offer important insights into the ways individuals' perceptions and responses are affected by ideological group websites. Prior research in non-ideological domains suggests that websites high in credibility cues such as expertise and that allow visitors to easily interact with the website would lead to high levels of agreement, which we saw. However, we also found that when the website was low on both credibility and interactivity, participants agreed more with the ideological view. This may be due to their alignment with visitor expectations for websites [39]. Visitors may expect groups with greater amounts of established credibility to also have more sophisticated, advanced websites [30]. This is underscored by the finding that the lowest agreement resulted when participants viewed websites low in credibility but high in interactivity, which may have violated expectations about the website. Website visitors may expect a group with the means to create a sophisticated website to also have the ability to establish their legitimacy through their content and history. Such an inconsistency may serve to distract the viewer, or the fancy website features such as interactive abilities may be perceived as the group attempting to mask its lack of actual group credibility. More importantly, credibility or interactivity alone may not be enough to foster agreement with an extreme ideological viewpoint as shifts in agreement may be difficult to achieve due to pre-existing beliefs on the topic. Unexpectedly, credibility actually boosted expressions of negative affect when participants responded to an anti-ideological prompt, regardless of agreement with the ideology. There are a few possible explanations for this. First, participants who did not agree with the ideology still saw the group's right to hold their viewpoint as legitimate and were upset that others were attacking it. Alternatively, those whose pre-existing beliefs aligned with the ideology rallied behind it and were upset when others disagreed. Another explanation is that they may have reacted negatively to the group's use of extreme measures, even when agreeing with the message itself. Or, the anti-ideology prompt simply primed more negative affect. Another unexpected finding was that interactivity led to

---

[3] As an example of this, part of one participant's comment stated: "While I agree with your point, you are going about it the wrong way. Name calling will not make a difference in our government."

greater negative affect. Interactive features may increase perceptions of legitimacy of the website, which can be a source of threat to non-believers, generating a negative response. Those who did agree with the group also experienced negative affect, possibly because they felt like the extreme way in which this group expressed the ideology was doing more to hurt than help the cause. However, the evocation of negative affect is not necessarily detrimental to the group's purpose. Negative affect can be a powerful source for motivation in terms of actions on behalf of the ideological group's cause [44].

Website visitors' strength of argument when responding to a pro-ideological prompt was also influenced by interactivity and credibility of the website. Low levels of interactivity boosted the effects of high credibility on argument strength while high levels of interactivity were detrimental to argument strength on the highly credible websites. When considered with the interaction for agreement, it appears arguments lower in strength were also highest in agreement with the ideology (i.e., when both credibility and interactivity are high or low). Therefore, ideological group websites that lack interactivity but present credible arguments may appear to be trying hard to seem legitimate through content even though their website is technologically unsophisticated, and those viewing the website may feel the need to articulate better arguments against the ideology to undermine the group. Additionally, websites higher in credibility but lower in interactivity may have allowed participants to read the information more thoroughly, boosting their ability to generate stronger arguments against the ideology due to higher processing of the information provided on the website.

These findings are critical as ideological groups aim to persuade, and their websites can have functional and contextual components that can influence their ability to draw and keep members. Hate groups in particular have generated a large internet profile [12], and research on this topic may be particularly important in educating the public on how to shield themselves or better understand persuasion attempts by these groups. This research also extends work on persuasive technology to a new realm – ideological group websites – and more research is needed to understand the various ways in which ideological group websites function to persuade others. Investigations into ideological groups' use of threat (e.g., emotional appeals) and how it functions with other persuasive components such as credibility and interactivity on websites would be an important line of research, as would researching the effects of violent content.

Future research could also look at global perceptions of credibility of websites, as interactivity may have enhanced the perceived legitimacy of the website and the group. The fact that our credibility manipulations were not explicitly noticed yet still affected the participants in various ways also offers an interesting line of future research, as credibility may function in a more heuristic manner, creating a cause for concern as individuals may be being impacted by these ideological group websites without even being aware. The interactivity manipulation in this study was also limited (e.g., the external links were present but were not fully functional), and research could expand this element to fully delineate its effects.

References

1. Ajzen, I.: Attitudes, Personality, and Behavior. Open University Press, Buckingham (2005)
2. Ajzen, I., Czasch, C., Flood, M.G.: From Intentions to Behavior: Implementation Intention, Commitment, and Conscientiousness. Journal of Applied Social Psychology 39, 1356–1372 (2009)
3. Allen, M.T., Angie, A.D., Davis, J.L., Byrne, C.L., O'Hair, H.D., Connelly, S., Mumford, M.D.: Virtual risk: The role of new media in violent and nonviolent ideological groups. In: Heath, R.L., O'Hair, H.D. (eds.) Handbook of Risk and Crisis Communication, pp. 446–470. Routledge, New York (2010)
4. Blazak, R.: White Boys to Terrorist Men: Target Recruitment of Nazi Skinheads. American Behavioral Scientist 44(6), 982–1000 (2001)
5. Campbell, D.E., Wright, R.T.: Shut-up I Don't Care: Understanding the Role of Relevance and Interactivity on Customer Attitudes toward Repetitive Online Advertising. Journal of Electronic Commerce Research 9(1), 62–76 (2008)
6. Chaiken, S., Maheswaran, D.: Heuristic Processing Can Bias Systematic Processing: Effects of Source Credibility, Argument Ambiguity, and Task Importance on Attitude Judgment. Journal of Personality And Social Psychology 66(3), 460–473 (1994)
7. Chen, Q., Griffith, D.A., Shen, F.: The Effects of Interactivity on Cross-Channel Communication Effectiveness. Journal of Interactive Advertising 5(2), N.PAG (2005)
8. Chung, X., Zhao, X.: Effects of Perceived Interactivity on Web Site Preference and Memory: The Role of Personal Motivation. Journal of Computer-Mediated Communication 10(1) (2004)
9. Danielson, D.R.: Web Credibility. In: Ghaoui, C. (ed.) Encyclopedia of Human-Computer Interaction, pp. 713–721. Idea Group, Inc., Hershey (2005)
10. Flanagin, A.J., Metzger, M.J.: The Role of Site Features, User Attributes, and Information Verification Behaviors on the Perceived Credibility of Web-Based Information. New Media & Society 9(2), 319–342 (2007)
11. Fogg, B.J.: Persuasive Technology: Using Computers to Change What We Think and Do. Morgan Kaufmann Publishers. San Francisco (2003)
12. Gerstenfeld, P.B., Grant, D.R., Chiang, C.: Hate Online: A Content Analysis of Extremist Internet Sites. Analyses of Social Issues and Public Policy (ASAP) 3(1), 29–44 (2003)
13. Ghose, S., Dou, W.: Interactive Functions and Their Impacts on the Appeal of Internet Presence Sites. Journal of Advertising Research 38(2), 29–43 (1998)
14. Glaser, J., Dixit, J., Green, D.P.: Studying Hate Crime with The Internet: What Makes Racists Advocate Racial Violence? Journal of Social Issues 58(1), 177–193 (2002)
15. Ha, L., James, E.L.: Interactivity Reexamined: A Baseline Analysis of Early Business Web Sites. Journal of Broadcasting & Electronic Media 42(4), 457–474 (1998)
16. Hovland, C.I., Janis, I.L., Kelley, H.H.: Communication and Persuasion; Psychological Studies of Opinion Change. Yale University Press, New Haven (1953)
17. Hovland, C.I., Weiss, W.: The Influence of Source Credibility on Communication Effectiveness. Public Opinion Quarterly 15, 635–650 (1951)
18. Jensen, M.L., Dunbar, N.E., Connelly, S., Hughes, M.G., Taylor, W.D., Adame, B.J., Rozzell, B.L.: Social Media on Violent Ideological Group Websites. Paper presented at the 19th America's Conference on Information Systems, Chicago, IL (August 2013)
19. Johnson, G.J., Bruner, G., Kumar, A.: Interactivity and Its Facets Revisited: Theory and Empirical Test. Journal Of Advertising 35(4), 35–52 (2006)

20. Kim, H., Stout, P.A.: The Effects of Interactivity on Information Processing and Attitude Change: Implications For Mental Health Stigma. Health Communication 25, 142–154 (2010)
21. Koenig, H.G., Büssing, A.: The Duke University Religion Index (DUREL): A Five-Item Measure For Use in Epidemiological Studies. Religions 1(1), 78–85 (2010)
22. Lee, E., Leets, L.: Persuasive Storytelling by Hate Groups Online Examining Its Effects on Adolescents. American Behavioral Scientist 45(6), 927–957 (2002)
23. Liu, Y.: Developing a Scale to Measure the Interactivity of Websites. Journal of Advertising Research 43(2), 207–216 (2003)
24. Liu, Y., Shrum, L.J.: What is Interactivity and is it always such a Good Thing? Implications of Definition, Person, and Situation for the Influence of Interactivity on Advertising Effectiveness. Journal of Advertising 31, 53–64 (2002)
25. Liu, Y., Shrum, L.J.: A Dual-Process Model of Interactivity Effects. Journal of Advertising 38(2), 53–68 (2009)
26. McCann, S.J.: Authoritarianism, Conservatism, Racial Diversity Threat, and the State Distribution of Hate Groups. The Journal of Psychology 144(1), 37–60 (2009)
27. McGinnies, E., Ward, C.: Better Liked than Right: Trustworthiness and Expertise as factors in Credibility. Personality and Social Psychology Bulletin 6, 467–472 (1980)
28. McCroskey, J.C.: Scales for the Measurement of Ethos. Speech Monographs 33, 65–72 (1966)
29. McCroskey, J.C., Teven, J.J.: Goodwill: A Reexamination of the Construct and Its Measurement. Communication Monographs 66(1), 90–103 (1999)
30. Metzger, M.J., Flanagin, A.J., Medders, R.B.: Social and Heuristic Approaches to Credibility Evaluation Online. Journal of Communication 60(3), 413–439 (2010)
31. Mumford, M.D., Bedell-Avers, K.E., Hunter, S.T., Espejo, J., Eubanks, D., Connelly, M.: Violence in Ideological and Non-Ideological Groups: A Quantitative Analysis of Qualitative Data. Journal of Applied Social Psychology 38(6), 1521–1561 (2008)
32. Ohanian, R.: Construction and Validation of a Scale to Measure Celebrity Endorsers' Perceived Expertise, Trustworthiness, and Attractiveness. Journal of Advertising 19(3), 39–52 (1990)
33. Petty, R.E., Cacioppo, J.T.: Attitudes and Persuasion: Classic and Contemporary Approaches. W. C. Brown Co. Publishers, Dubuque (1981)
34. Petty, R.E., Cacioppo, J.T.: Elaboration likelihood model. In: Berkowitz, L. (ed.) Advances in Experimental Social Psychology, vol. 19, pp. 123–205. Academic Press, Inc., Orlando (1986)
35. Pornpitakpan, C.: The Persuasiveness of Source Credibility: A Critical Review of Five Decades' Evidence. Journal of Applied Social Psychology 34(2), 243–281 (2004)
36. Rafaeli, S.: Interactivity: From New Media to Communication. In: Hawkins, R.P., Wieman, J.M., Pingree, S. (eds.) Advancing Communication Science: Merging Mass and Interpersonal Processes, pp. 110–134. Sage, Newbury Park (1988)
37. Ray, J.J.: A Scale to Measure Conservatism of American Public Opinion. The Journal of Social Psychology 119(2), 293–294 (1983)
38. Ruch, F., Ruch, W.W.: Employee Aptitude Survey Technical Report. Psychological Services, Incorporated, Chicago, IL (1983)
39. Sohn, D., Ci, C., Lee, B.: The Moderating Effects of Expectation on the Patterns of the Interactivity-Attitude Relationship. Journal of Advertising 36(3), 109–119 (2007)
40. Stanton, J.J.: Terror in Cyberspace: Terrorists will Exploit and Widen the Gap Between Governing Structures and the Public. American Behavioral Scientist 45(6), 1017–1032 (2002)

41. Sundar, S.S.: Exploring Receivers' Criteria for Perception of Print and Online News. Journalism and Mass Communication Quarterly 76, 373–386 (1999)
42. Sundar, S.S.: Theorizing Interactivity's Effects. Information Society 20(5), 385–389 (2004)
43. Sundar, S.S., Kim, J.: Interactivity and Persuasion: Influencing Attitudes with Information and Involvement. Journal of Interactive Advertising 5(2), 5–58 (2005)
44. Tausch, N., Becker, J.C., Spears, R., Christ, O., Saab, R., Singh, P., Siddiqui, R.N.: Explaining Radical Group Behavior: Developing Emotion and Efficacy Routes to Normative and Nonnormative Collective Action. Journal of Personality and Social Psychology 101(1), 129 (2011)
45. Van Dijk, T.A.: Ideology and Discourse Analysis. Journal of Political Ideologies 11(2), 115–140 (2006)
46. Vigil, J.D.: Urban Violence and Street Gangs. Annual Review of Anthropology, 225–242 (2003)
47. Wilson, E.J., Sherrell, D.L.: Source Effects in Communication and Persuasion Research: A Meta-Analysis of Effect Size. Journal Of The Academy of Marketing Science 21(2), 101–112 (1993)
48. Wu, G.: Conceptualizing and Measuring the Perceived Interactivity of Websites. Journal Of Current Issues & Research In Advertising (CTC Press) 28(1), 87–104 (2006)
49. Yoon, K., Kim, C.H., Kim, M.S.: A Cross-Cultural Comparison of the Effects of Source Credibility on Attitudes and Behavioral Intentions. Mass Communication and Society 1, 153–173 (1998)

Managing Depression through a Behavior Change Support System without Face-to-Face Therapy

Sitwat Langrial[1], Harri Oinas-Kukkonen[1],
Päivi Lappalainen[2], and Raimo Lappalainen[2]

[1] University of Oulu, Department of Information Processing Science
Rakentajantie 3, FIN-90570 Oulu, Finland
{sitwat.langrial,harri.oinas-kukkonen}@oulu.fi
[2] University of Jyväskylä, Department of Psychology, Finland
{paivi.k.lappalainen,raimo.lappalainen}@jyu.fi

Abstract. We present results from a study that examines impact of persuasive reminders and virtual rehearsal on the effectiveness of a Behavior Change Support System. Good Life Compass is a web-based BCSS aimed at supporting people with mild to moderate depression without face-to-face therapy. The content of virtual rehearsal were drawn from Acceptance and Commitment Therapy. Eligible participants were randomized into an intervention study and a control (wait-list) group. In this paper, both groups shall be reported as intervention group 1 and 2 respectively. For data collection, we employed semi-structured questionnaires and post-study interviews. As a result, participants acknowledged persuasive reminders as being helpful in completing weekly tasks and virtual rehearsal as an effective technique for learning new behaviors.

Keywords: Behavior Change Support Systems, Acceptance and Commitment Therapy, persuasive reminders, virtual rehearsal.

1 Introduction

Depression is among most common mental illnesses in modern society. It is expected that by the year 2030, it will contribute towards highest disease burden in developed countries [19, 24]. Depression has often been correlated with suicide, loss of productivity, social isolation, alcoholism and stigma [1]. Developing effective interventions for depression call for innovative solutions. Persuasive systems and behavioral psychology are well-studied research fields hence creating opportunities for intermediations based on amalgamation of cognitive behavioral techniques and information systems (IS).

Existing literature indicates that effectiveness of IS could improve if augmented with cognitive behavior therapy [24]. Noticeably, several hindrances have been reported that prevent people from using online as well as face-to-face treatments. For example, low motivation to reach experts, reluctance to discuss personal matters, lack of available professional services, distantly located health services, high treatment costs and stigma [1]. Human-Computer Interaction (HCI) researchers have shown

A. Spagnolli et al. (Eds.): PERSUASIVE 2014, LNCS 8462, pp. 155–166, 2014.

growing interest in studying behavior change interventions developed with intent to promote healthy behaviors [2]. Information systems have been developed to overcome said barriers by employing explicit or implicit persuasive techniques. Virtual rehearsal has been proposed as a key software feature that assists users to complete primary tasks [3], however relatively little research has been conducted on rehearsal in the fields of HCI and persuasive systems.

Keeping in mind the aforementioned challenges and the significance of improving mental well-being, we carried out this study using a web-based Behavior Change Support System (BCSS) [cf. 8]. The objective of the study was to evaluate impact of persuasive reminders and virtual rehearsal on the efficacy of a BCSS developed for people suffering from mild to moderate depressive symptoms.

2   Background

Existing literature indicates effectiveness of e-health interventions that are delivered over Internet and employ Cognitive Behavior Therapy (CBT) methods [4], however relatively few studies have reported use of value-based interventions incorporated with Acceptance and Commitment Therapy (ACT), the latest wave of CBT. ACT is known to increase psychological flexibility because it is positively correlated with better mental health [5].

Serious efforts have been made to understand the dynamics of IS for depression and mental disorders. Researchers have focused on evaluating effectiveness of IS in terms of task adherence [21], user satisfaction [20]. HCI researchers have emphasized designing systems that end up bringing intended change in behaviors. Consolvo et al. [6] propose using behavior change theories when designing interventions. Their design strategies [6] are valuable yet evaluating the effect of persuasive features has somewhat been vaguely described. This particular gap is clearly evident when it comes to software features such as virtual rehearsal [cf. 3]. Rehearsal has previously been used primarily in the field of CBT related studies. Psychology experts have acknowledged cognitive improvement through performance-based processes [7]. Significance of rehearsal as a behavior change technique has also been reported by [7] who argue that it is a useful method for improving self-efficacy. It is extraordinary to note that rehearsal, as a software feature, has not received due attention within the research field of persuasive systems [26].

Identifying this gap, we decided to study selected software features and their potential impact on effectiveness of a web-based BCSS for depression. A BCSS is defined as, "an information system designed to form, alter or reinforce attitudes, behaviors or an act of complying without using deception, coercion or inducements" [8]. BCSSs supplement the research field of behavior change interventions by emphasizing on creating desirable behavior/attitude change through non-coercive persuasion. As outlined by [8], interactive IS are expected to provide feedback and facilitate completion of target behaviors. In other words, we classify web-based IS as BCSSs [8] that are persuasive in nature, incorporated with augmented software features including but not limited to feedback, reminders and virtual rehearsal.

Building on Fogg's pivotal work [9], the Persuasive Systems Design model provides an opportunity to methodically design and evaluate persuasive systems [3]. According to [9], persuasive technology should prompt users to perform target behaviors when operating the system. Persuasive reminders could supplement BCSSs to facilitate task completion. Reminders might vary in design and form; for instance, they could be incorporated as guileless messages or feedback [18] and delivered via different means with varying frequencies. Previously, reminders have been employed in persuasive systems [10]. To date, different techniques have been studied to improve the effectiveness of reminders, for example, with tailored content [10]. Because our research employed questionnaires, we used Likert-scale to collect the responses. In addition, structured interviews were conducted. The reason to adopt this research approach is that it helps find common themes from the text using coding and indexing [23].

For this study, we formulated the following hypotheses:

H1. Persuasive reminders help users in task completion.
H2. Users would perceive persuasive reminders as a desirable feature.
H3. Virtual rehearsal helps users achieve improved self-confidence.
H4. Users with improved self-confidence continue to rehearse newly learned skills.
H5. The overall affect of the BCSS would lead to significant decrease in depression.

Both H1 and H2 were derived from the PSD model [3], H3 was based on the theory of Self-efficacy [16], and H4 was based on the Technology Acceptance Model [17].

3   Procedures

Recruitment. The study was conducted between September 2012 and January 2013. Recruitment advertisements were published on the 8th of September 2012. Participants were recruited through newspaper advertisements. It was stipulated in the advertisement that we were aiming to recruit those individuals who felt depressed. In response, 42 people contacted the university clinic via e-mail and/or telephone. Trained psychology student therapists performed initial screening. Keeping in mind professional code of conduct, ethical approval was granted by the Ethics Committee of the University of Jyväskylä and the Central Finland Healthcare District (Diary no: 15U/2012) on 27.08.2012. The application included research plan, measurements for the study, information for the participants about the research, informed consent and report of ethical aspects of the research. The study included no physical or psychological harm to the participants. Participants were provided intention of the study in detail and informed consent were received prior to the start of the study. It was also advised that the participants had no obligation to continue being part of the study. One participant decided to drop out before the screening process began. Consequently, 41 participants were interviewed over phone using a structured interview. Two participants did not meet the eligibility criteria and were dropped out from the study. Therefore, actual sample size comprised of 39 participants. Because the study included actual patients of depressive symptoms, approval was formally obtained from the Ethical Committee at the University of Jyväskylä, Finland. The inclusion criteria were: (1) self-reported depressive symptoms or depressed mood (2) no parallel psychological therapy at the time of the intervention, (3) possession of an email account, (4) access to computer and Internet, (5) access to telephone and (6) age 18 years or older.

Randomization. Randomization was performed on the 13th of September 2012 followed by pre-study interviews. Participants were randomized into two groups: (1) an intervention group 1 (n=19) that received measurements, automated weekly reminders (via email) and had access to weekly rehearsal exercises, and (2) an intervention group 2 (n=20) that first served as a waiting list control group and had to wait a period of six weeks before they could access the BCSS. The BCSS for intervention group 2 included the weekly rehearsal exercises (similar to those used in intervention group 1), but they did not receive automated weekly reminders. The intervention for group 1 commenced on the 28th of September 2012 and concluded on the 9th of November 2012 followed by final interviews with participants of intervention group 1. Treatment for intervention group 2 began from 17th of November 2012 and concluded in January 2013. Post measurements were taken between January 21 and January 25, 2013. A total of 28 (71.8%) females and 11 (28.2%) males with average age of 51 years comprised the sample. One participant from the intervention group dropped out before the post-measurement. Thus, the sample size consisted of 39 participants. The results reported in this paper are based on responses from participants of both groups.

The BCSS. Research team at the Department of Psychology, University of Jyväskylä, Finland developed the BCSS and the research team from the Department of Information Processing Science, University of Oulu, Finland integrated software features into it. ACT-based rehearsal exercises provided depression management skills. Virtual rehearsal as a software feature was used to enhance mindfulness, acceptance skills and commitment towards value-based actions among participants by utilizing a variety of metaphors, experiential exercises for mindfulness and behavioral activation [5]. ACT comprises of theoretical processes with an aim to enhance the psychological flexibility in people. Table 1 presents a brief overview of the modules used for the rehearsal content.

Persuasive Reminders and Virtual Rehearsal. Participants were required to complete one rehearsal module per week before moving on to the next level that was made available in the subsequent week. They were encouraged to practice newly learned skills including mindfulness, acceptance skills and to complete value based actions through email-based reminders. Therapists monitored whether participants completed weekly modules each Thursday. Those who did not complete weekly exercises in time were sent an additional reminder. In an event where a participant did not complete the task upon receiving two reminders, the assigned therapist contacted her via telephone. It is worth noting that there was only one client who was approached via telephone and that too for one time only.

Table 1. Acceptance Commitment Therapy Modules with brief descriptions

Week	ACT Modules	Brief explanation
1	Creative hopelessness and values	To offer specific verbal and experiential methods to help them determine their goals.
2	Value-based actions	Values are chosen qualities of purposive action that can never be obtained as an object but can be instantiated moment by moment.
3	Contact with the present moment	ACT promotes ongoing non-judgmental contact with psychological and environmental events as they occur.
4	Cognitive defusion	To alter the undesirable functions of thoughts and other private events, rather than trying to alter their form, frequency or situational sensitivity.
5	Self as context	It helps one become aware of his/her own experiences without any attachment leading to fostered acceptance.
6	Acceptance	It involves the ability to contact the present moment more fully as a conscious human being, and to change or persists in behavior.

Therapists. Graduate students of psychology performed the psychological therapy. Student therapists went through 10 hours of intensive training about ACT. Training sessions included lectures on general principles of ACT and core processes. During training sessions, students were provided with a handbook of ACT [11,12] highlighting detailed description of the therapy, its core processes, 32 metaphors, 18 exercises and practical forms that are commonly used in such therapies. Therapists received two hours of supervision during the first three and last three weeks of the program. The supervisor is an experienced clinician, licensed psychologist and psychotherapist with nearly 30 years experience of clinical work and supervision and 12 years of experience in ACT clinical practice.

Data Collection. Upon completion of the study, participants were asked questions about their experiences with the BCCS. The questionnaire consisted of two parts. The first part included demographic questions devised to collect information about the participants, their computing skills and familiarity with Internet. The second part involved questions about participants' views about system usefulness, ease of use, and impact of persuasive reminders on task completion, impact of virtual rehearsal on self-confidence and intention to rehearse newly learned behaviors. The questions used five-point Likert-type scale where 1 = strongly agree to 5 = strongly disagree. Finally they were interviewed in a post study satisfaction survey where experiences with the intervention were recorded, coded, and analyzed.

Psychological Measures. Symptoms of depression and self-reported confidence were assessed at the beginning and end of the study. For measuring depressive symptoms, Beck Depression Inventory-II [13] and Self-confidence were used as primary measures. Beck Depression Inventory (BDI-II) [13] includes 21 questions about depressive symptoms and their severity. The scale ranges from 0 – 63 (where 0 – 13 indicate no or very few depressive symptoms, 14 – 19 indicate mild depression, 20 – 28 indicate moderate depression and 29 – 63 indicate severe depression). BDI-II has been recognized to have reliability and validity [22, 25] in both nonclinical and clinical populations. To measure self-confidence of the participants, we used the Finnish Descriptive Visual Rating Scales, 0 – 100. The scale has shown good test and retest reliability [14].

4   Results

Researchers have paid significant attention to lack of task completion. For years high dropout rates have been a persistent problem for researchers and efforts have been made to find reasons behind it [15]. We hypothesized that persuasive reminders could lead to improved compliance. In this study, persuasive reminders were sent to the intervention group 1 only. At the end of first intervention period, participants were asked questions relating to their perceptions about the impact of persuasive reminders. Because intervention group 2 did not receive persuasive reminders, at the end of the intervention they were asked whether reminders could have helped them in completing required tasks.

At the end of the second intervention period, participants from both groups were invited to fill out questionnaires. In total 35 participants (Intervention group 1, n = 18; intervention group 2, n = 17) agreed to fill out the questionnaires. In response to the questions relating to virtual rehearsal and self-confidence, a high majority of participants (88.9%) reported that they felt confident in managing depression. Further a high number (86.1%) of participants not only felt self-confident in tackling depression but also showed intentions to practice newly learnt skills in future.

An overwhelming majority of the participants approved the system. H1 was based on the assumption that persuasive reminders would help users in task completion and H2 assumed that users would perceive persuasive reminders as a desirable software feature. Both H1 and H2 were derived from the PSD model [3], H3 anticipated a positive correlation between virtual rehearsal and self-confidence based on the theory of Self-efficacy [16], H4 assumed that users with improved self-confidence would intend continuous use of the BCSS. It was based on the Technology Acceptance Model [17] and H5 was based on the assumption that meaningful content of the rehearsal feature would be positively correlated with the overall effectiveness of the BCSS.

In response to questions relating to H1, a high majority of participants (83.3%) reported that persuasive reminders helped them in completing weekly exercises thereby supporting H1. Hypothesis 2 was developed assuming that participants from the intervention group 2 would perceive persuasive reminders as a desirable software feature. In response to the question, an overwhelming majority of participants (83.3%) from intervention group 2 expressed their wish to have received reminders. This finding supports H2. Hypothesis 3 assumed that virtual rehearsal would improve participants' self-confidence in managing depression. A high majority of participants from intervention group 1 (77.8%) and group 2 (100%) stated that virtual rehearsal improved their confidence in managing depression thus supporting H3. Hypothesis 4 was based on the assumption that participants with improved self-confidence would continue rehearsing newly acquired skills. Again, a high majority of participants from intervention group 1 (88.9%) and group 2 (88.2%) indicated intentions to rehearse newly learned skills in future. Thus, H4 is supported. Hypothesis 5 was based on the assumption that the overall affect of the BCSS would be such that participants' depression would decrease considerably. In order to verify Hypothesis 5, we analyzed mean scores for both BDI and Self-confidence. Outcomes from the analysis of pre- and post-measurements of BDI revealed significant decrease in both intervention group 1 (Mean score dropped by 8.72) and group 2 (Mean score dropped by 6.06). Similarly, promising results were prominent when self-confidence was analyzed. Outcomes from the analyses for pre and post-measurements revealed significant improvement in self-confidence in both intervention group 1 (mean increased from 48.11 to 61.83) and group 2 (mean increased from 49.00 to 60.00). Mean values for psychological measurements provide strong evidence for overall effectiveness of the BCSS thereby supporting H5. Table 2 exhibits scores for mean and standard deviations for both intervention groups.

Table 2. Mean scores and standard deviations for psychological measures

Measure Group	BDI Pre	BDI Post	Self-confidence Pre	Self-confidence Post
Intervention Group 1	22.11 (8.00) n = 19	13.39 (10.72) n = 18	48.11 (18.98) n = 19	61.83 (18.03) n = 18
Intervention Group 2	18.00 (7.44) n = 20	11.949 (7.95) n = 16	49.00 (18.19) n = 20	60.00 (23.16) n = 16

Post study questions focused on system usefulness, impact of persuasive reminders on task completion, whether reminders were obtrusive, influence of virtual rehearsal on participants' behaviors, whether rehearsal improved participants' self-confidence and would they continue using the rehearsal exercises in future.

Tables 3 and 4 exhibit validated responses; Mean scores and Standard Deviations from participants of Intervention group 1 and 2 respectively.

Participants generally approved persuasive reminders with a majority giving positive feedback acknowledging that in today's overwhelmingly busy lifestyle, it is easy to overlook important tasks. Participants from intervention group (83.3%) highly approved the use of reminders. Below are some exemplary comments:

Table 3. Responses from participants from Intervention Group 1

Themes for Intervention Group I	Validated Responses	Mean	Std. Deviation
System was useful	Yes (15) (83.3%) No (3) (16.7%)	1.17	.383
Reminders helped complete weekly tasks	Yes (15) (83.3%) No (3) (16.7%)	1.61	.778
Reminders did not interrupt me	Yes (17) (94.4%) No (1) (5.6%)	1.28	.575
Rehearsal influenced my behavior in a positive way	Yes (15) (83.3%) No (3) (16.7%)	1.56	.784
Rehearsal improved my confidence	Yes (14) (77.8%) No (4) (22.2%)	1.22	.428
I intend to rehearse in future	Yes (16) (88.9%) No (2) (11.1%)	1.39	.698

Table 4. Responses from participants from Intervention Group 2

Themes for Intervention Group II	Validated Responses	Mean	Std. Deviation
System was useful	Yes (17) (100%) No (0) (0.0%)	1.00	.000
Reminders would have been a desirable feature	Yes (14) (82.4%) No (3) (17.6%)	1.18	.393
Reminders should be unobtrusive	Yes (15) (88.2%) No (2) (11.8%)	1.41	.712
Rehearsal influenced my behavior in a positive way	Yes (15) (88.2%) No (2) (11.8%)	1.12	.332
Rehearsal improved my confidence	Yes (17) (100%) No (0) (0.0%)	1.00	.000
I intend to rehearse in future	Yes (15) (88.2%) No (2) (11.8%)	1.12	.322

P1. "Reminders assured me to remember doing the assignments; I use email very often."
P2. "They reminded me of doing my homework and I found the link (to be) very handy."
P3. "Reminders give (gave) you the feeling that you are not alone. They encouraged and gave a boost for replying to the assignments. It felt personal."
P4. "In addition to email-based reminders, SMS could be beneficial."
P5. "Add supportive criticism; enveloping criticism in a way that it won't depress (discourage) the person."

Participants of intervention group 2 received the same intervention though reminders were not sent out. A high majority (82.4%) stated that reminders would have been have been desirable. Some of the exemplary comments are stated below:

P6. "Yes, if one has a tendency towards forgetting things that need to be done (reminders would have helped)."
P7. "Yes, because I forgot, since there were no reminders; the due dates were hard to remember."

Some mixed remarks were also noted. Below are a few representative comments:

P8. "I did not need to be reminded. I was already committed to the program".
P9. "I would try to make reminders and rehearsal (exercises) less demanding".

A high majority of participants approved the rehearsal feature and acknowledged it as a technique to learn new skills. Some of the representative comments are stated below:

P10. "Exercises (rehearsals) were good. All in all, the interaction was excellent".
P11. "Weekly themes (rehearsals) were very good. They (rehearsal exercises) brought me in touch with my (core) values and I learned to be consciously present in the moment".
P12. "I found rehearsal content to be supportive. It kept me on track".

Based on the qualitative feedback from the participants, we identified following themes to further improve users-system interaction.

(1) Provide Positive Criticism/Feedback. Provision of positive feedback is vital for developing effective BCSSs. The PSD model [3] advocates implementing positive feedback. This augments interactivity and user-system dialogue. Previously, the impact of feedback has been studied. One study has been reported that users expressed a desire for meaningful and positive feedback [18].

(2) Supplement Email-Based Reminders with SMS. We propose that email-based reminders could be made more effective when supplemented with SMS. Use of SMS-based reminders has been suggested for e-Health interventions. Similarly, [10] promote the use of mobile reminders for health behavior change. They support their argument by stating that mobile phones are like constant partners therefore making it easier for the persuasive messages to be delivered.

(3) Add Supportive Content in Reminders. It is vital that people suffering from depressive symptoms are not left in a situation where they feel unassisted. One of the emerging themes from the open-ended questions was that reminders should be designed in a way that they make users feel *"important"*. We therefore suggest that adding empathy and supportive content to reminders could have a positive influence on users.

(4) **Remind People of Their Values.** The content of rehearsals could further be made effective if it helps people to reflect upon their values. This would mean that the content of rehearsals is developed in a way that people are reminded of their values and goals thereby supporting them to commit to actions that reduce disparity between their values/beliefs and actual actions. Such content could help people in overcoming different situations, for example, unpredictable changes in everyday situations.

5   Discussion

The objective of the study was to analyze the impact of persuasive reminders and virtual rehearsal on the effectiveness of a web-based BCSS. Participants' reflections about its usefulness, persuasive reminders and virtual rehearsal reveal that it was well received. Significant improvements were observed in post study psychological measurements where depressive symptoms decreased noticeably while in parallel participants' self-confidence improved considerably. However, reminders seem not to have an added effect on the efficacy of the BCSS (compared rehearsal only) as measured by observing changes in depression and self-confidence scores. This is an interesting finding. One reason for lack of effect of reminders could be that the ACT-based rehearsals were so effective, engaging and intrinsically motivated the participants. Responses from the participants indicate that they learned new skills for managing depression. We suggest that this is critical for behavior change process. In addition, a high majority of participants felt self-confident in tackling depressive symptoms at their own and indicated their intention to continue practicing newly learned skills. These findings are in line with the theory of Self-Efficacy as proposed by [16].

Our work has several contributions for researchers of persuasive systems in particular and healthcare in general. First, to the best of our knowledge, it is the only study where a web-based BCSS incorporated with ACT-based virtual rehearsals was evaluated involving patients suffering from mild to moderate depression without face-to-face therapy. Second, the findings reveal that although persuasive reminders were positively perceived however they did not have any additional influence on task completion. This study has some limitations. First, the sample size is relatively low therefore it is relatively hard to generalize the results. However, it must be noted that recruiting people with depression is a hard task. Second, the intervention did not include a follow up. In future studies a research setting where a post intervention follow-up is included is recommended.

6   Conclusions

We have presented qualitative evaluation of a web-based BCSS assimilated with value, acceptance and mindfulness-based rehearsal techniques for treating depression without face-to-face therapy. First we studied persuasive reminders and their effect on task completion. Second, virtual rehearsal was evaluated in terms of learning new behaviors leading to potentially higher self-efficacy. Lastly, we evaluated usefulness of the BCSS and its benefits as experienced by participants. The findings reveal interesting inferences. It is surprising to note that persuasive reminders did not have an added effect on task completion, which calls for further investigation. Virtual rehearsal was well received by the participants and helped them learn new skills and behaviors. The findings are promising because the entire intervention was performed without face-to-face therapy. We believe that the in-depth insights gained through post study questionnaires and interviews have contributed towards existing knowledge relating to behavior change interventions. Presented results are a good starting point for researchers to implement information systems for people with depression and other mental disorders.

Acknowledgements. This research is part of OASIS research group of Martti Ahtisaari Institute, University of Oulu. This study was supported by the SalWe Research Program for Mind and Body (Tekes – The Finnish Funding Agency for Technology and Innovation grant 1104/10). We would like to thank Liisa Kuonanoja from OASIS research group, University of Oulu, and Riikkasisko Kirjonen and the entire team of student therapists from Department of Psychology, University of Jyväskylä for their valuable contribution in the study.

References

1. Aromaa, E., Tolvanen, A., Tuulari, J., Wahlbeck, K.: Personal stigma and use of mental health services among people with depression in a general population in Finland. BMC Psychiatry 11(1), 52 (2011)
2. Consolvo, S., Klasnja, P., McDonald, D.W., Landay, J.A.: Goal-setting considerations for persuasive technologies that encourage physical activity. In: Proceedings of the 4th International Conference on Persuasive Technology, p. 8. ACM (2009)
3. Oinas-Kukkonen, H., Harjumaa, M.: Persuasive Systems Design: Key Issues, Process Model, and System Features. Communications of the Association for Information Systems 24, Article 28, 485–500 (2009)
4. Andersson, G., Cuijpers, P.: Internet-based and other computerized psychological treatments for adult depression: a Meta-analysis. Cog. Behav. Ther. 38(4), 196–205 (2009)
5. Hayes, S.C., Luoma, J.B., Bond, F.W., Masuda, A., Lilles, J.: Acceptance and Commitment Therapy: Model, Processes and Outcomes. Behavioral Research and Therapy 44, 1–25 (2005)
6. Consolvo, S., McDonald, D.W., Landay, J.A.: Theory-driven design strategies for technologies that support behavior change in everyday life. In: Proceedings of the SIGCHI Conference on Human Factors in Computing Systems, pp. 405–414. ACM (2009)
7. Thorpe, G.L., Hecker, J.E., Cavallaro, L.A., Kulberg, G.E.: Insight Versus Rehearsal in Cognitive-Behavior Therapy: A Crossover Study with Sixteen Phobics. Behavioural Psychotherapy 15(4), 319–336 (1987)
8. Oinas-Kukkonen, H.: A foundation for the study of behavior change support systems. Personal and Ubiquitous Computing 17(6), 1223–1235 (2013)
9. Fogg, B.J.: Persuasive technology: using computers to change what we think and do. Ubiquity, 5 (December 2002)

10. Fry, J.P., Neff, R.A.: Periodic Prompts and Reminders in Health Promotion and Health Behavior Interventions: Systematic Review. Journal of Medical Internet Research 11(2), e16 (2009)

11. Haynes, S.N., O'Brien, W., Kaholokula, J.: Behavioral assessment and case formulation. Wiley. com (2011)

12. Lappalainen, R., Lehtonen, T., Skarp, E., Taubert, E., Ojanen, M., Hayes, S.C.: The Impact of CBT and ACT Models Using Psychology Trainee Therapists A Preliminary Controlled Effectiveness Trial. Behavior Modification 31(4), 488–511 (2007)

13. Beck, A.T., Ward, C., Mendelson, M.: Beck depression inventory (BDI). Arch. Gen. Psychiatry 4(6), 561–571 (1961)

14. Sjögren-Rönkä, T., Ojanen, M.T., Leskinen, E.K., Mustalampi, S.T., Mälkiä, E.A.: Physical and psychosocial prerequisites of functioning in relation to work ability and general subjective well-being among office workers. Scandinavian Journal of Work, Environment & Health, 184–190 (2002)

15. Kelders, S.M., et al.: Persuasive system design does matter: a systematic review of adherence to web-based interventions. Journal of Medical Internet Research 14(6) (2012)

16. Bandura, A., Adams, N.E.: Analysis of self-efficacy theory of behavioral change. Cognitive Therapy and Research 1(4), 287–310 (1977)

17. Legris, P., Ingham, J., Collerette, P.: Why do people use information technology? A critical review of the technology acceptance model. Information & Management 40(3), 191–204 (2003)

18. Arroyo, E., Bonanni, L., Selker, T.: Waterbot: exploring feedback and persuasive techniques at the sink. In: Proceedings of the SIGCHI Conference on Human Factors in Computing Systems, pp. 631–639. ACM (April 2005)

19. Williams, A., Manias, E., Walker, R.: Interventions to improve medication adherence in people with multiple chronic conditions: a systematic review. Journal of Advanced Nursing 63(2), 132–143 (2008)

20. Delone, W.H.: The DeLone and McLean model of information systems success: a ten-year update. Journal of Management Information Systems 19(4), 9–30 (2003)

21. Bickmore, T.W., Mauer, D., Crespo, F., Brown, T.: Persuasion, task interruption and health regimen adherence. In: de Kort, Y.A.W., IJsselsteijn, W.A., Midden, C., Eggen, B., Fogg, B.J. (eds.) PERSUASIVE 2007. LNCS, vol. 4744, pp. 1–11. Springer, Heidelberg (2007)

22. Segal, D.L., Coolidge, F.L., Cahill, B.S., O'Riley, A.A.: Psychometric properties of the Beck Depression Inventory—II (BDI-II) among community-dwelling older adults. Behavior Modification 32(1), 3–20 (2008)

23. Miles, M.B., Huberman, A.M.: Qualitative data analysis: An expanded sourcebook. Sage (1994)

24. Warmerdam, L., van Straten, A., Twisk, J., Riper, H., Cuijpers, P.: Internet-based treatment for adults with depressive symptoms: randomized controlled trial. Journal of Medical Internet Research 10(4) (2008)

25. Beck, J.S.: Cognitive behavior therapy: Basics and beyond. Guilford Press (2011)

26. Tørning, K., Oinas-Kukkonen, H.: Persuasive System Design: State of Art and Future Directions. In: Proceedings of the Fourth International Conference on Persuasive Technology, Claremont, CA, USA, April 26-29. ACM International Conference Proceeding Series, vol. 350 (2009)

Using Ambient Lighting in Persuasive Communication: The Role of Pre-existing Color Associations

Shengnan Lu, Jaap Ham, and Cees J.H. Midden

Human-Technology Interaction, Eindhoven University of Technology, P.O. Box 513,
5600 MB, Eindhoven, Netherlands
{s.lu,j.r.c.ham,c.j.h.midden}@tue.nl

Abstract. Earlier research indicated that ambient persuasive lighting can have persuasive effects on energy-efficiency behavior. However, why would this kind of ambient feedback be effective? The current research investigated the influence of the strength of associations (of colors used for giving feedback) on the effectiveness of ambient feedback. Two color sets were chosen from a pretest to represent strongly- and weakly-associated with energy consumption, i.e. red versus green and yellow vs. purple, respectively. Results indicated that lighting feedback that was strongly associated with energy consumption had stronger persuasive effects than weakly-associated lighting feedback. Moreover, participants who received weakly-associated feedback needed more time to program the thermostat when performing the additional cognitive task (as compared to participants without additional task), while this difference was not found in strongly-associated feedback condition. This research reveals that the persuasive potential of ambient persuasive lighting can be enhanced by making use of pre-existing color associations.

Keywords: Ambient persuasive technology, Ambient lighting, Color association, Color perception.

1 Introduction

Over the last few decades, the exhaustion of natural resources and the threats of growing green-house gases and consequently, global warming, have been frequently discussed within interdisciplinary studies. This concern has urged nations worldwide to seek for substantial reductions in energy consumption.

Although such technological solutions as efficient systems and the development of renewable energy sources are of great importance, recent studies show that consumer behavior could play a crucial role in reducing the level of energy consumption, especially for household energy conservation. Abrahamse et al. have evaluated the effectiveness of tailored feedback about their energy consumption to encourage people to reduce energy consumption [1]. Interventions have been employed with varying degrees of success. Therefore, influencing consumer behavior to stimulate energy-efficiency behavior has become an important target of nation and international policy efforts.

A. Spagnolli et al. (Eds.): PERSUASIVE 2014, LNCS 8462, pp. 167–178, 2014.
© Springer International Publishing Switzerland 2014

Recent reviews have provided new opportunities for feedback by embedding feedback in user-system interaction. For example, by adding an energy bar to the user interface of a washing machine [2], there was an 18% increase in energy conservation both in lab and field studies.   Basically, the approach of [2] entailed giving factual feedback in terms of kWh. More recent research suggested that social feedback could even more effectively influence energy consumption behavior. For instance, Midden and Ham [3] increased the persuasiveness of energy feedback when using a washing machine system through a smart robotic agent that provided social feedback. They found that social feedback can promote more pro-environmental behaviors than factual, evaluative feedback. Also, Jahn et al. [4] present a novel smart home system that uses intuitive user interfaces that show energy consumption data, e.g. energy price, energy source, standby consumption etc.. This kind of feedback allowed users to observe not only the overall household consumption but also each device's consumption in a meaningful context.

However, both factual feedback and social feedback might not be suited for many situations. For example, both types of feedback might lose their persuasive power in situation in which there are no reference values that lack emotional appeal, in which recognition of facial expressions is hampered, etc. In addition, in many day-to-day situations people might not be motivated or lack the cognitive capacity to consciously process relatively complex information [5].

To deal with this problem, earlier research proposed to use ambient feedback that might employ ambient media such as light, airflow, and sound to act as background influences, working at the periphery of human perception [6]. In a paper by Wilson et al. [7], heating system feedback in tandem with information about windows being open (or closed) was provided in the form of two output mechanisms: light (i.e., color) and sound. For instance, if a window is opened in tandem with a detected increase in radiator surface temperature, the light color corresponding to temperature immediately displays a warning light (i.e., red) to indicate waste. Also, Arroyo et al. [8] presented various feedback and persuasion techniques of augmented physical interfaces with value-added design, which sought to return a sense of value to water exiting the tap, and provide useful information about the temperature of the water without altering the function of the sink. For example, one of their designs was called Heat-Sink, and consisted of colored LEDs mounted around the faucet aerator that could illuminate the stream of water with a red-colored lighting when water was hot, and blue when water was cold. Feedback given through this kind of persuasive technology might be easier to process, and therefore still effective in various situations in which more focal persuasive technology might lose its effectiveness, or when users lack the cognitive capacity or motivation to spend cognitive attention to the influencing attempt. This was confirmed by [9]. That is, Maan et al. [9] shed light on fundamental characteristics of ambient feedback. They tested the effect of feedback through a lamp that could gradually change color dependent on the amount of energy consumption of the participant in a certain task, and compared these effects to more widely used factual feedback. Results indicated that feedback though ambient lighting was more effective than numerical feedback. In addition, processing ambient lighting feedback seemed easier in the sense that performing an additional cognitive task did not interfere with it.

However, it remains unclear why this form of ambient persuasive technology was effective. In the current paper we argue that an important reason for this kind of lighting feedback being so effective is that people have pre-existing associations with the ambient lighting colors that were used in [9]. That is, the colors used were red and green, and these colors are generally associated with high and low energy consumption. And therefore ambient lighting feedback that uses such colors might be more effective: easier to process and leading to stronger persuasive effects. In contrast, we argue that for people to process factual feedback, much more cognitive processing capacity is needed, amongst others because of the lack of pre-existing association of factual feedback information.

Therefore, we performed a study on the influence of the strength of associations (of colors used for giving feedback with high and low energy consumption) on the effectiveness of ambient feedback.

Indeed, earlier research suggested that colors may have different meanings, and even might have different meanings in different association settings. For example, red (vs. blue) could induce avoidance (vs. approach) motivation [10]. Also, as indicated by [11], people in red surroundings scored higher on stress and anxiety measures, and other research reported a strong effect of lighting on arousal [12]. Eiseman concluded in [13] that red is the most viscerally alive hue, the symbolic color of strong-willed and expresses strong emotions. The color red may command us to stop but at the same time encourages movement, which included both positive effect (e.g. exciting and powerful) and negative effect (e.g. overly aggressive and violent).

Importantly, for current purposes we needed two color sets with different strengths of associations with energy consumption: one set of colors having strong associations to high and low energy consumptions, and one set of colors for which these associations were weak. Therefore, a pre-test assessing color meaning was conducted. Based on this pre-test (described below), we chose the color set of red and green as strongly-associated with energy consumption, and yellow and purple as a set of two colors weakly-associated with energy consumption. Bases on this pretest we ran our experiment, assessing the effectiveness of these two sets of feedback colors as ambient lighting feedback. Although some publications seem to treat the types of color meanings as universal [14], there also appear to be significant variations induced by cultural differences [15]. Therefore, next to our main research questions, we wanted to investigate whether the color's meaning (with respect to energy consumption) would be cross-culturally recognized.

We expected lighting feedback with strong associations to be most effective (H1): that is, participants who received lighting feedback that is strongly-associated with energy consumption would save more energy than participants who received lighting feedback that is weakly-associated with energy consumption. We also expected that strongly-associated lighting feedback could be processed faster than weakly-associated feedback, resulting in a decrease in the time used to complete tasks.

Because we were also interested in whether or not the persuasive power of the two types of lighting feedback was independent of user attention, we manipulated cognitive load of the participants. That is, half of the participants were distracted by an additional cognitive task which consisted of a random number recognition task while performing the trials in the experiment (comparable to the successful cognitive load manipulation used in [13]).

Overall, we expected participants in high cognitive load conditions to use the most energy (H2): participants who performed an additional cognitive task would save less energy than participants who did not performed an additional cognitive task because they were distracted and could process the given feedback less optimally. Also, performing an additional cognitive would slow the processing of task completion. This main effect is not directly related to our research question which focusses on the effects of type of lighting feedback.

Finally, as argued above, we expected that the effectiveness (in terms of lower energy consumption and faster task completion times) of lighting feedback for participants receiving *strongly-associated* lighting feedback would not be diminished by those participants performing the additional cognitive task, whereas the effectiveness of lighting feedback for participants receiving *weakly-associated* lighting feedback would be diminished by those participants performing the additional cognitive task (H3). That is to say, only in weakly-associated lighting conditions would participants spend more time on task completion, and save less energy if they were put under high cognitive load.

2   Pre-test

2.1   Method

2.1.1   Participants

Fifty-two participants (26 Chinese and 26 Dutch) were invited to fill in a survey of different colors. These participants were students (at several Chinese Universities or at Eindhoven University of Technology; mean age $M = 23.0$, $SD = .40$) and they filled out the questionnaire on their own computer at diverse locations.

2.1.2   Materials

After an introduction to the study, participants' color evaluations were assessed. That is, participants were asked to rate various colors on two questions: "Please indicate whether you think a specific color is strongly related to HIGH energy consumption", and the same question was posed about relationship to low energy consumption. Seven rainbow color blocks, attached by corresponding English and Dutch names, were listed following each question. In addition, we used 7-point rating scale, from 1 "Not at all associated" to 7 "Very strongly associated" (see in Figure 1). Then, in phase 3 about evaluating pairs of colors, we listed the full combination of each two (out of seven) colors, 21 color pairs in total. Every color set was presented as two color blocks with "vs." between them, and followed by their English name.

1. For the following **seven colors**, please indicate whether you think a specific color is strongly related to **HIGH** energy consumption.

	Not at all associated	Very weakly associated	Weakly associated	Not weakly/not strongly associated	Moderately associated	Strongly associated	Very strongly associated
■ Red/Rood	○	○	○	○	○	○	○
▨ Orange/Oranje	○	○	○	○	○	○	○
☐ Yellow/Geel	○	○	○	○	○	○	○
■ Green/Groen	○	○	○	○	○	○	○
▨ Blue/Blauw	○	○	○	○	○	○	○
■ Dark Blue/Donker Blauw	○	○	○	○	○	○	○
■ Purple/Paars	○	○	○	○	○	○	○

Fig. 1. Online Survey

The last phase of this survey is about demographic information. Age, gender and country of birth were collected. The whole survey lasted approximately 5 minutes.

2.2   Result and Discussion

In general, results showed no difference of color meanings between Dutch and Chinese group, with respect to associating with the level of energy consumption.

For the individual color evaluation, red was ranked as the color mostly associated with high energy consumption (rating scores, $M = 6.85$, $SD = .05$) in both groups, and the mean of red scores between Chinese and Dutch group was not different, $t(50) = -.76$, $p = .45$. By contrast, green was rated as the color mostly associated with low energy consumption (rating scores, $M = 6.38$, $SD = 1.36$) in both groups. Specifically, Dutch group rated green a higher score on low-energy-consumption scale ($M = 6.77$, $SD = .71$) than Chinese group ($M = 6.00$, $SD = 1.72$), $F(1, 50) = 4.44$, $p = .04$, which indicated that green in Dutch group had a stronger association with low energy than green in Chinese group.

For the individual colors of yellow and purple, both were rated in the middle of the scales (not weakly/strongly associated with energy consumption), which are ($M = 4.67$, $SD = 1.10$) and ($M = 3.02$, $SD = 1.58$), respectively.

Of the color sets, red vs. green ranked on the first place, which meant this color set was most strongly associated with energy consumption ($M = 6.12$, $SD = 1.53$). To control for hue difference, all color pairs should have a hue difference of an approximately similar distance on color circle. Then, yellow vs. purple was chosen as the other color set which was weakly-associated with energy consumption, with a low score ($M = 2.93$, $SD = 1.47$) on the rating scale. Furthermore, the scores of these two color sets were differently, $t(51) = 10.44$, $p < .001$.

Using these two sets of colors, we had a basis for a manipulation of feedback type (i.e. colors strongly-associated with energy consumption vs. weakly-associated with energy consumption) that we will use in our experimental design.

3   Experiment

3.1   Method

3.1.1   Participants

Ninety-nine native Dutch participants (54 male and 45 female) took part in this experiment. Most of them were university students from 18 to 30 years old, but eight participants were from outside the university and were over 30 years old. We invited only participants who were not color blind, and also made sure all participants could recognize red, green, yellow and purple. All of them were randomly assigned to one of four experimental conditions: 2 (feedback type: Red vs. Green, vs. Yellow vs. Purple) × 2 (cognitive load: no load vs. load). The experiments lasted 30 minutes, for which participants were paid €5 at the end.

3.1.2   Materials and Procedure

All the tasks we used in this experiment were fully computerized and the lighting feedback was provided via the peripheral LED light (see in Figure 2a). The LED was ambient and it was projected on the side walls (Figure 2b). The participants could perceive the feedback at periphery of their perception, while paying focal attention on a computer-based task.

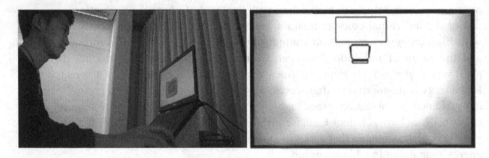

Fig. 2. (a). Ambient feedback through red lighting from the ceiling; (b). LED projected on the side walls

Upon arrival, participants were requested to sit in front of the computer. All of them were asked to read and sign a consent form if they agreed to participate in this research before participating in the experiment. Participants could also stop the experiment at any time without reason. There was no pain or discomfort during the whole experimental procedure.

A simulated programmable thermostat panel was presented on the computer screen (see in Figure 3). This virtual LCD thermostat panel, a model of an available central heating interface in Dutch households, was used to gather data about participants' energy consumption behavior while performing tasks. The temperatures they set during each scenario (described below) were used to determine the lighting colors.

In the strongly-associated-lighting feedback condition, the LED light (on the side walls) was given a red color in the peripheral environment when energy consumption was at a high level, and a green color when at a low level. When a participant's thermostat settings lead to energy consumption between the high and low level, the peripheral light emitted was set to a color between green and red in different saturations with the same brightness. White was set as the neutral color corresponding to medium energy consumption level in this experiment. In the weakly-associated-lighting feedback condition, yellow lighting represented high energy consumption and purple represented low energy consumption.

Before they began to run the trials, all participants were given two specific goals to strive during the whole programming of the thermostat: (1) to program the thermostat such that the house would be comfortable to live in; and (2) to use as little energy as possible. The first goal was to motivate participants to use enough energy to reach a comfortable level. If we only included the second goal, all the participants have chosen to use as little energy as possible by simply not turning the heating on at all, which was irrelevant to any kind of feedback about energy consumption.

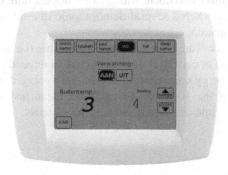

Fig. 3. The simulated programmable heating system interface

All the participants had the same two practical trials, followed by ten test trials in random orders. For each of the ten trials, the different scenario description was presented above the virtual thermostat panel, such as "It is night and you are going to bed. It is -10°C outside"; it is Sunday afternoon and you are at home. Outside temperature is 18°C". All the scenarios were used only once for each participant. People received feedback after each continuous change of settings, until they pressed the "Ready" button. The default temperature of thermostat in each scenario was randomized between 16°C and 24°C. We also explained that the lighting feedback reflected the energy consumption level of all the six rooms, not one specific room, so as to prevent misunderstanding the comprehensive meaning of the ambient lighting. For each task, we collected the energy consumption, and the total amount of time a participant used for that task.

Participants in the cognitive load conditions performed an additional cognitive task while setting the thermostat. This cognitive task was comparable to the successful cognitive load manipulation in [13], and was presented during all ten test trials. Participants heard a random series of recorded spoken numbers from 1 to 30 with a 3 seconds interval. We registered the number of correct responses (pressing the space bar whenever they heard an odd number through a speaker next to their laptop).

After completing all the trials, a manipulation check was done in terms of color recognition. For the each four colors, we kept the hue and brightness constant, dividing saturation into five levels from maximum to white. In strongly-associated lighting feedback condition, ten colors between intensive red and intensive green would be presented one by one in random order on the side walls. Participants were asked to evaluate the color meanings with respect to high or low energy consumption. We collected their recognition time and rating scores. The procedure in the weakly-associated lighting condition was the same, and lighting would change between intensive yellow and intensive purple.

Next, participants were asked to answer four questions with which we assessed their emotional state during the experiment. These questions (all posed in Dutch) consisted of: "To do these 10 tasks, I had..." (1 – not enough time to 7 – more than enough time), "During the execution of the tasks, I was..." (1 – very nervous to 7 – not nervous at all), "I do not feel very at ease." (1 – strongly disagree to 7 – strongly agree), "Taking part in this experiment was..." (1 – not exciting to 7 – very exciting).

Finally, participants answered several demographic questions, were debriefed and thanked for their participation.

The scores of energy consumption and completing time (i.e. a participant needed to program the control unit) in each trial were collected, as dependent variables.

To calculate mean energy consumption scores, we averaged a participant's energy consumption in each of the 10 trials. To calculate mean task completion time, we averaged a participant's time duration in each of the 10 trials.

3.2   Result

3.2.1   Main Effect Analyses

The mean energy consumption scores were submitted to a 2 (feedback type: strongly-associated vs. weakly-associated) × 2 (cognitive load: low vs. high) between-subject analysis of variance (ANOVA). As expected, participants who received strongly-associated lighting feedback used less energy ($M = 647$, $SE = 198.0$) than participants who received weakly-associated lighting feedback ($M = 727$, $SE = 198.2$), $F(1,95) = 4.01$, $p = .048$. This indicated that participants could save 11% more energy when they received the ambient lighting feedback whose colors were strongly-associated with energy consumption (i.e. red vs. green), than when they received lighting feedback whose colors were weakly-associated with energy consumption (i.e. yellow vs. purple).

Different from what we had expected, we found no interaction effect on energy consumption scores, $F < 1$. That indicated there is no difference between strongly-associated and weakly-associated lighting feedback within high and low cognitive load level. Furthermore, the energy consumption of participants who performed the additional cognitive load task when they setting temperature showed no difference from the energy consumption of participants who did not have cognitive load task, $F = 1.12$, $p = .29$.

To investigate whether the feedback is easy to process, the average completing time per each trial was submitted to the same 2 × 2 ANOVA. As advised by Ratcliff [16], the response times should exclude outliers (more than two SDs from the average response time). Therefore, we removed these (six out of 99) participants from this analysis. Our expectations were confirmed. That is, first, we found a main effect of cognitive load on time to solve a task, $F(1,89) = 4.89$, $p = .03$. The participants who performed the additional cognitive load task needed more time to solve a task ($M = 37.2s$, $SE = 11.19$) than participants who did not perform this additional load task ($M = 32.7s$, $SE = 10.00$). More importantly, results also showed the expected interaction effect of feedback type × cognitive load, $F(1,89) = 4.33$, $p = .04$. That is to say, participants who received yellow vs. purple lighting feedback needed more time to program the thermostat in high cognitive load condition ($M = 39.5s$, $SE = 13.42$) than participants in low cognitive load condition ($M = 30.2s$, $SE = 5.41$), $F(1,89) = 8.72$, $p = .004$. Whereas, this difference was not found between participants who received strongly-associated lighting feedback with an additional cognitive task ($M = 35.3s$, $SE=8.65$) and participants without additional cognitive task ($M = 35.0s$, $SE = 12.54$), $F(1,89) = .01$, $p = .92$.

However, we did not find the main effect of feedback type on trial time to solve a task, $F < 1$.

3.2.2   Exploratory Analysis

For color recognition task after 10 trials, participants who received strongly-associated lighting feedback could recognize this color set (i.e. red and green in 10 saturation levels) more accurate (error distance, $M = 7.1$, $SE = 3.94$) than people who received weakly-associated lighting feedback (i.e. yellow and purple in 10 saturation levels) (error distance, $M = 9.3$, $SE = 4.93$), $F(1,89) = 6.51$, $p = .012$. According to [10], some red in the field of view could enhance performance on focused detail-oriented task. This might explain why in our study participants perform better when red and green are used to give feedback in a task.

And in terms of manipulation check on "nervous", the results showed that participants in yellow vs. purple lighting condition felt more nervous ($M = 5.2$, $SE = 1.47$) than participants in red vs. green lighting condition ($M = 5.7$, $SE=1.68$), $F(1,95) = 4.25$, $p = .042$. We also found the main effect of cognitive load indicating that participants who did the additional cognitive task felt more nervous ($M = 4.5$, $SE = 1.68$) than participants who did not perform the additional cognitive task ($M = 6.4$, $SE = 1.24$), $F(1,95) = 52.41$, $p < .001$. No interaction effect on "nervous" was found, $F < 1$. It might have been the case that participants in cognitive load conditions (especially also in weakly-associated lighting feedback condition) overloaded the finite amount of working memory one possesses, and felt nervous to perform the task at a good level.

4   Conclusion and Discussion

In this study, ambient lighting feedback in strongly-associated condition could be generally recognized more accurately than lighting feedback in weakly-associated condition. And results indicated that participants who received feedback through ambient colored lighting which was strongly associated with energy consumption saved more energy through the thermostat programming tasks than participants who received weakly-associated lighting feedback. Thereby, in line with our expectation, this current research suggests that ambient lighting feedback with colors strongly associated with energy consumption had larger persuasive effects than ambient lighting feedback of which colors were weakly associated with energy consumption (approximately 11%). However, the main effect of feedback type on completion time was not found.

Furthermore, results provided mixed evidence for our interaction hypothesis. That is, in contrast to our expectation, the current results did not show evidence for an interaction effect on *energy consumption*, which means that there was no difference between strongly-associated and weakly-associated lighting feedback within each cognitive load level. However, results showed the interaction effect on *task completion time*, which indicated that participants in weakly-associated lighting feedback condition need more time to program the thermostat when performing an additional task than participants without an additional task. This difference was not found in the strongly-associated lighting feedback condition, which means that adding cognitive load did not lead to slower processing when participants received strongly-associated lighting feedback. It seems quite straightforward that participants in the weakly-associated lighting condition used more time to reach a good level of energy consumption, especially in high cognitive load. If we collect the dynamic energy consumption based on seconds during each trial, we may find the interaction effect on energy consumption at the early stage. Another reason could be that participants might be well-trained after first several trials, which they can easily understand and process the ambient lighting feedback in the rest trials. We only analyzed the average scores of energy consumption of all the trials in this study. What we can do in the further study is to record the dynamic scores of energy consumption based on their actions. Then, we may find the interaction effect on energy consumption at the beginning of their actions.

A further reason for the lacking interaction effect on energy consumption might be that the strength of the color association was not high enough. For instance, color set in weakly-associated-lighting condition (i.e. yellow vs. purple) could still be associated with energy consumption in an ecological, according to debriefing after experiment. Some participants indicated that yellow looked like sun, and felt as a warmer color. While purple was a dark color and felt cold. If ambient lighting became yellow, participants could intuitively realize high energy consumption. To test whether or not the colors (in yellow vs. purple lighting condition) could be intuitively (or easily) linked to energy consumption, future research might test the strength of color associations, when the colored lighting is presented in a reversed combination (i.e. purple means high energy consumption, while yellow represents low energy consumption).

Additionally, the measuring of scores of energy consumption might be biased by the default setting of temperature in each six rooms. In the current program, the default status of the heating system in each room was "OFF". It could be turned on only when clicking the button "ON" on the programming thermostat. This might have caused a positive link between low action and low energy consumption. For instance, if participants performed the trials very fast and did not change the default settings, the lower energy consumption, which we recorded did not mean that people saved more energy. Thereby, further studies should avoid this situation and set the default status of heating system in each room on "ON". In this case, if participants forgot to control the thermostat in one room, the total energy consumption still kept default high level in that room. Thus future study a default low energy level should be avoided

Finally, as shown in the analysis of the participant's emotional state (e.g. whether you are nervous when performing the 10 trials), participants in the weakly-associated lighting condition felt more nervous than participant in the strongly-associated lighting condition. Concerning the effect of cognitive load on "nervous", participants were more nervous in high cognitive load condition than in low cognitive load condition. This may have meant that nervous participants ignored changing the default energy state (i.e. OFF), and saved more energy coincidently, which were even not their original purposes. This might also be the reason why there was no interaction effect on energy consumption. Furthermore, exploratory results of color recognition suggested that the training on color's association with energy consumption might play an important role in ambient lighting feedback perception.

Overall, the current research indicates that the persuasive potential of ambient persuasive lighting can be enhanced by linking to pre-existing color associations.

References

1. Abrahamse, W., Steg, L., Vlek, C., Rothengatter, T.: A review of intervention studies aimed at household energy conservation. Journal of Environmental Psychology 25, 273–291 (2005)
2. McCalley, L., Midden, C.: Energy conservation through product-integrated feedback: The roles of goal-setting and social orientation. Journal of Economic Psychology 23, 589–603 (2002)
3. Midden, C., Ham, J.: Using negative and positive social feedback from a robotic agent to save energy. In: Proceedings of the 4th International Conference on Persuasive Technology, p. 12. ACM (2009)
4. Jahn, M., Jentsch, M., Prause, C.R., Pramudianto, F., Al-Akkad, A., Reiner, R.: The energy aware smart home. In: 2010 5th International Conference on Future Information Technology (Future Tech), pp. 1–8. IEEE (2010)
5. Bargh, J.: The automaticity of everyday life. In: Wyer Jr., R.S. (ed.) The Automaticity of Everyday Life: Advances in Social Cognition, vol. 10, pp. 1–61 (1997)
6. Ishii, H., Ullmer, B.: Tangible bits: Towards seamless interfaces between people, bits and atoms. In: Proceedings of the ACM SIGCHI Conference on Human Factors in Computing Systems, pp. 234–241. ACM (1997)
7. Wilson, G.T., Lilley, D., Bhamra, T.A.: Design feedback interventions for household energy consumption reduction (2013)
8. Arroyo, E., Bonanni, L., Selker, T.: Waterbot: exploring feedback and persuasive techniques at the sink. In: Proceedings of the SIGCHI Conference on Human Factors in Computing Systems, pp. 631–639. ACM (2005)

9. Maan, S., Merkus, B., Ham, J., Midden, C.: Making it not too obvious: the effect of ambient light feedback on space heating energy consumption. Energy Efficiency 4, 175–183 (2011)

10. Mehta, R., Zhu, R.: Blue or Red? Exploring the effect of color on cognitive task performances. Science 323, 1226–1229 (2009)

11. Baron, R., Rea, M., Daniels, S.: Effects of indoor lighting (illuminance and spectral distribution) on the performance of cognitive tasks and interpersonal behaviors: the potential mediating role of positive affect. Motivation and Emotion 9, 1–33 (1992)

12. Kwallek, N., Lewis, C., Robbins, A.: Effects of office interior color on workers' mood and productivity. Perceptual and Motor Skills 66, 123–128 (1988)

13. Eiseman, L.: Color-Messages & Meanings: A PANTONE Color Resource. North Light Books (2006)

14. Finkelstein, E.: Use the right colors for maximum impact: Understanding color. Inside Microsoft PowerPoint 10, 7–10 (2003)

15. Carroll Childress, D.D.: The power of color: Shades of Meaning. Master, The University of Houston Clear Lake, Houston (2008)

16. Marsh, R., Hicks, J.: Event-based prospective memory and executive control of working memory. Journal of Experimental Psychology. Learning, Memory, and Cognition 24, 336–349 (1998)

'This Is Your Life!'

The Design of a Positive Psychology Intervention Using Metaphor to Motivate

Geke D.S. Ludden, Saskia M. Kelders, and Bas H.J. Snippert

University of Twente, Faculty of Engineering Technology,
Department of Product Design, De Horst, Drienerlolaan 5, 7522NB, Enschede
{g.d.s.ludden,s.m.kelders}@utwente.nl,
info@snipdesign,nl

Abstract. 'This Is Your Life' is a training aimed at personal growth, or 'flourishing', and is based on the science of positive psychology. The objective of this project was to create a design for a digital version of a book with theory and exercises about positive psychology. The target group for the digital version were primary school teachers. A user-centered design approach was used together with persuasive and gameful design frameworks. More specifically, a metaphorical design was used to motivate the target group to start using the training and to continue using and complete the training. Several metaphors were explored and tested with the target group. Finally, a working prototype of the digital training was developed and tested by the target user group. From this final test we found that the chosen metaphorical design indeed motivated people to (1) start working on the training and (2) continue working on the training.

Keywords: persuasion, positive psychology, motivation, adherence, design.

1 Introduction

Positive psychology is the study of the positive functioning and resilience of individuals. Central to this is the research on the influence of psychological flexibility, positive emotions, finding and using personal talents, optimism and hope, compassion, values and goals and positive relationships on the well-being of human beings. The premise is that enhancing these capabilities leads to a better psychological health: a greater capacity to lead a pleasant, successful, social and meaningful life. This can also be named optimal functioning or 'flourishing' (see e.g., Lyubomirsky, 2008; Seligman & Csikszentmihalyi, 2000). A new positive psychology intervention (a training or therapy that participants can execute mostly independently) was recently developed by Ernst Bohlmeijer to improve the 'flourishing' of teachers in primary education (Bohlmeijer & Hulsbergen, 2013).

The content of positive psychology interventions is mostly focused on active participation of the user. The general structure for positive psychology interventions

A. Spagnolli et al. (Eds.): PERSUASIVE 2014, LNCS 8462, pp. 179–190, 2014.

is a series of themes with different exercises, which aim to teach positive psychology principles and offer guidelines to use them practically in everyday life. These exercises can be divided in at least two major groups: reflective exercises and activity based exercises. Reflective exercises generally contain questions which facilitate a process of self-inquiry by the user. For example an intervention can contain exercises in which the intervention user investigates his or her life to discover what his or her strengths and talents are. These exercises are mostly constructed in multiple sub-questions, which guide the user through the process of searching and discovering.

The other type of exercises are based on activities to which the user should dedicate at least a few minutes up to hours per day, week or month. In many interventions the importance of repetition is stressed, to receive the full benefits of the exercise(s). The importance of repetition and of active participation in order for the intervention to be effective illustrates that adherence is an important topic when it comes to this type of interventions. This is even more true for a digital interventions, which is the topic of this project. Adherence or actually the lack thereof, is one of the major challenges when it comes to digital interventions. Non-adherence is defined as 'the fact that not all participants use or keep using the intervention in the desired way'. The problem with non-adherence is that participants may not receive the full benefits of an intervention, or worse, no benefit at all (S. M. Kelders et al., 2012). Therefore, it is of utmost importance for digital interventions that they are motivating to use.

In the field of persuasive technology, motivating techniques have been explored by a variety of researchers. For example, Ham & Midden (2010) have argued that providing feedback through ambient light instead of through numbers could be experienced as more motivating because less cognitive effort is needed. In the field of gamification and serious games, it has been argued that a diverse range of gaming elements could have a motivational effect (Deterding et al., 2011). To some extent, the effect of the use of game elements in innovative products within the (mental) health domain has been shown in case studies (see e.g., Consolvo et al., 2008; Visch et al., 2011). Merry et al found positive effects on adherence with the use of a serious game for adolescents seeking help for depression (Merry et al., 2012). However, empirical experimental research on the motivational effects of specific game elements is often lacking in such case studies. In this paper, we would like to present a case-study that illustrates the motivating effect of using metaphors in the design of online interventions.

The demonstration project that is the topic of this paper was the individual graduation project of the 3rd author at the Faculty of Engineering (master in Industrial Design Engineering) at the University of Twente. The project demonstrates a digital intervention for primary school teachers based on positive psychology. The intervention was designed using persuasive elements and gaming elements. In particular, the intervention makes use of metaphor to motivate. We will describe the user centered design process of the intervention and an evaluation of metaphor as a motivational element with end users based on a first-encounter trial.

2   Using Metaphor to Motivate

One of the key challenges in designing web-based applications is how to give shape in words and visuals to challenges, goals, and feedback provided during interaction. In many traditional applications, emphasis is on concrete textual input (i.e., instructions or numbers signifying scores or tasks left to accomplish) or concrete images (e.g., desktop like wallpapers or avatars). However, in addition to such concrete elements, other design techniques, that are relatively new to the field of online interventions, could improve the experience of using such an intervention. Making use of metaphors is one of those techniques.

Lakoff and Johnson (1980) describe the essence of metaphor as understanding and experiencing one kind of thing (target) in terms of another (source). In her thesis, Nazli Cila (2013) gives an overview of the use of metaphor in design and of how designers communicate with users of products through metaphors. She for example describes that designers can use metaphors as a means to convey meaning in a product. In her definition, a product metaphor is "Any kind of product that is shaped to reference the physical properties (e.g., form, sound, movement, smell, and so on) of another distinct entity for particular expressive purposes." As such, any property of one entity (the source) that is mapped on a design (the target) can be seen as a product metaphor. Indeed, Ludden et al (2012) have shown that product designers can create products incorporating metaphors that people understand by making mind maps that show common associations from source to target. In interface design, metaphors have been used frequently to make items of the interface easier to understand and use. Think for example of the metaphor of the desktop. Since this metaphor was introduced, people have been able to find things on their monitor much as they were used to finding items on their desk. Other examples are the directory (folder), looking like a physical folder and the file, looking like a piece of paper with a folded corner.

The examples above illustrate the use of very simple, direct metaphors. A 'deeper' metaphor, a metaphor for which the distance between target and source is further (implying that the relationship between the two is less easy to see) could also facilitate attribution of the meaning of the source onto the target. This aspect of metaphors could be used to transfer a motivating element from a source onto a target (the design). To illustrate how this works, we will use Figure 1. In this figure, an illustration is presented that describes how the online intervention 'Superbetter' works. Superbetter is an intervention that, much like the intervention that this project describes, is set up to increase flourishing in people's lives; allow them to be a 'superbetter' version of themselves. In the image in figure 1, progress towards end-goals is visualized in terms of a steep road (and hence, not in terms of meaningless numbers or textual elements). In daily life, we commonly talk about tasks we undertake in terms of progress along a path ('I'm almost there', 'We're making progress', and 'I was sidetracked for a while'). Therefore, the metaphor of the steep road makes intuitive sense. When (as in 'Superbetter') coupled to the notion of going upwards and reaching the top (e.g., 'Rising to the occasion', 'I reached the top'), an element of prideful achievement is added upon successful completion. Finally, obstacles are presented along the way such as a bridge to cross and hurdles to overcome, further adding elements of playful challenge and hence as an opportunity for mastery and gaining of self-confidence.

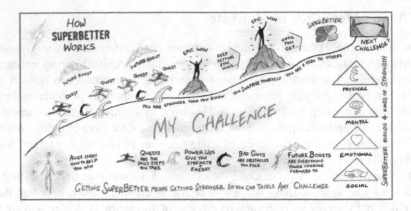

Fig. 1. Illustration describing the online intervention 'Superbetter

Taken together, this suggest that employing metaphors in web-based applications may not just be used for fun or to ensure a usable interface, but that they may actually be used to communicate value and meaning to a user and may contribute to elicitation of positive affect during interaction. As such, making use of a metaphor can be seen as a persuasive and motivational element in an intervention.

3   User Centered Design of a Digital Intervention

The design case discussed here was a re-design of a web-based intervention based on a book training (S.M. Kelders et al., 2013). The training from the book 'This is your life' was adapted for primary school teaching staff into six chapters with different themes, containing both exercises and background information, all on paper. The re-design discussed here was aimed at digitizing the training for primary school teaching staff. The design of the digital intervention was carried out in a user-centered design manner (see e.g., Gould & Lewis, 1985), i.e., in close interaction with the proposed target group. With this aim, two interactive focus group sessions with representatives of the target group were organized.

Next to their interaction with the user group, the designers of the interactive part of the intervention worked in close collaboration with the psychologists who designed the content of the intervention.

3.1   First Focus Group Session and Design of First Concepts

In the first focus group session with the target group, both designers and psychologists participated. Next to this, teachers from several schools were present (n = 8 age 25-45.) This first session was focused on the target groups previous experience with the paper version of the intervention and on their daily habits and use of technology.

From the first focus group session, we found that teachers did not use some of the exercises regularly because they could not motivate themselves to do so. Teachers claimed that more reminders for exercises could help them to make doing the exercises a routine behavior. It was also mentioned that audio or video instructions (more interactivity) would be beneficial. Another finding was that there is a difference between younger teachers and older teachers with respect to their use of technology and willingness to adopt trainings or interventions such as 'This is your life'. Therefore, it was decided to direct the digital intervention at green schools (schools with teachers with an average age of 30).

After this focus group, the project team (of designers and psychologists) decided that using metaphors in the design of the concepts of the digital intervention could be a way to motivate teachers to make the intervention easier to understand and more fun to use. Three concept directions were developed in which metaphors were used on different levels. Figure 2, 3, and 4 show the three concepts; in each of these figures, an overview screen of the training (image on the left) as well as a view of a chapter / lesson (image on the right) can be seen. The first concept (Figure 2) uses a 'library' as a metaphor for the training. In this concept, 'opening a book in a library' is used as a metaphor for opening a new chapter of the training. The lesson view looks like a book while still holding reference to the library. This can be seen as a very direct, almost literal metaphor: target (the online training with different chapters) and source (the library) are from the same domain, it is very easy to see the relationship between the two.

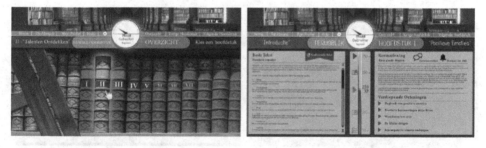

Fig. 2. Concept using 'library' as a metaphor

The second concept (see Figure 3) uses a tree as a metaphor for the training. For this metaphor, the distance from target to source is larger; the relationship between a tree and a training is less easy to understand. Here, the metaphor of 'picking apples from a tree' is used for the concept of using different lessons (chapters) from the training. With this metaphor, the *meaning* and motivating element of picking apples as something that is beneficial for someone is also visualized by the basket (the more apples I have collected in my basket, the better). This might motivate users of this concept to open the different chapters of the training and perform the exercises in order to fill their basket.

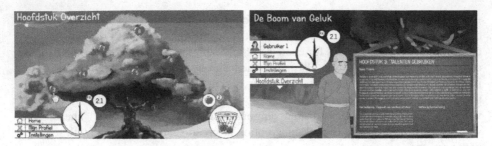

Fig. 3. Concept using 'tree' as a metaphor

The last concept (Figure 4) shows the intervention presented as a journey on a map. Here, the concept of a journey and the 'discovery' of different places on a map along the way is again used to transfer the motivating aspect of a journey of 'wanting to discover new things' and 'wanting to complete a journey'. Again, this is an example of a 'deeper' metaphor; target and source are not from the same domain. However, in this case, the relationship between target and source may still be quite easy to understand because of the conventionality of the metaphor. The intervention is about improving people's lives and it is not uncommon to look upon life as a journey. In fact, in English, there are many words and phrases connected to life that use the metaphor of a journey. Someone might for example say "After university I was *at a crossroads*, and I didn't know *which way to go*." Or "You have to *move on* and forget about what has happened."

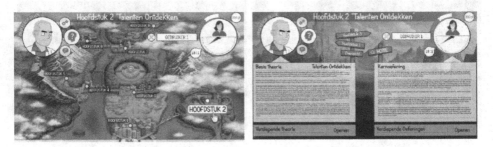

Fig. 4. Concept using 'journey' as a metaphor

3.2   Second Focus Group Session; Evaluation and Co-creation

The three concepts as presented in Figure 2, 3, and 4 were used in a second focus group. In this focus group, potential end users of the concept (N=5, ages between 25-35) offered feedback on the concepts and they gave suggestions for improvements. To facilitate this, several co-creation exercises were used (Stickdorn & Schneider, 2010).

The participants were handed a booklet of A3 posters with the concepts and separate elements that required feedback. The participants were first allowed to browse through their booklet and explore what was there. Next, several elements of the concepts were systematically reviewed. Each concept was marked with several points of interests (POI) which would serve as a guide for the evaluation. Each POI was introduced with some information what it resembled and what it would do in a live interface. After that, the participants were asked to stick a post-it to the corresponding POI number with their comments for that POI. The participants were encouraged to write down anything that would come to mind. At some of the POI's a short discussion sparked and participants generated input such as possible improvements. The discussions were moderated by the designer to stay within time limits and after a few minutes participants were asked to write down all their input on the discussed element, without forcing a group decision on the discussed ideas or improvements. After all POI's had been discussed, participants were encouraged to clearly mark their favorite concept. Finally, participants created a collage of their ideal concept. They were allowed to cut and paste anything from the concept booklet or to draw their own ideas if they so desired. The last A3 poster (of the A3 booklet) showed a template they could use.

From this focus group, there was a clear winner amongst the concepts. All participants listed the concept that used the metaphor of a journey on a map as their favorite. One of the participants elaborated that it would feel like a journey to make yourself happy, which he imagined to fit the training perfectly. The other participants agreed and gave similar comments. This implies that the participants of the focus group recognized and understood the metaphor of the journey that was presented in this concept very well. Next to this, gaming elements that were represented in this and other concepts were recognized and appreciated. Further, the colorfulness of the journey concept was found to be most closely related to the overarching subject of the training (positive psychology). Furthermore, participants of the focus group mentioned that they would like to see as little text as possible and a clear interface with subtle elements that give insights in what is coming next or what is left for them to do.

3.3   Final Design

Because the results of the focus group clearly indicated that the target group showed a preference for the concept of the intervention presented as a journey on a map, this concept was further developed into a working prototype.

The main storyline for the final design is that of the user following a journey towards a flourishing life, guided by a Professor. Two screens (the home or overview screen and a view of a lesson/chapter) of the final working prototype are presented in Figure 5 and 6. The journey leads through eight locations (chapters) where knowledge (lessons) can be found to teach the user the 'secrets' (theory) to flourishing. In the final design, the typical terminology from trainings or school-like activities (i.e. lessons, exercises, chapters, etc.) was changed into terminology that was more relevant to the metaphor of the journey that was used. For instance: 'chapters' are 'locations' on the map and each location has 'challenges' which are the 'exercises' of the training. When a user completes the challenges for a specific location, he or she can get the 'key' to a next location. Locations also have names that are related to the 'life is a journey' metaphor, such as 'The island of broken dreams' and 'The river of flow'. The image at the top of the screen with the puzzle icons shows a user's progress within the current location.

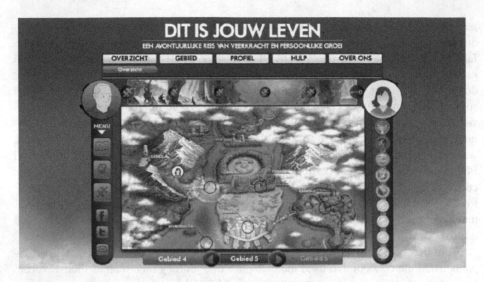

Fig. 5. The final prototype – overview map

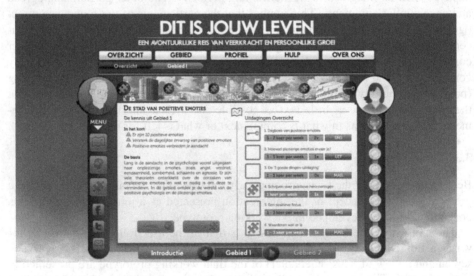

Fig. 6. The final prototype – lesson view

4   User Test with Prototype

In order to test and evaluate the final prototype, individual test sessions with primary school teachers (n=13, 3 male, mean age=38) were organized. The test was designed to measure both the ability of the intervention to motivate as well as several usability factors. Next to this, we collected feedback on the visualizations, the training structure and general remarks. For this paper, we will report on the questions that measured the ability of the design to motivate only.

4.1   Method

The sessions were structured in two parts: a pre-evaluation and post-evaluation.[1] Sitting in front of a computer, the participant would first look at the training website. The participant was asked a set of pre-evaluation questions by the researcher. These questions were about their first impressions on the motivational factor of the training (e.g., 'Can you tell to what extent the design of the website motivates you to start with the training, 1 being completely unmotivated and 9 being completely motivated?' and 'Can you tell to what extent the design of the website excites you, on a similar scale as the previous question?')

Next, the participant was asked to complete the prototype of the training. This took about 10 minutes. The introduction core exercise, which was to read the introduction theory, was completed. After that, a key was presented that unlocked location two (The City of Positive Emotions). In this location participants could again read the theory and complete the core exercise. After finishing the training in location two the prototype ended and a next set of questions was asked through a digital form. Questions that tested the motivational aspect of the training were the following: 'After this introduction I would like to continue with the full   training' , 'I am motivated to continue the training', 'The design of the training is challenging' and 'The design of the training is playful.'

During the entire session observations were made of (unexpected) user behavior, for example, the preferred usage of navigation elements (i.e. top, side or bottom navigation),   exploration of menus and content and moments during the usage in which the participants required help (i.e. when they asked the observer for explanations).

4.2   Results

To the question about their first impression of the website, all participants reacted that the website looked good and professional. Also, they reported that their curiosity was sparked or that they were excited about discovering the landscape of the map overview. Eight participants found the interface unclear or cluttered on first experiencing it. Responses to the question that asked participants to rate to what extent the design of the website motivated them showed that generally, the design motivated participants to a reasonable extent ($m = 7.3$, $sd = 0.6$). Comments were that the first impression made them curious, and that it invited or challenged them to continue on the supposed 'journey' or 'adventure'. Four participants found the website playful or 'like a game' and two participants explicitly mentioned they did not fancy games. Respondents reported to be excited about the design of the website ($m = 7.5$, $sd = 1.1$). Comments resembled those for the first two questions: the site looks good, and was perceived as a professional website. Some participants repeated that they would like some more color or a different style altogether.

Responses to questions after finishing the prototype showed similar results; Participants reported that they would like to continue the training after having finished the

---

[1] Before the start of the test, participants were informed of the purpose of the test and signed a consent form.

prototype (m = 6.9, sd = 1.2) and that the training motivated them to continue (m = 6.2, sd = 2.2), the design of the training was found challenging (m = 7.3, sd = 1.0) and playful (m = 7.2, sd = 1.0).

5   Discussion

From the user evaluation of the prototype we found that the final design of the intervention that was the topic of this study was seen as motivating and stimulating by users. Moreover, the metaphorical element of the design (the presentation of the intervention as a journey on a map) was seen as motivating. However, in this study we only let users use a prototype of the intervention for a short time. To determine whether (the motivating aspect of) this design will indeed lead to better adherence to the intervention we are planning a Randomized Controlled Trial that will compare effects on adherence of this design to that of the (more traditional) design of 'Voluit Leven' online.

Participants in the second focus group showed a clear preference for the concept that used a journey on a map as a metaphor. In our explanation of the concepts, we have stated that this is an example of a deep metaphor that is conventional. We would like to argue that these elements together (the depth of the metaphor and its conventionality) have led to this choice. While a deeper metaphor is often found more interesting (Cila, 2012), a deep metaphor that people do not understand will never work. In this case, where a (training about) life is seen as a journey, the metaphor will be easy to understand because of its conventionality. Therefore, the metaphor works and is still interesting, it fits the purpose (this training about life) very well.

In this paper, our main argument is on metaphor working as a motivational element in the design of an online intervention. As can been seen in Figure 5 and 6, the eventual design of this training used other motivating elements (mostly inspired on gaming) as well. For example, during the training, pieces of a puzzle can be 'earned' to reach new locations (levels). Also, completing the exercises in a particular area will result in that area being presented as more colorful. Eventually, all these elements will work together to motivate a user of such an intervention. Using too many motivating elements would not be an advisable strategy, rather, a sensible and balanced selection has to be made. Therefore, further research into the capacities to motivate that different elements have in separation and in combination is in order.

As a motivating element, it was also mentioned by participants that a walkthrough at the start of the training could very well serve for setting goals. Indeed, if participants know from the start what the map will look like after they have finished all elements of the training, this may motivate them to reach this goal.

The differences in scores on motivation before and after completing the prototype were small; however it is worth noticing that the score for motivation seems to be somewhat lower in the post-evaluation questions. An explanation for this may be the interest in this type of intervention in itself, rather than the design of the training. Upon first viewing the design of the intervention, respondents were not aware of the aim of the training. Whereas after completing the prototype they were. During the post-evaluation some of the participants mentioned they actually did not have interest in the subject of the training, although if they would have had an interest in it, they would be motivated by the design. Remarks of respondents after the individual sessions seem to reveal that especially the male participants (relatively few men participated in our evaluation sessions) lack affinity with the theme of the training. This concurs with findings that most web-based interventions are mainly used by women (S. M. Kelders et al., 2011). Apparently, the appealing design of this intervention did not overcome the lack of interest in the subject of the training.

Making use of metaphors is not necessarily a gamification technique. In the case study presented here, we have used both a metaphor and gamification elements. Recently, there has been some debate about using gamification because elements of gaming would only extrinsically motivate people and are in many cases not meaningfully designed (Gartner, 2012). Using metaphors to motivate may be a good way to create meaningful design, resulting in enduring involvement with the intervention. However, controlled studies comparing metaphor based interventions with standard interventions and/or with gamified interventions are necessary to support this claim.

References

1. Bohlmeijer, E.T., Hulsbergen, M.L.: Dit is jouw leven. Ervaar de effecten van de positieve psychologie. Uitgeverij Boom, Amsterdam (2013)
2. Cila, N.: Metaphors we design by. The use of metaphors in product design. Delft University of Technology, Delft (2013)
3. Consolvo, S., McDonald, D.W., Toscos, T., Chen, M.Y., Froehlich, J., Harrison, B., Landay, J.A.: Activity Sensing in the Wild: A Field Trial of UbiFit Garden. In: CHI 2008: 26th Annual CHI Conference on Human Factors in Computing Systems Vols 1 and 2, Conference Proceedings, pp. 1797–1806 (2008)
4. Deterding, S., Dixon, D., Khaled, R., Nacke, L.: From game design elements to gamefulness: defining gamification. Paper presented at the 15th International Academic MindTrek Conference: Envisioning Future Media Environments (2011)
5. Gartner, http://www.gartner.com/newsroom/id/2251015 (accessed February 2, 2012)
6. Gould, J., Lewis, C.: Designing for usability - Key principles and what designers think. Commun. ACM 28, 300–311 (1985)
7. Ham, J., Midden, C.: Ambient Persuasive Technology Needs Little Cognitive Effort: The Differential Effects of Cognitive Load on Lighting Feedback versus Factual Feedback. In: Ploug, T., Hasle, P., Oinas-Kukkonen, H. (eds.) PERSUASIVE 2010. LNCS, vol. 6137, pp. 132–142. Springer, Heidelberg (2010)
8. Kelders, S.M., Kok, R.N., Ossebaard, H.C., Van Gemert-Pijnen, J.E.W.C.: Persuasive System Design Does Matter: A Systematic Review of Adherence to Web-Based Interventions. Journal of Medical Internet Research 14(6), 2–25 (2012)
9. Kelders, S.M., Pots, W.T.M., Oskam, M.J., Bohlmeijer, E.T., van Gemert-Pijnen, J.E.W.C.: Development of a web-based intervention for the indicated prevention of depression. BMC Medical Informatics and Decision Making 13(26), 1–11 (2013)

10. Kelders, S.M., Van Gemert-Pijnen, J.E.W.C., Werkman, A., Nijland, N., Seydel, E.R.: Effectiveness of a Web-based intervention aimed at healthy dietary and physical activity behavior: a randomized controlled trial about users and usage. Journal of Medical Internet Research 13(2), e32 (2011)
11. Lakoff, G., Johnson, M.: Metaphors we live by. The University of Chicago Press, Chicago and London (1980)
12. Ludden, G.D.S., Kudrowitz, B.M., Schifferstein, H.N.J., Hekkert, P.: Surprise and humor in product design Designing sensory metaphors in multiple modalities. Humor-International Journal of Humor Research 25(3), 285–309 (2012)
13. Lyubomirsky, S.: The how of hapiness: a new approach to getting the life you want. The Penguin Press, New York (2008)
14. Merry, S.N., Stasiak, K., Shepherd, M., Frampton, C., Fleming, T., Lucassen, M.F.G.: The effectiveness of SPARX, a computerised self help intervention for adolescents seeking help for depression: randomised controlled non-inferiority trial. BMJ 344(apr18 3), e2598 (2012)
15. Seligman, M.E., Csikszentmihalyi, M.: Positive psychology. An introduction. American Psychologist 55(1), 5–14 (2000)
16. Stickdorn, M., Schneider, J.: This is Service Design Thinking: Basics, Tools, Cases. BIS Publishers, Amsterdam (2010)
17. Visch, V.T., de Wit, M., Dinh, L., van den Brule, D., Melles, M., Sonneveld, M.H.: Industrial design meets mental healthcare: designing therapy-enhancing products involving game-elements for mental healthcare - three case studies. Paper presented at the IEEE Proceedings of SEGAH Serious Games and Applications for Health, Braga (2011)

Investigating the Influence of Social Exclusion on Persuasion by a Virtual Agent

Peter A.M. Ruijten, Jaap Ham, and Cees J.H. Midden

Eindhoven University of Technology, School of Innovation Sciences,
Eindhoven, Netherlands, P.O. 513
p.a.m.ruijten@tue.nl

Abstract. Persuasive agents may function as a tool to induce changes in human behavior. Research has shown that human-likeness of such agents influences their effectiveness. Besides characteristics of the agent, other characteristics may also have strong influences on persuasive agents' effectiveness. One such characteristic is social exclusion. When people feel socially excluded, they are more sensitive to social influence. In two studies, we investigated this effect in a human-agent interaction. Results show stronger behavior changes for socially exclusion compared to social inclusion. This effect seems stronger for females than for males.

Keywords: Social exclusion, Social influence, Virtual agent.

1   Introduction

Artificial agents are becoming more prevalent in our society. Most of those artificial agents have in common that they are designed to make our life more comfortable. Another possible employment of such agents is to help us being more sustainable and reduce our carbon footprint. In this context artificial agents are used to persuade consumers into changing their behavior. *Persuasive* artificial agents may function as an effective tool to induce changes in human behavior [1].

As such, a persuasive artificial agent may function as an effective tool to induce changes in human behavior [1]. It has been argued that anthropomorphism is a key concept in the effectiveness of social feedback from artificial agents [2]. Research has shown that anthropomorphic artificial agents are evaluated more positively [3], and are experienced as more socially present [4] compared to non-anthropomorphic artificial agents. However, the effectiveness of artificial agents is not only dependent on agent characteristics, but also on human characteristics [5]. The tendency to anthropomorphize agents or other objects can differ between individuals. Epley and colleagues' theoretical framework [5] described sociality motivation (the desire for social contact and affiliation) as one of the major factors that cause people to have a higher tendency to anthropomorphize non-human objects. Furthermore, the tendency to anthropomorphize objects or artificial agents is thus larger for people who are chronically lonely compared to those who are chronically connected with others

A. Spagnolli et al. (Eds.): PERSUASIVE 2014, LNCS 8462, pp. 191–200, 2014.

[e.g., 6, 7]. Research has shown that lonely people anthropomorphize a robot more than people in a control group [8]. Furthermore, people who are experimentally induced to feel lonely perceive an artificial agent as more social [9].

The effectiveness of a persuasive message from an artificial agent is thus likely to differ with the extent to which this agent is perceived as human-like (i.e., anthropomorphized). Therefore, we expect that a persuasive message from an artificial agent will more strongly influence the behavior of socially excluded people compared to those who feel socially connected. This hypothesis will be investigated in two studies. Study 1 is designed to measure the effects of social inclusion or exclusion on the effectiveness of a virtual agent's persuasive message. Study 2 replicates the setup of Study 1 and adds one factor: the virtual agent's gender.

2   Study 1

In this study, we investigate the effect of being socially excluded on susceptibility to social feedback from a virtual agent. Research has shown that socially excluded people are more likely to attribute socialness to virtual agents [e.g.; 6, 8, 9]. As a response to this, people may be more sensitive to feedback given by such agents. We hypothesize that people that have been socially excluded will change their behavior more according to feedback from a virtual agent compared to those who have been socially included.

2.1   Method

Participants and Design
Sixty-three participants (38 males and 27 females; $M_{age} = 26.1$, $SD_{age} = 11.1$) were randomly assigned to one of three experimental conditions of a between-subjects design. Two of the three conditions were designed to make participants feel either socially included ($n = 21$) or excluded ($n = 22$). A third condition was designed as explorative control condition ($n = 20$) without exclusion manipulation. All participants were native Dutch speakers. The experiment lasted 30 minutes for which participants were paid €5.

Materials and Procedure
At the beginning of the experiment, the participants were informed via the computer screen that all collected data would be analyzed anonymously, and their rights to stop at any time (without consequences for payment) were explained. By pressing a button, they would agree to participate in the experiment. To make participants feel socially included or excluded, they played the Cyberball game [10]. In this game, participants played a virtual ball tossing game with two computerized players. The game instructions were the following: when the ball is tossed to you, you need to click on one of the other two players to toss the ball to that player. Participants in the inclusion condition received the ball roughly 30% of the throws. Participants in the exclusion

condition received the ball a few times in the beginning of the game, after which the computerized players tossed the ball to each other only during the rest of the game. The participants were told that this game was necessary to practice mental visualization of a situation. This game is often used to experimentally induce participants to feel socially excluded [e.g., 10-13].

After playing the Cyberball game, participants were introduced to a virtual agent that would provide feedback about choices they made during the main task. The agent was presented on a second monitor and was programmed to respond to every choice participants made in the following task with evaluative statements.

Next, participants started with the main experimental task: the washing machine task as used in earlier research by [14]. In this task, a simulated washing machine panel was presented on the screen and participants were asked to complete ten laundry tasks (e.g., wash four dirty jeans) on the computer. The ten tasks were randomly picked from a set of 23 different tasks.

During the setting of the simulated washing machine, participants received social feedback from the virtual agent. This feedback was based on the simulated energy that was used by the chosen settings and had six levels, three of which positive (e.g., "Fantastic!") and three negative (e.g., "Terrible!"). All participants received feedback based on the energy use of their settings. The main dependent variable was created by following these steps: first, energy use scores were standardized to be able to compare the settings between laundry tasks. Next, the difference on this standardized value between every setting and the previous setting (caused by an action of the participant, e.g., increasing the washing temperature) was calculated. This value precisely shows the effect of feedback on energy use, and will be referred to as the Energy Difference Score (EDS) in the remainder of this paper. A positive EDS indicates that the participant uses more energy than in the previous action, and a negative EDS indicates that the participant saves energy compared with the previous action.

After performing the washing machine task, participants completed two questionnaires about their perception of the virtual agent. For this, we used the 5-item anthropomorphism scale adapted from the Godspeed questionnaire developed by [15] (7-point scale, $\alpha = 0.76$) and a 7-item questionnaire based on [7] (7-point scale, $\alpha = 0.863$). The responses on these questionnaires were averaged and used as explicit measurements of anthropomorphism. They will be referred to as the Bartneck scale and the Waytz questions respectively.

Hereafter, participants were asked a series of questions to check if the manipulation was successful. The first question was what percentage of the balls they thought were thrown at them during the game (referred to as Ball percentage), followed by questions related to their evaluation of the game and the other players (referred to as Game evaluation), 13 items ($\alpha = 0.93$).

For explorative reasons, we also measured perceived intelligence of the agent (adapted from [15], 5 items, 7-point scale, $\alpha = 0.87$), perceived agent knowledge (adapted from [16], 8 items, 7-point scale, $\alpha = 0.87$), and need to belong (adapted from [17], 10 items, 7-point scale, $\alpha = 0.87$). No effects were found on any of these scales, and they will not be included in the results section.

At the end of the session, participants were debriefed about the goal of the cyber-ball game and the feedback provided by the virtual agent. If there were no further questions, participants were paid and thanked for their contribution.

2.2   Results

To check whether the manipulation was successful, results on the two manipulation checks (Ball percentage and Game evaluation) were submitted to independent sam-ples t-tests with the two Cyberball conditions as groups. Results showed a significant difference between the groups on the Ball percentage, $t(41) = 8.15$, $p < 0.001$, $r^2 = 0.60$. Participants in the inclusion condition ($M = 39.90$, $SD = 16.62$) reported having received a higher percentage of the balls in the game than participants in the exclusion condition ($M = 9.41$, $SD = 5.56$). Also, a significant difference on Game evaluation between the inclusion condition ($M = 4.07$, $SD = 1.03$) and the exclusion condition ($M = 2.51$, $SD = 0.79$) was found, $t(41) = 5.59$, $p < 0.001$, $r^2 = 0.42$.

Our main hypothesis was tested with a Linear Mixed Model[1] with a single factor (Cyberball: Inclusion vs. Exclusion) between subjects design with EDS as dependent variable and the specific washing task as random factor[2]. This analysis showed a sig-nificant main effect of Cyberball, $F(1, 942.34) = 7.81$, $p = 0.01$. Participants who were excluded had a lower EDS ($EMM = -0.63$, $SE = 0.06$) than participants who were included ($EMM = -0.49$, $SE = 0.05$). The average EDS of participants in the control group ($M = -0.66$, $SE = 0.04$) was comparable to the exclusion group.

To check whether the manipulation had an effect on explicit anthropomorphism measurements, the averaged scores on both the Bartneck scale and the Waytz ques-tions were submitted to an independent samples t-test with the two Cyberball condi-tions as groups. Results showed no significant difference on either the Bartneck scale ($t < 1$, $p > 0.05$) or the Waytz questions ($t < 1.6$, $p > 0.05$).

Exploratory Analysis

Because earlier research suggested that for understanding the interaction between a human and an artificial social agent it is important to take the gender of the artificial agent into account [18, 19], we also included participant gender to the model. In this analysis, EDS was submitted to a 2 (cyberball: inclusion vs. exclusion) X 2 (partici-pant gender: male vs. female) Linear Mixed Model with the specific washing task as random factor. Interestingly, the results showed a main effect of participant gender, $F(1, 1539.13) = 7.27$, $p < 0.01$. More specifically, female participants had a lower EDS ($EMM = -0.67$, $SE = 0.06$) than male participants ($EMM = -0.52$, $SE = 0.05$). Results provided no evidence for an interaction between Cyberball and Gender, $F < 1$, $p > 0.80$.

---

[1] We used a Linear Mixed Model because the data consisted of multiple measurements per participant that were dependent of each other. The LMM method is designed to take this into account. The values for degrees of freedom are obtained by a Satterthwaite approximation.
[2] Recall that the washing task in each trial was randomly chosen from a set of 23 tasks.

2.3   Discussion

This study was designed to investigate the effect of being socially excluded on susceptibility to social feedback from a virtual agent. As expected, results showed that people who were experimentally induced to feel socially excluded were more sensitive to the social feedback from an agent compared to those who were included. Furthermore, female participants appeared to be more sensitive in general to the feedback than male participants. This discrepancy between male and female participants could be explained in two ways.

The agent that was used in the experiment was female, and this may have caused differences in responses between males and females. Earlier research has shown that virtual agents can have a greater influence on people's attitudes when those agents have the same gender as the participant [18]. On the other hand, females may be more persuasible in general [19]. A meta-analytic study has already suggested this effect to be present in the context of social influence studies [19]. Furthermore, females may more able to adapt to feedback in a presumably stereotypical task [20]. In Study 2 we will elaborate on these explanations and investigate which of the two explanations above is most probable.

3   Study 2

In Study 1 we found an expected main effect of Cyberball on susceptibility to social feedback from a virtual agent. We also found an unexpected effect of participant gender. That is, female participants appeared to be influenced more by the social feedback than male participants. This effect may have occurred because of different reasons. First, the effect may have occurred because female participants are more sensitive to female virtual humans, whereas male participants show a greater attitude change when persuaded by a male virtual agent [18]. On the other hand, a meta-analytic review has shown that women in general are more susceptible to social influence than men [19]. This may have been caused by contextual features of the experimental setups [20]. Nevertheless, our experimental setup (programming a washing machine interface) can be seen as a stereotypical female task. In this study, we investigated the effect of being socially excluded on susceptibility to social feedback as provided by a male versus a female virtual agent. We hypothesize, in line with Study 1, that social exclusion in the Cyberball game will promote behavior change as a result of feedback from a virtual social agent. Furthermore, we investigate whether the gender effect found in Study 1 is more likely to be explained by the *gender of the participant* or by the *interaction* with a *same-sex* virtual agent.

3.1   Method

Participants and Design
Eighty-nine participants (60 males and 29 females; M_{age} = 24.0, SD_{age} = 10.1) were randomly assigned to one of four experimental conditions of a 2 (cyberball: inclusion vs. exclusion) X 2 (gender combination: same sex vs. opposite sex) between-subjects design. The Cyberball conditions were identical to those in Study 1. They were

designed to make participants feel either socially included ($n = 44$) or excluded ($n = 45$). The gender combination conditions (same sex $n = 49$, opposite sex $n = 40$) were created by having participants interact with a male or a female virtual agent (as depicted in Figure 1). All participants were native Dutch speakers. The experiment lasted 30 minutes for which participants were paid €5.

Materials and Procedure
At the beginning of the experiment, the participants were informed via the computer screen that all collected data would be analyzed anonymously, and their rights to stop at any time (without consequences for payment) were explained. Like in Study 1, participants played the Cyberball game [10] to make them feel socially included or excluded. They were told that this game was necessary to practice mental visualization.

After playing the Cyberball game, participants were introduced to one of the virtual agents (as depicted in Fig. 1), dependent on the experimental condition. The agent would provide feedback on participants' choices during the main task. The agent was presented on a second monitor and was programmed to respond to every choice participants made in the following task. Next, participants played the laundry task as explained in Study 1. Both the feedback levels and the main dependent variable (EDS) remained the same.

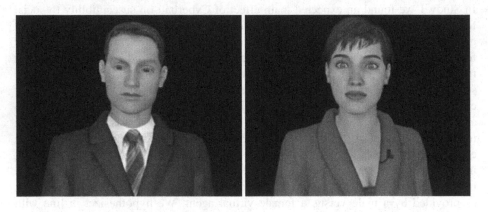

Fig. 1. The male agent (left) used in Study 2 and the female agent (right) used in both studies

After completing the washing trials, participants completed two questionnaires about their perception of the virtual agent. For this, we again used the Bartneck scale (5 items, 7-point scale, $\alpha = 0.75$) and the Waytz questions (7 items, 4-point scale, $\alpha = 0.84$) as explicit measurements of anthropomorphism.

Next, participants were asked the manipulation check questions[3]. The first question again asked participants the percentage of the balls they thought were thrown at them

---

[3] Due to a programming error, data from one of the four conditions was not properly saved, leading to the exclusion of data from 22 participants. The Cronbach's α's and results on the manipulation check are based on data from the remaining 67 participants.

during the game (referred to as Ball percentage). Next, there were 14 items in total (one item from Study 1 was split up into two items in Study 2), which were combined into to one manipulation check score ($\alpha = 0.92$), referred to as Game evaluation.

For explorative reasons, we also asked participants' evaluations of the agent's usefulness, attractiveness, likability, and pleasantness. This questionnaire consisted of 9 items ($\alpha = 0.86$), referred to as Agent evaluation. No effects were found on this questionnaire, and therefore it will not be included in the results section.

At the end of the session, participants were debriefed about the goal of the cyberball game and the feedback provided by the virtual agent. If there were no further questions, participants were paid and thanked for their contribution.

3.2   Results

To check whether the manipulation was successful, results on the two manipulation check scores (Ball percentage and Game evaluation) were submitted to independent samples t-tests with the two Cyberball conditions as groups. Results showed a significant difference between the groups on the Ball percentage, $t(65) = 11.68$, $p < 0.001$, $r^2 = 0.63$. Participants in the inclusion condition ($M = 48.82$, $SD = 20.08$) reported having received a higher percentage of the balls in the game than participants in the exclusion condition ($M = 10.57$, $SD = 6.00$). Also, a significant difference on Game evaluation between the inclusion condition ($M = 4.02$, $SD = 0.94$) and the exclusion condition ($M = 2.27$, $SD = 0.52$) was found, $t(65) = 9.82$, $p < 0.001$, $r^2 = 0.57$.

Our main hypothesis was tested with a Linear Mixed Model with a single factor (cyberball: inclusion vs. exclusion) between subjects design with EDS as dependent variable and the specific washing task as random factor. The analysis showed a significant main effect of Cyberball, $F(1, 2282.78) = 4.01$, $p = 0.05$. Participants who were excluded saved more energy ($EMM = -0.64$, $SE = 0.03$) than participants who were included ($EMM = -0.56$, $SE = 0.03$).

To investigate whether the gender effect found in Study 1 is more likely to be explained by the *gender of the participant* or by the *interaction* with a *same-sex* virtual agent, we submitted EDS to a 2(Cyberball: Inclusion vs. Exclusion) X 2(Participant gender: Male vs. Female) X 2(Gender combination: Same sex vs. Opposite sex) Linear Mixed Model with the specific washing task as random factor[4]. This analysis revealed a main effect of Participant gender, $F(1, 2587.14) = 9.15$, $p < 0.01$. More specifically, female participants saved more energy ($M = -0.69$, $SE = 0.03$) than male participants did ($M = -0.57$, $SE = 0.02$). Results provided no evidence for an effect of Gender-combination, and no significant interaction was found between any of the variables, all F's < 1, all p's > 0.5.

To check whether the manipulation had an effect on explicit anthropomorphism measurements, the scores on the Bartneck scale and the Waytz questions were submitted to independent samples t-tests with the two Cyberball conditions as groups.

---

[4] Due to restrictions of the statistical package SPSS, the analysis could only be performed on the first 151 actions of each participant. Two participants had more actions in the task, causing the exclusion of 17 actions (0.2% of the total data).

Results showed no significant difference on the Bartneck scale ($t < 1$, $p > 0.05$). However, a significant difference between the Cyberball conditions was found on the Waytz questions, $t(87) = 2.18$, $p = 0.03$, $r^2 = 0.05$. Participants in the inclusion condition ($M = 2.03$, $SD = 0.74$) reported higher anthropomorphic values than participants in the exclusion condition ($M = 1.71$, $SD = 0.67$).

3.3   Discussion

This study was designed to investigate the effect of social exclusion on susceptibility to social feedback from a virtual agent of the same sex versus opposite sex. Our main hypothesis that people who are experimentally induced to feel socially excluded are more sensitive to the social feedback compared to those who were included was supported. Furthermore, we investigated whether female participants are more sensitive to the feedback than male participants, or whether the discrepancy is found only in same-sex conditions. Results suggested that participant's gender had an influence on energy use, whereas gender combination did not have an influence on energy use. It should be noted, however, that many of our participants were males, and this skewed distribution may have altered the results. Nevertheless, the gender effect shown in this study matches that of Study 1, which strengthens our confidence in the effect.

One surprising finding in this study is that socially excluded people seem to score lower on an explicit anthropomorphism measurement than socially included people. This finding is the opposite of what we would expect. When taking a closer look at the questions of the anthropomorphism questionnaire, it can be noted that items are very explicit and dominantly about highly cognitive features (i.e.; having free will, consciousness). This explains the low averages as well (the highest average is still below the scale's midpoint). We argue that it is unlikely that a virtual agent's behavior on a computer screen evokes such strong impressions of humanness, and that participants' responses on these questions are mainly their personal opinions about virtual agents. Individual differences have been shown to be a strong determinant of anthropomorphic perceptions in various contexts [7]. To be able to measure subtle changes in people's perceptions of humanlike virtual agents or robots in both higher cognitive features and more appearance related features, a less explicit measurement may be more suitable [21].

4   General Discussion

People's motives for agreeing with others or changing their behavior accordingly may depend on both agent and human (or: sender and receiver) characteristics (for an overview, see [22]). In two studies, we investigated the effects of a human characteristic, being socially excluded, on susceptibility to social feedback from an external trigger, a virtual agent. Results in both studies showed a main effect of exclusion on energy use in a simulated washing machine task. This indicates that social exclusion can determine part of the effectiveness of social feedback of a virtual agent. Furthermore, we consistently found an effect of participant gender in both studies. That is female participants appeared to save more energy than male participants. This effect may have been caused by the context of the task, which was quite stereotypical (doing laundry). Follow-up research could investigate the importance of this experimental context, which has been identified before as an important determinant of gender effects in experimental studies [20].

Several limitations of this research should be taken into account. First, the results are lab based. Our participants performed a simulated washing task on a computer. Although the lab procedure has been validated in field research through previous studies [23], this is different from a real-life situation. Furthermore, we manipulated participants to feel socially excluded, but we could not assess to what extent they experienced the negative consequences of being socially excluded. Nevertheless, we found confirmation for the hypothesis that socially excluded people are more sensitive to social persuasion. To investigate the effects of social exclusion on behavior change in a broader context, different settings can be used where not everything is strictly controlled in a laboratory environment.

Second, the experimental context of a washing machine task may have strongly influenced the effects of participant gender. As [20] stated, when the design of the experiment itself induces stronger effects for one sex compared to the other sex, this difference may not be part of the general nature of social influence. More research is needed to investigate whether the effect of participant gender will hold in different contexts.

Third, we expected anthropomorphism to be the link between social exclusion and persuasion, but we found no evidence for this. Either our claim is invalid, or the measurements do not measure the right aspects of anthropomorphism. Care needs to be given to adequate measurement of anthropomorphism.

Overall, our results are promising and adding to the body of literature in the field of persuasive social agents. We showed that an agent's persuasiveness can be influenced by a specific social-emotional state of a target person, which suggests that adaptive properties of the agent that can take account of these personal states will contribute to the effectiveness of the agent. This adaptivity could be an important design challenge for the development of future persuasive agents.

References

1. Ham, J., Midden, C.: A persuasive robotic agent to save energy: The influence of social feedback, feedback valence and task similarity on energy conservation behavior. In: Ge, S.S., Li, H., Cabibihan, J.-J., Tan, Y.K. (eds.) ICSR 2010. LNCS, vol. 6414, pp. 335–344. Springer, Heidelberg (2010)
2. Fong, T., Nourbakhsh, I., Dautenhahn, K.: A survey of socially interactive robots. Robotics and Autonomous Systems 42(3), 143–166 (2003)
3. Qiu, L., Benbasat, I.: Evaluating anthropomorphic product recommendation agents: a social relationship perspective to designing information systems. Journal of Management Information Systems 25(4), 145–182 (2009)
4. Choi, Y.K., Miracle, G.E., Biocca, F.: The effects of anthropomorphic agents on advertising effectiveness and the mediating role of presence. Journal of Interactive Advertising 2(1) (2001)

5. Epley, N., Waytz, A., Cacioppo, J.T.: On seeing human: a three-factor theory of anthropomorphism. Psychological Review 114(4), 864 (2007)
6. Epley, N., Akalis, S., Waytz, A., Cacioppo, J.T.: Creating Social Connection Through Inferential Reproduction Loneliness and Perceived Agency in Gadgets, Gods, and Greyhounds. Psychological Science 19(2), 114–120 (2008)
7. Waytz, A., Cacioppo, J., Epley, N.: Who sees human? The stability and importance of individual differences in anthropomorphism. Perspectives on Psychological Science 5(3), 219–232 (2010)
8. Eyssel, F., Reich, N.: Loneliness makes the heart grow fonder (of robots)? On the effects of loneliness on psychological anthropomorphism. In: Proceedings of 8th ACM/IEEE Conference on Conference on Human-Robot Interaction, pp. 121–122. IEEE (2013)
9. Jung, Y., Lee, K.M.: Effects of physical embodiment on social presence of social robots. In: Proceedings of PRESENCE, pp. 80–87 (2004)
10. Williams, K.D., Jarvis, B.: Cyberball: A program for use in research on interpersonal ostracism and acceptance. Behavior Research Methods 38(1), 174–180 (2006)
11. Van Beest, I., Williams, K.D.: When inclusion costs and ostracism pays, ostracism still hurts. Journal of Personality and Social Psychology 91(5), 918 (2006)
12. Bernstein, M.J., Claypool, H.M.: Social exclusion and pain sensitivity why exclusion sometimes hurts and sometimes numbs. Personality and Social Psychology Bulletin 38(2), 185–196 (2012)
13. Zadro, L., Williams, K.D., Richardson, R.: How low can you go? Ostracism by a computer is sufficient to lower self-reported levels of belonging, control, self-esteem, and meaningful existence. Journal of Experimental Social Psychology 40(4), 560–567 (2004)
14. Midden, C., Ham, J.: The persuasive effects of positive and negative social feedback from an embodied agent on energy conservation behavior. In: Proceedings of the AISB 2008 Symposium on Persuasive Technology, pp. 9–13. AISB (2008)
15. Bartneck, C., Croft, E., Kulic, D.: Measuring the anthropomorphism, animacy, likeability, perceived intelligence and perceived safety of robots. In: Metrics for HRI Workshop, Technical Report, pp. 37–44. IEEE (2008)
16. Powers, A., Kiesler, S.: The advisor robot: tracing people's mental model from a robot's physical attributes. In: Proceedings of the 1st ACM SIGCHI/SIGART Conference on Human-Robot Interaction, pp. 218–225. ACM (2006)
17. Baumeister, R.F., Leary, M.R.: The need to belong: desire for interpersonal attachments as a fundamental human motivation. Psychological Bulletin 117(3), 497 (1995)
18. Guadagno, R.E., Blascovich, J., Bailenson, J.N., Mccall, C.: Virtual humans and persuasion: The effects of agency and behavioral realism. Media Psychology 10(1), 1–22 (2007)
19. Eagly, A.H., Carli, L.L.: Sex of researchers and sex-typed communications as determinants of sex differences in influenceability: a meta-analysis of social influence studies. Psychological Bulletin 90(1), 1–20 (1981)
20. Eagly, A.H.: Sex differences in influenceability. Psychological Bulletin 85(1), 86 (1978)
21. Ruijten, P.A.M., Bouten, D.H.L., Rouschop, D.C.J., Ham, J., Midden, C.J.H.: The Development of a Rasch-Type Anthropomorphism Scale (2013) (under review)
22. Wood, W.: Attitude change: Persuasion and social influence. Annual Review of Psychology 51(1), 539–570 (2000)
23. Midden, C.J.H., Ham, J.: Persuasive Technology to promote pro-environmental behaviour. In: Steg, L., van den Berg, A.E., de Groot, J.I.M. (eds.) Environmental Psychology an Introduction, pp. 243–254. BPS Blackwell, West-Sussex (2013)

An Empirical Comparison of Variations
of a Virtual Representation of an Individual's Health

Andreas Schmeil and L. Suzanne Suggs

Università della Svizzera Italiana (USI), Lugano, Switzerland
{andreas.schmeil,suzanne.suggs}@usi.ch

Abstract. In this paper we present a study that empirically compares the effects of different variations of a virtual representation of health (VRH) on an individual's motivation and intention to improve their health behavior. We aimed to understand how the approach of a 3D virtual character can be most effective for positively influencing an individual's motivation and intention to engage in a healthier diet and more physical activity. Four variations of this vicarious virtual character were tested: (1) holding a still pose, (2) mimicking health behavior, (3) personifying a possible future health status, and (4) both mimicking health behavior and personifying a possible future health status. The results from data collected from 512 participants in three European countries indicate that in particular juxtaposing the current VRH to a possible future version has a positive effect. Subjective satisfaction measurements imply that that the approach is well received by a general population.

Keywords: Virtual character, VRH, health behavior, behavior change, 3D, physical activity, nutrition, visual communication.

1 Introduction

While simple in theory, in reality, maintaining a healthy lifestyle is an ever-growing challenge for individuals worldwide. Modern society and infrastructures can make it difficult to follow current recommendations for eating healthy and getting regular physical activity (PA). These two health behaviors are related to the prevention of some of the most severe health problems, including overweight and obesity, diabetes, cancer, and heart diseases. However, having the knowledge about the risks of low physical activity and poor dietary habits is not enough to change health behaviors.

In order to improve health behavior (or maintain good health behavior) individuals need support. Behavioral theory suggests that being motivated and having an intention to change are determinants of actual behavior change [1, 2]. Information and communication technologies (ICT) are increasingly being used as support for (semi-) automatic 'health behavior support tools', including providing coaching and feedback mechanisms. Some systems use "health profiles" where users can overview, update, and read about their overall health status, based on self-reported or objective data [15]. Feedback about that health status and ways to improve it are showing real

A. Spagnolli et al. (Eds.): PERSUASIVE 2014, LNCS 8462, pp. 201–223, 2014.

promise in motivating health behaviors [15, 1, 6]. However, novel approaches to providing such personalization and support are increasingly possible and accessible.

The following section gives an overview of related work, which is followed with our research question and design. The paper continues with a presentation of our Virtual Representation of Health (VRH), followed by a detailed description of the experiment, including the hypotheses and the experimental conditions. Finally, we present the results, discuss the findings, and close with remarks and an outlook to future research directions in this field.

1.1   Related Work

Outside of games, the value and effects of virtual characters (i.e., animated, human-like, visual characters, often displayed in three-dimensional environments) on health behavior change have rarely been investigated, despite the positive findings of the few published studies [3].

An examination of eating behaviors found positive results when testing whether behavior change occurs from a virtual setting to the real world [8]. Virtual representations of individuals that perform physical activity were found to increase the likelihood of the individuals themselves engaging in physical activity within 24 hours after the exposure [7]. This effect was particularly strong if there was a high similarity between individual and their virtual representation. Virtual representations of physical selves have also been found to serve as valuable reinforcement instruments: in order to prevent their VRH from gaining weight, individuals engaged in more physical activity [7].

In the first study to demonstrate social influence effects with virtual mimickers (i.e., virtual characters that partly or fully imitate their real counterpart's behavior), Bailenson and Yee found that mimicking characters were more persuasive and were generally regarded higher than non-mimickers, despite the fact that participants did not notice the mimicry [1]. Virtual doppelgängers – virtual characters that authentically reflect the visual appearance of individuals, using photo textures – showed an even higher persuasive potential, one application for which could be health behavior change [9]. Increase in motivation can also been accomplished through the use of vicarious virtual characters [5].

Studies to date have investigated virtual characters in virtual reality lab settings, yet no published work has investigated virtual characters online, which are always-accessible. Moreover, studies have not examined variations of virtual characters online and their effects on determinants of health behavior.

2   Research Question and Hypotheses

We investigated the following research question: *Which variation of the VRH has the most positive effect on motivation and intention to improve health behavior?*

We also aimed to understand which variation of the VRH do participants wish to see again and how satisfied participants were with the VRH.

In this study, health behavior refers to diet and physical activity behaviors. Further, following the terms and abbreviations coined by Bailenson et al., namely those of the 'virtual representation of one's physical self' (VRS) and the 'virtual representation of others' (VRO) [4], we use the term 'virtual representation of one's health' (VRH) to describe the personification of an individual's health in form of a virtual character. These terms are to be understood as clearly distinct from the notion of avatar.

To answer this research question, we developed a virtual character that reflects an individual's health status and health behavior, and tested its effects on motivation and intention through an experimental study with adults from three European countries.

2.1 Hypotheses

The related research presented above provides evidence of the value and feasibility of using virtual characters as representations of selves for health behavior change. Findings further imply that persuasiveness can be increased either by a strong visual similarity of the virtual representation and the physical person (i.e., model identification, see [7, 9]), or through mimicking of an individual's behavior (e.g. [1, 7]). We transfer this concept of mimicking that has been used for virtual representations of self (VRS) to a virtual representation of one's health (VRH).

Further, persuasiveness could be increased by displaying the future virtual self in an age –rendered process. As this has shown positive effects on motivating financial behavior about retirement savings [10], this could also motivate health behavior change. Thus, our hypotheses for this research were the following:

1. Viewing one's VRH juxtaposed to a possible future version and mimicking their health behavior has the most positive impact on motivation and intention to engage in (a) more physical activity and (b) a healthier diet.
2. All versions of the VRH will result in participants expressing motivation and intention to return to the VRH, but condition 4 will have the greatest positive effect on motivation and intention.
3. Users will be generally satisfied with using a VRH as a support mechanism for changing their health behavior and subsequent health status.

3   Virtual Representation of Health

The virtual representation – or personification – of one's health (VRH) was developed as a 3D virtual character in a WebGL canvas that can be embedded into any website. WebGL (Web Graphics Library) is the first graphics standard for the web, allows for fast, native 3D graphics in the browser, and is supported by all modern browsers. The VRH embeds the canvas in a regular web page, accompanied by textual explanations.

The development of the VRH was preceded by a pre-study that investigated *what health looks like*. In this pre-study, 172 adult participants from 11 countries were asked to describe the physical and behavioral characteristics of healthy and non-healthy people. These characteristics were used to inform the appearance of the VRH, including body posture, skin color, skin complexion, and body size.

The VRH is thus *not* a representation of an individual, but a personification of an individual's health status and health behavior. Data used to inform the appearance of the VRH in our experimental study were collected in a questionnaire taken just before exposure to the VRH and included height and weight, gender, last 7-day physical activity behavior and eating behavior. The VRH was developed in both male and female versions, each disposing of three different body shapes and three different poses or animations, as well as three different skin textures, for a total of 54 variations. The following subsections describe these three main dimensions of variation.

Body Shapes. The body shape of the VRH reflects the body mass index (BMI) of an individual. BMI is an indication of body fat. The VRH tool calculates the BMI from the height and weight (BMI = weight in kg divided by the squared height in m [12]) and categorizes BMI values below or equal to 25 as normal weight, values between 25 and 30 as overweight, and values of 30 and over as obese (for simplicity, this first prototype of the tool aggregates underweight into the normal BMI level).

Figure 1 illustrates the three different body shapes of the female VRH: the left image shows the normal body shape, the center image the overweight body shape, and the right image the obese body shape.

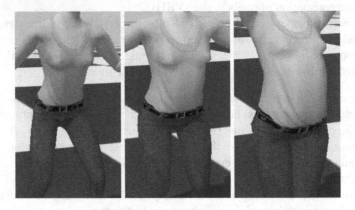

Fig. 1. Illustration of the normal (left), overweight (center), and obese (right) versions of the (female) VRH

Poses and Animations. The available poses and animations represent the level of physical activity of an individual. The VRH displays one of three different physical activity levels, ranging from sedentary to a very active level. The VRH illustrates the PA levels either as still poses or as continuously repeating animations. This feature was implemented in order to test the effects of an animated character against those of a still one (more details on the experiment design in the next section).

Informed by the findings of the pre-study on what health looks like, we modeled the inactive pose as a closed stance (i.e., crouching, bent back, bowed head), whereas for the active pose we modeled an open stance (i.e., open arms, straight back, steady on the legs). Similarly, the animated inactive PA level was modeled as slow sitting/crouched animation, whereas the active PA level was implemented as an energetic workout including push-ups, twists, and bends. For the average PA level the poses and animations were correspondingly averaged.

Skin Texture. The skin texture of the VRH conveys health status by means of three different manifestations of skin complexion and skin issues, based on the pre-study findings. We designed healthy skin as having a slightly sun-tanned complexion without notable skin blemishes. We rendered the unhealthy skin using a more colorless (i.e., pale) skin complexion and added wrinkles and rings under the eyes; we also desaturated the hair color. For the average skin level, the skin texture was averaged.

Figure 2 shows the different variations of skin complexions to personify health status. In order to ensure a visible effect, the different tones in skin complexion and the facial skin issues were exaggerated. This way, the changes are also visible on a fast-moving VRH (e.g. when the VRH performs a very active workout). A neutral face expression was used throughout all versions of the VRH.

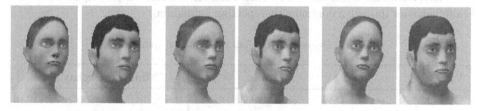

Fig. 2. Illustration of the healthy (left), average (center), and unhealthy (right) variations of the skin of the VRH, for both gender versions

4   Experimental Design

A controlled experiment was used to examine the effects of the different variations of the VRH on adults in three European countries. The objective was to investigate which variation of VRH has the most positive effects on an individual's motivation and intention to improve health behavior.

We implemented the experiment with the variation of the VRH as two between-subject factors, one being the variation of showing still or mimicking characters, the other the variation of displaying a possible future health status. The four experimental conditions were as follows: a VRH that does not model behavior or personify possible future health status (Exp1), a VRH that does not model behavior but personifies possible future health status (Exp2), a VRH that models behavior but does not personify changes in future health status (Exp3), and a VRH that both models behavior and personifies possible changes in health status (Exp4).

The following dependent variables were measured: motivation to engage in more PA, intention to engage in more PA, motivation to engage in a healthier diet, and intention to engage in a healthier diet. Each behavior was asked in reference to the coming week (e.g., motivation to engage in a healthier diet in the coming week). Further, we measured motivation and intention to access the VRH tool again.

4.1   Experimental Conditions

The four experimental conditions are illustrated in Table 1 using screenshots of the intervention participants were exposed to during the experiment.

We designed the first experimental condition (Exp1) as the simplest condition. In this condition, the VRH, representing a participant's health status, is displayed in a still pose, which models their health behavior.

Exp2 shows two virtual characters. On the left side of the screen, the personification of the current health status and behavior is shown, whereas on the right it shows the personification of a probable future health status, if the participant continues the current health behavior (self-reported PA and nutrition behavior). The body shape and skin complexion for the personification of a possible future health are calculated by the tool using a formula that factors in the reported levels of PA and nutrition behavior and decides which body shape and which skin complexion and facial issue level to apply for the personification of the estimated future health.

Instead of showing an additional personification of future health, Exp3 shows only one VRH, but an animated one – the virtual character models the participant's current health behavior through a continuously repeating animation.

Table 1. Overview of the four experimental conditions

VRH	Still pose	Mimicking behavior
No display of change of appearance	Exp1	Exp3
Displaying personification of possible future health status	Exp2	Exp4

Exp4 combines Exp2 and Exp3 and so displays two animated virtual characters side by side: the left VRH represents a participant's current health status and health behavior, while the right VRH represents a probable future, in case the participant continues their current health behavior (PA and nutrition). The body shape and skin complexion for the personification of the probable future health status are calculated by the tool as in Exp2, and the animation is the same for both present and future.

5   Measures

Participants completed both a pre and post-questionnaire immediately before and after exposure to the VRH. In the pre-test participants were asked for their age, gender, email, education level, country of origin, country of residency, height, and weight. They were also asked to report how many days in the last week they got at least 30 minutes of physical activity and how many days they met the guidelines for a healthy diet (with those guidelines displayed) in the last seven days. At both pre and post-test, participants were asked to state how motivated they were to improve each behavior (nut/PA) by choosing one point on a 7 point likert scale (from extremely motivated to not at all motivated). They were also asked if they intended to meet the recommendations for each health behavior on most days of the coming week, also using a 7 point likert scale ranging from completely disagree to completely agree. At post-test, participants were asked about their motivation and intention to access the VRH tool again as well as to provide feedback about their satisfaction with and thoughts about the VRH tool.

6   Participant Recruitment and Procedures

Participants. The participants were recruited online through an online recruitment agency and participation in the study was voluntary. The study respects professional code of conduct and research ethics. The eligible population was composed by individuals with the following characteristics:

- Interested in improving their physical activity and/or nutrition behavior
- Ability to complete questionnaires in English
- Using a modern web browser supporting WebGL (e.g. Firefox, Chrome, Maxthon, etc.); participants were asked to test their browser prior to taking part in the study

A total of 512 adults participated in the study (186 from Germany, 177 from Poland, and 149 from the UK). There were 293 men and 219 women with a mean age of 33 years. 55% were of healthy weight, 28% overweight, 11% obese, and 6% underweight. In Europe, approximately 50% of adults are overweight or obese [14].

Procedure. The experimental study was conducted fully online. The VRH was embedded in a webpage between the pre- and post-questionnaires. After a browser compatibility test was conducted and after the individual confirmed their informed consent, participants were asked to complete the baseline (pre-test) questionnaire. Upon completion of the pre-test, they were randomly assigned to one of the four experimental conditions.

The intervention itself, the exposure to the VRH, which was constructed using information the participant had reported in the pre-test (height, weight, gender, and past 7-day PA and nutrition behavior). On average, participants viewed their VRH(s) for just over 1 minute. After the exposure the participant was asked to fill in the post-test.

7   Results

For data analysis, we conducted paired t-tests and F tests, both showing the same results. We ran comparison tests using a true latent score with 15% assumed measurement error, allowing for pairwise comparisons between conditions and the results of our reported paired t-tests were confirmed.

7.1   Motivation and Intention to Improve Health Behavior

Results of paired t-tests showed significant positive changes in motivation to be more physically active for participants in all conditions. There were significant, positive changes for participants in Exp2, Exp3, and Exp4. Exp4 showed the most positive and most significant effects overall. Paired t-tests showed that the pre-post changes in motivation to improve nutrition behavior were positive and significant only for participants in Exp4. Those in Exp2 and Exp3 also showed positive changes, but were not statistically significant. Exp1 reported a non-significant decrease in nutrition motivation. For intention to improve their nutrition behavior the next week, all experimental conditions showed positive and significant changes. Exp4 showed the largest positive change. Additionally significant differences in changes were found for all pairwise comparisons except Exp4-Exp3. While Figure 3 presents a means comparison of the change (pre- to post-exposure) in motivation and intention to engage in (a) more PA and (b) a healthier diet, Table 2 reprints the t-values from the conducted tests, indicating significance levels.

7.2   Motivation and Intention to Return to the VRH Tool

All Experimental groups showed a high level of motivation to return to the VRH tool again (mean of 5 to 5.5, out of 7-point scales). While there were no significant differences between groups or between genders in motivation to return to the VRH tool, there were differences between countries: UK participants had a significantly higher motivation to access the tool again than the German participants, which in turn had a significantly higher motivation than participants from Poland.

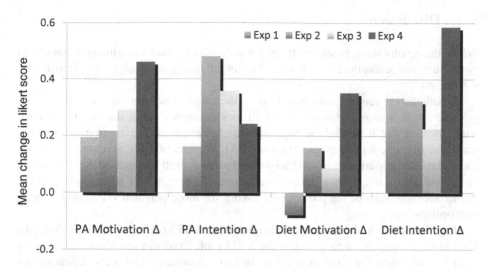

Fig. 3. Means comparison of the changes in motivation and intention to engage in more physical activity (left) and in a healthier diet (right)

Table 2. The t-values from the conducted paired t-tests

	Exp1 t(128)	Exp2 t(132)	Exp3 t(136)	Exp4 t(127)
Motivation to improve PA behavior	1.94, p=.05	2.32, p<.05	2.90, p<.01	3.81, p<.001
Intention to improve PA behavior	1.58, n.s.	4.54, p<.001	3.22, p<.001	1.97, p<.05
Motivation to improve nutrition behavior	-1.14, n.s.	1.72, n.s.	0.86, n.s.	3.94, p<.001
Intention to improve nutrition behavior	3.71, p<.001	3.60, p<.001	2.29, p<.05	5.55, p<.001

7.3   Satisfaction with the VRH Tool

Of the 512 participants, 362 provided qualitative feedback about the VRH tool. Overall, participants across countries and genders were satisfied with the tool. The majority of the comments (65%) provided suggest that the VRH was a "great idea", "innovative", "intriguing", "love it", and "helpful". 11% of the comments expressed negative impressions, including the VRH being "ugly", "robot-like" and not an accurate representation of themselves. Interestingly, and importantly, 9% of the respondents clearly showed that they identified with their VRH, by mentioning it as representing 'themselves' and using reflexive pronouns, (e.g., „am I that big", „cool seeing my prototype work out"). The comments did not notably differ between conditions.

8   Discussion

While the results show positive effects for all measures and experimental conditions (with just one exception, see Figure 3), not all positive changes are statistically significant.

Hypothesis H1 can be confirmed: Exp4 is the single condition for which significant positive changes were measured across all four outcomes. Also, the means comparisons illustrate that it yielded the largest positive changes, with exception of one measurement (the intention to engage in more PA). We identify this as a tendency that a more elaborate variation of a VRH might lead to an overall stronger positive effect for health behavior change than simpler variations. This argument is supported by the numerous comments of the participants asking for more personalization and interaction options.

Hypothesis H2 can be partially confirmed: while all Experimental groups showed a high level of motivation to return to the VRH tool, Exp4 did not show significantly higher results than the other conditions. In fact, measured differences depending on country of residence imply that the popularity, or success, of such a tool might depend more on culture than on its features in detail.

Regarding H3, the mostly positive feedback left by the participants suggests that users are generally satisfied with using a VRH. This finding, however, should be treated with caution, as it reflects a snapshot after a brief first exposure to a VRH. In order to draw more generic conclusions, a longitudinal study will be required.

8.1   Limitations

One of the major limitations of this study is the fact that the tested prototype exclusively uses body mass index to understand the body shape of a user. BMI is a vague measurement method to classify a person into the underweight, normal weight, overweight, and obese categories, but it is not accurate for muscular bodies. People with a significant amount of muscular mass are mistakenly classified as overweight or obese. This shortcoming of the BMI approach is where the most negative comments received from participants stem from, and could be eradicated by supporting the BMI measurement with a visual selection of body shapes, out of which the user could pick the one most similar to their actual body shape.

In this study, we exclusively modeled physical activity behavior (exercise) and did not model nutrition behavior, by for example, having the VRH eat different types of food for the different nutrition behavior levels (e.g. a healthy salad vs. unhealthy fries). This shortcoming of the current study should be considered in the design of future studies.

Finally, the lack of a control condition is another limitation of this study. While our aim to understand the differing effects of four versions of a VHR did not require a control condition, the lack of a control group prohibits understanding the magnitude of the effects of viewing a VRH at all. Future investigations will include a control condition so to address this research question.

9   Conclusion

We have presented an experimental study that investigated the effects of a customized virtual character – serving as a personified representation of an individual's health – on the participants' motivation and intention to improve their health behavior. We have also described our developed prototype in detail.

While the experiment did not provide empirical evidence to fully confirm all hypotheses, the results suggest that the approach is worthwhile for further investigation. Two main tendencies, the juxtaposition of a present with a possible future VRH and the elaboration of the VRH using tailored animations both show promise to improve two antecedents of behavior change, that is motivation and intention. In other words, the results of this study imply that visually displaying one's current VRH and the future VRH side by side serve best as triggers to motivate change. This goes in line with the literature on tailoring health communication, which shows that individualized communication that is interactive and gives feedback can be effective in influencing motivation and intention to change health behaviors [13, 11].

10   Future Work

The results of the experiment and the comments of the participants are encouraging for further development of the prototype and investigations in various directions. Future studies should investigate the following research questions:

- Does personifying an individual's health (i.e., using a VRH) have a more positive impact on health behavior than visualizing a virtual representation or doppelgänger of an individual (VRS)?
- Do individuals perceive the virtual characters as representations of health or as representations of themselves? What are the distinguishing factors?
- Is mimicking better for PA behavior or for nutrition behavior?
- How far into the future should possible health status portray to be effective at motivating change?
- How much personalization is needed to initiate change, improve motivation and intention and keep people engaged?
- How much interaction is most effective for behavior change?
- How much gaming (incentives, rewards, feedback) is effective, if at all?
- How well can the concept of anticipated effect be used as a determinant of behavior change?

For future studies we plan to gather data from larger samples and in more countries. We also plan to include more qualitative data, so to better understand the strengths and weaknesses of the approach. We also plan to examine the effects of VRH on actual behavior change using objective measures.

Acknowledgements. This study was funded by Merck & Co., Inc. The authors thank in particular Per Andersen and Alan Lowenstein and his team for their collaboration. We further thank Dr. Emil Coman for the great help in analyzing the results.

References

1. Abraham, C., Michie, S.: A taxonomy of behavior change techniques used in interventions. Health Psychology 3, 379–387 (2008)
2. Ajzen, I.: The Theory of Planned Behavior. Organizational Behavioral and Human Decision Processes 50, 179–211 (1991)
3. Bailenson, J.N., Yee, N.: Digital Chameleons: Automatic assimilation of non-verbal gestures in immersive virtual environments. Psychological Science 16, 814–819 (2005)
4. Bailenson, J.N., Blascovich, J., Guadagno, R.E.: Self-representations in im-mersive virtual environments. Journal of Applied Social Psychology 38(11), 2673–2690 (2008)
5. Baylor, A.L.: Promoting motivation with virtual agents and avatars: role of visual presence and appearance. Phil. Trans. R. Soc. B 364, 3559–3565 (2009)
6. Fjeldsoe, B.S., Marshall, A.L., Miller, Y.D.: Behavior Change Interventions Delivered by Mobile Telephone Short-Message Service. Am. J. Prev. Med. 6(2), 165–173 (2009)
7. Fox, J., Bailenson, J.N.: Virtual self-modeling: The effects of vicarious rein-forcement and identification on exercise behaviors. Media Psychology 12, 1–25 (2009)
8. Fox, J., Bailenson, J.N., Binney, J.: Virtual experiences, physical behaviors: The effect of presence on imitation of an eating avatar. PRESENCE: Teleoperators & Virtual Environments 18(4), 294–303 (2009)
9. Fox, J., Bailenson, J.N.: The use of doppelgängers to promote health behavior change. CyberTherapy & Rehabilitation 3(2), 16–17 (2010)
10. Hershfield, H.E., Goldstein, D.G., Sharpe, W.F., Fox, J., Yeykelis, L., Car-stensen, L.L., Bailenson, J.N.: Increasing saving behavior through age-progressed renderings of the future self. Journal of Marketing Research 48, S23–S37 (2011)
11. Krebs, P., Prochaskab, J.O., Rossi, J.S.: Preventive Medicine 51(3-4), 214–221 (2008)
12. National Health Service UK. How can I work out my body mass index (BMI) (2014), http://www.nhs.uk/chq/Pages/how-can-i-work-out-my-bmi.aspx
13. Noar, Benac, Harris: Does Tailoring Matter? Meta-Analytic Review of Tai-lored Print Health Behavior Change Interventions. Psychological Bulletin 133(4), 673–693 (2007)
14. OECD. Health at a Glance: Europe 2012: Overweight and obesity among adults (2012), http://dx.doi.org/10.1787/888932704076
15. Webb, T.L., Joseph, J., Yardley, L., Michie, S.: Using the internet to promote health behavior change: a systematic review and meta-analysis of the impact of theo-retical basis, use of behavior change techniques, and mode of delivery on effi-cacy. Journal of Medical Internet Research 12(1) (2010)

Appendix: Questionnaires

Pre-survey (1/4)

Please answer the following questions honestly.

   1. Email:

   2. Age:

   3. Are you? ☐ Male ☐ Female

   4. In what country were you born?

   5. In what country do you live now?

   6. What is your highest level of education attained so far?

   7. Height: m   -or-   ft in

   8. Weight: kg   -or-   st lb

Physical Activity

Adults should aim to be active daily. It is recommended to do at least 30 minutes of moderate physical activity on at least 5 days a week. Moderate-intensity physical activity requires a moderate amount of effort and noticeably accelerates the heart rate and moderately increases the breathing rate.

   9. In the last 7 days, how many days did you engage in physical activity?

   0 ☐   1 ☐   2 ☐   3 ☐   4 ☐   5 ☐   6 ☐   7 ☐

Thinking about the coming week (<u>next</u> 7 days), how would you answer the following questions?

10. I intend to meet the recommendations for weekly PA this coming week.

completely   ☐   ☐   ☐   ☐   ☐   ☐   ☐   *completely*
disagree   *agree*

11. Currently, how motivated are you to meet the recommendations for weekly PA this coming week?

not at all   ☐   ☐   ☐   ☐   ☐   ☐   ☐   *extremely*
motivated   *motivated*

Diet

A healthy diet is defined as follows:
• 1.5-2 liters of *liquid*, preferably water, and avoiding sugared drinks • 3 or more portions of *vegetables* • 2 or more portions of *fruit* • 3 portions of *flour products*, preferably whole grain • 2-3 portions of *milk and dairy* (unless vegan diet is followed) • 1 portions of meat, fish, egg, or other *protein* sources (tofu, corn) • 2-3 tsp. of olive oil, canola oil, or butter • In moderation: sweets, sugared drinks, alcohol, salted snacks

12. In the <u>last</u> 7 days, how many days did you come close to meeting the above <u>dietary</u> recommendations?

0 ☐   1 ☐   2 ☐   3 ☐   4 ☐   5 ☐   6 ☐   7 ☐

Thinking about the coming week (<u>next</u> 7 days), how would you answer the following questions?

13. I intend to meet the recommendations for a healthy diet on most days this coming week

completely   ☐   ☐   ☐   ☐   ☐   ☐   ☐   *completely*
disagree   *agree*

14. How motivated are you to meet the recommendations for a healthy diet on most days in this coming week

not at all   ☐   ☐   ☐   ☐   ☐   ☐   ☐   *extremely*
motivated   *motivated*

Pre-survey (2/4)

Please answer the following questions honestly.

15. To what extent do you agree with the following statements?

| In un-certain times, I usually expect the best. | *com-pletely disagree* | ☐ ☐ ☐ ☐ ☐ ☐ ☐ | *com-pletely agree* |

| It's easy for me to relax. | *com-pletely disagree* | ☐ ☐ ☐ ☐ ☐ ☐ ☐ | *com-pletely agree* |

| If some-thing can go wrong for me it will. | *com-pletely disagree* | ☐ ☐ ☐ ☐ ☐ ☐ ☐ | *com-pletely agree* |

| I am always optimis-tic about my future. | *com-pletely disagree* | ☐ ☐ ☐ ☐ ☐ ☐ ☐ | *com-pletely agree* |

| I enjoy my friends a lot. | *com-pletely disagree* | ☐ ☐ ☐ ☐ ☐ ☐ ☐ | *com-pletely agree* |

| It's im-portant for me to keep busy. | *com-pletely disagree* | ☐ ☐ ☐ ☐ ☐ ☐ ☐ | *com-pletely agree* |

I hardly ever expect things to go my way.

com-pletely disagree ☐ ☐ ☐ ☐ ☐ ☐ ☐ *com-pletely agree*

I don't get up-set too easily.

com-pletely disagree ☐ ☐ ☐ ☐ ☐ ☐ ☐ *com-pletely agree*

I rarely count on good things happen-ing to me.

com-pletely disagree ☐ ☐ ☐ ☐ ☐ ☐ ☐ *com-pletely agree*

Overall, I expect more good things to happen to me than bad.

com-pletely disagree ☐ ☐ ☐ ☐ ☐ ☐ ☐ *com-pletely agree*

Pre-survey (3/4)

Please answer the following question honestly.

16. How do you perceive yourself regarding the following attributes?

Try to describe yourself as accurately as possible. Describe yourself on the following scales as you see yourself at the present time, not as much as you wish to be in the future. Describe yourself as you are generally or typically, as compared with other people you know of the same sex and of roughly your age

silent	☐	☐	☐	☒	☐	☐	☐	*talkative*
unassertive	☐	☐	☐	☒	☐	☐	☐	*assertive*
unadventurous	☐	☐	☐	☒	☐	☐	☐	*adventurous*
unenergetic	☐	☐	☐	☒	☐	☐	☐	*energetic*
timid	☐	☐	☐	☒	☐	☐	☐	*bold*
unkind	☐	☐	☐	☒	☐	☐	☐	*kind*
uncooperative	☐	☐	☐	☒	☐	☐	☐	*cooperative*
selfish	☐	☐	☐	☒	☐	☐	☐	*unselfish*
distrustful	☐	☐	☐	☒	☐	☐	☐	*trustful*
stingy	☐	☐	☐	☒	☐	☐	☐	*generous*
disorganized	☐	☐	☐	☒	☐	☐	☐	*organized*
irresponsible	☐	☐	☐	☒	☐	☐	☐	*responsible*
impractical	☐	☐	☐	☒	☐	☐	☐	*practical*

careless	☐	☐	☐	◉	☐	☐	☐	thorough
lazy	☐	☐	☐	◉	☐	☐	☐	hardworking
relaxed	☐	☐	☐	◉	☐	☐	☐	tense
at ease	☐	☐	☐	◉	☐	☐	☐	nervous
stable	☐	☐	☐	◉	☐	☐	☐	unstable
contented	☐	☐	☐	◉	☐	☐	☐	discontented
unemotional	☐	☐	☐	◉	☐	☐	☐	emotional
unimaginative	☐	☐	☐	◉	☐	☐	☐	imaginative
uncreative	☐	☐	☐	◉	☐	☐	☐	creative
inquisitive	☐	☐	☐	◉	☐	☐	☐	curious
unreflective	☐	☐	☐	◉	☐	☐	☐	reflective
unsophisti-cated	☐	☐	☐	◉	☐	☐	☐	sophisti-cated

Pre-survey (4/4)

Please answer the following questions honestly.

Internet & Technology
17. How would you describe your Internet use?
Please tell us to what extent the following statements describe you well.

18. When I get a new electronic device, I usually need someone to set it up or show me how to use it.

completely disagree ☐   ☐   ☐   ☐   *completely agree*

19. I often feel annoyed by having to respond to intrusions from my electronic devices.

completely disagree ☐   ☐   ☐   ☐   *completely agree*

20. How much, if at all, have communication and information devices improved the following?

The way you pursue your hobbies or interests	*not at all*	☐	☐	☐	☐	☐	☐	☐	*a lot*
Your ability to do your job	*not at all*	☐	☐	☐	☐	☐	☐	☐	*a lot*
Your ability to learn new things	*not at all*	☐	☐	☐	☐	☐	☐	☐	*a lot*
Your ability to keep in touch with friends and family	*not at all*	☐	☐	☐	☐	☐	☐	☐	*a lot*

Your ability to share ideas and creations with others	*not at all*	☐	☐	☐	☐	☐	☐	☐	*a lot*
Your ability to work/collaborate with others	*not at all*	☐	☐	☐	☐	☐	☐	☐	*a lot*
Keeping a good (or improving your) health behavior	*not at all*	☐	☐	☐	☐	☐	☐	☐	*a lot*

Post-survey

Now that you have viewed your digital persona, please answer to the following final questions.

Physical Activity

> Adults should aim to be active daily. It is recommended to do at least 30 minutes of moderate physical activity on at least 5 days a week. Moderate-intensity physical activity requires a moderate amount of effort and noticeably accelerates the heart rate and moderately increases the breathing rate.

Thinking about the coming week (next 7 days), how would you answer the following questions?

1. I intend to meet the recommendations for weekly PA this coming week.

completely   ☐   ☐   ☐   ☐   ☐   ☐   ☐   *completely*
disagree   *agree*

2. Currently, how motivated are you to meet the recommendations for weekly PA this coming week?

not at all   ☐   ☐   ☐   ☐   ☐   ☐   ☐   *extremely*
motivated   *motivated*

Diet

> A healthy diet is defined as follows:
> - 1.5-2 liters of liquid, preferably water, and avoiding sugared drinks
> - 3 or more portions of vegetables
> - 2 or more portions of fruit
> - 3 portions of flour products, preferably whole grain
> - 2-3 portions of milk and dairy (unless vegan diet is followed)
> - 1 portions of meat, fish, egg, or other protein sources (tofu, corn)
> - 2-3 tsp. of olive oil, canola oil, or butter
> - In moderation: sweets, sugared drinks, alcohol, salted snacks

Thinking about the coming week (next 7 days), how would you answer the following questions?

3. I intend to meet the recommendations for a healthy diet on most days this coming week.

completely   ☐   ☐   ☐   ☐   ☐   ☐   ☐   *completely*
disagree   *agree*

4. How motivated are you to meet the recommendations for a healthy diet on most days in this coming week?

not at all   ☐   ☐   ☐   ☐   ☐   ☐   ☐   *extremely*
motivated   *motivated*

Digital Persona

If given the opportunity to see your Digital Persona again in one week, how would you answer the following questions?

5. I intent to come back to this site again next week and view changes in my Digital Persona.

completely   ☐   ☐   ☐   ☐   ☐   ☐   ☐   *completely*
disagree   *agree*

6. How motivated are you to come back to this website again and view changes in your digital persona?

not at all   ☐   ☐   ☐   ☐   ☐   ☐   ☐   *extremely*
motivated   *motivated*

7. Please share your impressions about the Digital Persona with us.

8. Do you have any suggestions for the further development of the Digital Persona?

Using Social Influence for Motivating Customers to Generate and Share Feedback

Agnis Stibe and Harri Oinas-Kukkonen

Oulu Advanced Research on Software and Information Systems
Department of Information Processing Science
P.O. Box 3000, FI-90014 University of Oulu, Finland
{agnis.stibe,harri.oinas-kukkonen}@oulu.fi

Abstract. A combination of high tech environments and social influence concepts holds great potential to positively effect behaviors and attitudes of individuals. Drawing upon socio-psychological theories, this study explores how social influence design principles change customer engagement in sharing feedback. For that purpose, an information system consisting of social influence design principles was implemented on situated displays and examined with 77 Twitter users. The results reveal interplay between the design principles and their capacity to explain 52% of the variance in perceived persuasiveness of the system, which can further predict 40% of the variance in behavioral intention of participants to provide feedback through the system in the future. The findings could be instrumental in progress towards a richer understanding of how to further harness social influence for customer engagement through socio-technical environments and how it effects the development of novel persuasive systems.

Keywords: Customer engagement, social influence, persuasive systems design.

1   Introduction

Customers experience greater engagement with organizations when they are able to exchange feedback. It creates a sense of community that encourages open communications [17]. In turn, emerging technologies empower businesses to approach customers in innovative ways [24]. The social web provides the necessary infrastructure for such interaction, and mobile devices enable organizations to gather customer feedback [23]. For example, situated displays nowadays are increasingly entering public places and are being used to draw peoples' attention [12], while individuals evidently use their social media accounts on smart computing devices to interact with them. Such environments create opportunities for ongoing interaction at almost any location [2]. The integral parts of these technology-enhanced environments are information systems that are linked with social media and designed for large displays to support the aforementioned interactivity. Now, the real challenge would be to design operational software features that encourage customer engagement in this kind of setting.

According to Oinas-Kukkonen and Harjumaa [22], information systems can facilitate social influence when augmented with relevant persuasive principles. This

A. Spagnolli et al. (Eds.): PERSUASIVE 2014, LNCS 8462, pp. 224–235, 2014.
© Springer International Publishing Switzerland 2014

implies that people in public places could experience social influence not only from others around them, but equally through information systems that are equipped with persuasive design principles. Furthermore, persuasive systems could be classified as social actors [10], and would therefore be capable of retaining their social influence potential even in the absence of other people. Such persuasive systems are helpful in facilitating behavioral and attitudinal change within the novel social context described earlier. For example, publicly displayed systems (screens) could harness social influence design principles to engage people in generating and sharing feedback.

Earlier research about similar environments merely concentrates either on interaction through public screens [21] or on behavior changes urged by interactive environments [18]. There is a need to gain deeper knowledge about how social influence could be further harnessed to engage people through publically displayed systems. Accordingly, the present study attempts to answer the following research question:

RQ: How can social influence design principles persuade people to engage with publically displayed systems that are integrated with social media?

According to Chatterjee and Price [4], studying the ability of persuasive technologies to engage users is a pivotal future research direction. The objective of the present study is to examine how social influence design principles affect the perceived persuasiveness of a publicly displayed system and the behavioral intention of users to engage with it in the future. For that purpose, an information system composed of social influence design principles was developed and empirically examined with 77 Twitter users. The results reveal that the design principles are intricately interconnected and altogether they can explain more than half of the variance in the persuasiveness of the system, which can further predict forty percent of the variance in the behavioral intention of participants to provide feedback through the system in the future.

2   Background

Social influence has a long history in the field of psychology research, where it encompasses several forms of potential influences on human behaviors by way of the actual, imagined, or implied presence of others [26]. Historically, social influence has often been associated with compliance, identification, internalization, obedience, and persuasion, although it is considered distinct from conformity, power, and authority. Current research on social influence falls mainly under areas of minority influence in group settings, dynamic social impact theory, social influence in expectation states theory, and persuasion [5, 6]. The latter is broadly defined as changes in behaviors or attitudes due to information received from others. It focuses on the interaction between source and recipient, thus underpins the theoretical background for this study.

In line with the socio-technical context of this study, Fogg [10] suggests that computers are effective persuaders because of their capacity to maintain a high level of interactivity and adjust influence strategies as situations develop. In addition, they can be more persistent and be accessed ubiquitously. Technologies typically do not seek to influence users on their own, but, through services that can be designed on top of them, they facilitate and simplify the behavior change process.

3   Social Influence Design Principles

As an extension of Fogg's [10] work on persuasive technologies, Oinas-Kukkonen and Harjumaa [22] proposed the Persuasive Systems Design model, which describes the key issues, the process model, and the design principles for developing and evaluating persuasive information systems. The model has previously been examined in various contexts. However, there is limited knowledge about the relations between the model's seven design principles, listed under the social support category [14]. For this research, all seven principles were considered, based on the study context.

Social science theories related to persuasion suggest multiple sources of reference for every social influence design principle that is proposed by the model. When people use information about others to evaluate themselves, they engage in social comparison [9]. More precisely, social comparison is defined as the process of thinking about others in relation to the self [33]. This process influences motivation, as people look for self-enhancement when comparing themselves with others who are worse off, or they look for self-improvement when seeking a positive example for comparison [32].

The influence of others also leads people to conform in order to be liked and accepted [7]. This specific human behavior is guided by perceptions of the popularity of certain behaviors, that is, by social norms. Studies emphasize that both injunctive and descriptive norms are particularly effective in altering peoples' behaviors and attitudes. Injunctive norms inform people about what ought to be done, whereas descriptive norms refer to what most people actually do [5].

Interpersonal factors of cooperation, competition, and recognition provide important intrinsic motivations that would not be present in the absence of other people [16]. Competition and cooperation are directed toward the same social end by at least two individuals [19]. On a social level, people cooperate when they are striving to achieve the same goals or are working together, but compete when they are trying to achieve the same goal that is scarce or are seeking to gain what others are endeavoring to gain at the same time [20]. With independent tasks, combining the scores of different people can encourage cooperation, but providing some salient metric for people to compare their performances could promote competition [16]. Next, recognition could be experienced after competing or cooperating with others [28] or can simply be enjoyed when gaining acceptance and approval from others.

Within a social context, people learn from others by observing their behaviors [3]. This implies that the transmission of information from one individual to another happens through imitation, teaching, and spoken or written language. According to Bandura [3], social learning is ubiquitous and potent because it allows people to avoid the costs of individual learning.

Finally, the mere or imagined presence of people in social situations creates an atmosphere of evaluation, which enhances the performance, speed, and accuracy of well-practiced tasks, but reduces the performance of less familiar tasks. These social facilitation effects occur in the presence of both passive onlookers and people who are actively engaged in the same activity [34].

4   Research Hypotheses and Methodology

The review of related theoretical foundations demonstrates that all seven social influence design principles embrace, in one form or the other, an effect on human attitude and behavior. Attitude, according to Ajzen [1], is defined as peoples' positive or negative feelings about performing a target behavior, and it is the central perspective that must be considered when reflecting on persuasion, as it represents an evaluative integration of cognitions and affects [6]. This implies that peoples' attitudes towards generating and sharing feedback, that is, towards the perceived persuasiveness [15] of the system in this study, are altered by social influence design principles. Thus, hypothesis H1 is formulated for this study as follows: *Social influence design principles positively affect perceived persuasiveness.*

Furthermore, Ajzen [1] suggests that peoples' attitudes towards behaviors are primary determinants of their behavioral intentions and are immediate and important predictors of their actual behavior. This means that people are likely to also share feedback in the future if they retain or develop a positive attitude towards such contribution behavior through persuasive experiences. Thus, hypothesis H2 is formulated as follows: *Perceived persuasiveness positively affects behavioral intention.*

To explore the hypothesized effects of social influence on human attitude and behavior, a persuasive system (hereinafter, the system) was developed with all seven social influence design principles (hereinafter, features) at its core. The system was integrated with Twitter, a popular micro-blogging social media platform that has been found to influence actions outside the virtual world [29].

According to the specified context of the present study, the system was designed for projection on large public screen displays, with an aim to engage users in generating and sharing feedback. Its interface attracted peoples' attention by posing questions at the top of the display (Fig. 1), and users were able to provide feedback using Twitter messages, that is, tweets. As people started using the system, it automatically showed all updates on the screen display, so everyone could follow their own actions and what others were tweeting.

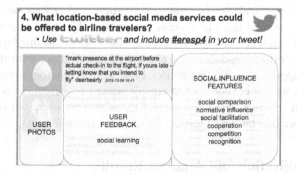

Fig. 1. System display

Feedback provided by users was displayed in the form of a newsfeed on the left side of the display. This feature provided a means for social learning, as it allowed users to observe how others generated tweets and to continuously learn from that [3]. On the right side of the display, the remaining six social influence features were implemented (Fig. 2), rotating in 15-second intervals when the system was used.

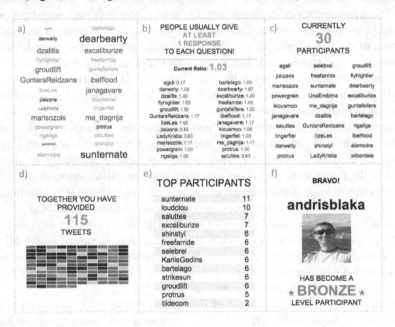

Fig. 2. Social influence features: a) social comparison, b) normative influence, c) social facilitation, d) cooperation, e) competition, and f) recognition

Initially, all features were blank, and, after the first successful tweet, they began to operate and form patterns. Based on the number of tweets provided by each individual, their usernames a) grew in size and changed color to enable social comparison; e) were arranged hierarchically to facilitate competition; and f) were accompanied with their pictures and special titles to express recognition. The total number of provided tweets, that is, of generated and shared feedback messages, was displayed as the result of d) cooperative efforts; and the total number of contributors with their usernames were listed to support c) social facilitation. Finally, b) injunctive norm was provided in the form of a statement (above) and complemented by calculations representing a descriptive norm (below). The implemented features were pretested by three groups of people to assure that they emphasized the intended meaning.

5   Data Collection and Analysis Results

The system was demonstrated in several seminars both in Latvia and Finland. The demonstrations were performed to empirically test the effect of the designed social influence features. Prior to the demonstrations, the participants were provided a brief description of the system and advised that participation was not obligatory. In all, 77 participants volunteered and used the system. After each demonstration, users filled out an online questionnaire about their experiences using seven-point Likert-type scale indicators (Appendix A). The gender distribution of the participants was 57% female and 43% male. The majority of participants were 25–34 years old (53%), with the next largest group being 35–44 years old (29%).

The collected data was analyzed with partial least squares structural equation modeling (PLS-SEM) using WarpPLS 4.0 software. This method was selected because it is well suited to exploratory research and is appropriate when the purpose of the research is to predict rather than to test established theory [11]. Data analysis with PLS-SEM includes both assessment of the reliability and validity of the measurement model and assessment of the structural model. The measurement model includes the relationships between the constructs (Table 1) and the indicators used to measure them (Appendix A). The measurement instrument for this study was developed based on the theory-driven items, which were pretested with four scholars from the same field of research before the study. Further, the properties of the scales were assessed in terms of item loadings, discriminant validity, and internal consistency, where item loadings and internal consistencies greater than .70 are considered acceptable.

Table 1. Latent variable coefficients and correlations

	COR	CR	AV	VIF	SL	SC	NI	SF	C	CT	RE	PP	BI
SL	.84	.73	.64	1.3	**.80**								
SC	.84	.72	.64	1.5	.05	**.80**							
NI	.89	.82	.73	1.8	.31	.18	**.86**						
SF	.84	.71	.63	1.2	.17	.39	.20	**.79**					
CR	.85	.74	.66	1.6	.33	.19	.54	.16	**.81**				
CT	.87	.78	.69	1.8	.19	.46	.23	.25	.29	**.83**			
RE	.87	.77	.69	1.5	.16	.32	.31	.17	.30	.47	**.83**		
PP	.86	.76	.68	2.5	.42	.12	.58	.17	.50	.45	.31	**.82**	
BI	.96	.94	.90	1.9	.37	.07	.49	.20	.38	.30	.42	.62	**.95**

COR = Composite Reliability; CRA = Cronbach's Alpha; VIF = variance inflation factor (full collinearity); Bolded diagonal = square root of Average Variance Extracted (AVE)

The constructs in the model display good internal consistency, as evidenced by their composite reliability scores, which range from .84 to .96. Inspection of the latent variable correlations and square root of the average variance extracted (AVE) in Table 1 demonstrate that all constructs share more variance with their own indicators than with other constructs, demonstrating adequate internal consistency.

To explore how the designed social influence features affect the perceived persuasiveness of the system, the structural model for this study (Fig. 3) originated from and was shaped upon the strongest correlations between constructs that were observable from the measurement model (Table 1). In the analysis of the model, a PLS mode M regression algorithm was used, in which the measurement model weights are calculated through a least squares regression, where the latent variable score is the predictor and the indicators are the criteria [13]. In addition, the jackknifing resampling procedure was applied to test the significance of the path coefficients.

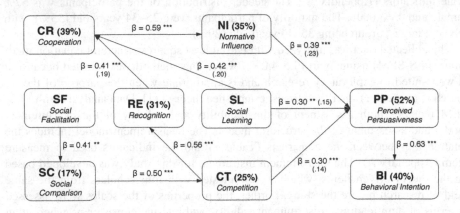

Fig. 3. The structural model with results of PLS-SEM analysis

As can be observed from Figure 3, the results of the PLS-SEM analysis provide substantial support for the structural model. They reveal that the social influence features are intricately interconnected and that altogether they can explain 52% of the variance in perceived persuasiveness of the system, which can further predict 40% of the variance in the behavioral intention of participants to provide feedback through the system in the future. The main direct contributors to explain the variance in perceived persuasiveness were found to be normative influence (23%), social learning (15%), and competition (14%). Social learning and recognition together can explain 39% of the variance in cooperation, which in turn can explain 35 % of the variance in normative influence. Social facilitation can explain 17% of the variance in social comparison, which can further explain 25% of the variance in competition, while it can explain 31% of the variance in recognition. Finally, the β values demonstrate the strength of relationships between the constructs and the asterisks mark their statistical significance, while the R-squared contributions are presented in brackets.

For a more elaborate view of the structural model, total effects and effect sizes for total effects are presented in Table 2. Effect sizes (f^2) determine whether the effects indicated by the path coefficients are small (.02), medium (.15), or large (.35). Additionally, the results of PLS-SEM analysis provide fit and quality indices that support the structural model [13]. Besides reporting the values of average path coefficient (APC = .450, p < .001) and average adjusted R-squared (AARS = .329, p < .001), the model demonstrates a large explanatory power (GoF = .486). Moreover, both Sympson's paradox ratio (SPR = 1.000) and the nonlinear bivariate causality direction ratio (NLBCDR = 1.000) provide evidence that the model is free from Sympson's paradox instances, and the direction of causality is supported.

Table 2. Total effects and effect sizes

	SF	SC	CT	RE	SL	CR	NI	PP
SC	.41** (.17)							
CT	.21** (.05)	.50*** (.25)						
RE	.11* (.02)	.28*** (.09)	.56*** (.31)					
CR	.05* (.01)	.11** (.02)	.23*** (.07)	.41*** (.19)	.42*** (.20)			
NI	.03* (.01)	.07** (.01)	.13** (.03)	.24*** (.07)	.25*** (.08)	.59*** (.35)		
PP	.07* (.01)	.18*** (.02)	.35*** (.16)	.09** (.03)	.40*** (.20)	.23*** (.12)	.39*** (.23)	
BI	.05* (.01)	.11*** (.01)	.22*** (.07)	.06** (.03)	.25*** (.09)	.15** (.06)	.25*** (.12)	.63*** (.40)

*** $p < .001$; ** $p < .01$; * $p < .05$; (f^2) = Cohen's f-squared
SF has no inbound arrows (row is empty) and BI has no outbound arrows (column is empty)

6   Discussion

The results of this study reveal the strength and prominence of social influence features in designing persuasive systems for user engagement in sharing feedback through situated displays. The findings provide empirical evidence for the pertinence of the research model, and therefore contribute to the existing body of knowledge.

It is remarkable to discover that the seven social influence design principles can explain more than half of the variance in the perceived persuasiveness of the system (supporting H1), which further can predict forty percent of the variance in the behavioral intention of participants to provide feedback through the system in the future (supporting H2). This implies that social influence design principles affect peoples' behaviors not only when they are using the system, but also affects their attitudes about their future behaviors, indicating that there is a long lasting effect. These findings demonstrate several advances compared to previous research in which, for example, only three features were explored and less variance was explained [30].

The main direct contributors to explain the variance in perceived persuasiveness were found to be normative influence, social learning, and competition. The effects of the first two design principles have been discovered and verified previously [30], while the latter adds another significant contribution that better explains the persuasiveness of the system. According to the relevant theories described earlier, all three design principles, namely social learning [3], normative influence [5, 7], and competition [16, 19, 20, 28], should promote favorable impressions of the given system; that is, they should influence how much people felt persuaded to engage in feedback generation and sharing, and this study confirms that.

The remaining four social influence design principles also indicate substantial effects on perceived persuasiveness, as can be observed from their total effects and effect sizes (Table 2). However, in contrast to the three aforementioned design principles, they correlated more with other design principles than with perceived persuasiveness (Table 1). Accordingly, it was found that cooperation [16, 19, 20, 28] correlates with and positively affects normative influence [5, 7]. This implies that people in novel contexts tend to acquire and shape social norms through ongoing cooperation [8], that is, through collective feedback generation and sharing, in this study. At the same time, people learn new behaviors by observing others [3]. So, if people can monitor how others contribute, they can learn new ways of collaborating in a certain social context. This explanation provides support for the direct positive effect of social learning on cooperation in the model. Concurrently, cooperation is also positively affected by recognition [16], as indicated in the model. This implies that people appreciate being recognized, which fosters their participation and contribution [25]. As such, recognition motivates individuals to produce more content, and therefore facilitates cooperative efforts.

In competition [16, 19, 20, 28], people strive to achieve more than others and, if successful, they can reach a level where their accomplishments are appreciated and recognized by others [16, 31]. People have a preference for general social recognition, which is scarce by nature, and intensified competition unsurprisingly drives people towards achieving it [27]. This explains the direct positive effect of competition on recognition in the model. Further, humans have a fundamental need to compare their behaviors with those of other people in order to evaluate their abilities and opinions [9, 32, 33]. Additionally, Festinger [9] suggested that social comparison leads to competition and not to matching when abilities and behaviors are evaluated. Consequently, this underpins the finding of a direct positive effect of social comparison on competition in previous studies [31] as well as in the present study. Additionally, the three theoretical concepts, namely, social comparison, competition, and recognition, are already intertwined on the conceptual level, as each of them enables people to determine their individual performance [27, 31], which is not explicitly inherent in the other constructs in the model (Fig. 3).

Finally, social facilitation was found to be in correlation with and to have a direct positive impact on social comparison, which could be explained by social facilitation theory [34], suggesting that people are influenced when surrounded by others. So, the larger the number of users interacting with the system, the more opportunities there are for people to compare their own behaviors with those of others. In summary, the present study revealed the strongest correlations between the seven social influence design principles and their predictive powers to account for the persuasiveness of the system. However, the obtained research model needs to be further investigated and tested in other settings and with various combinations of the design principles.

7   Conclusions

Studies presented in this paper are highly relevant, as they advance the design of future information systems. Along these lines, this study provides both researchers and practitioners with richer insights on how social influence principles could be designed as persuasive software features in information systems aimed at facilitating behavior change. Drawing upon socio-psychological theories and interconnecting them through the Persuasive Systems Design model [22], the paper explores the effects of social influence design principles on users of the system with respect to their engagement in feedback sharing through social media integrated with situated displays.

The main contributions of this study include the designed social influence features, and the developed measurement instrument and constituted research model, as they supplement the existing body of knowledge and could be instrumental for scholars focusing on research related to social influence effects on user behavior mediated by information systems. Limitations of the study include the setting, where users were able to watch others sharing feedback, and a relatively narrow sample size of respondents. Nevertheless, the obtained research model, the reviewed theoretical concepts, and the design of particular social influence features could be applied and tested in multiple contexts.

This study provides valuable input for further research related to social influence on user behavior and highlights several useful features for designers of persuasive systems. At the same time, organizations could gain direct benefits by designing and launching similar systems on their premises in order to collect feedback from their customers. For example, a screen in a coffee room could potentially engage employees to share feedback about concerns and ideas related to their work.

In the future, where countless screens are increasingly entering public places, including supermarkets, museums, hospitals, schools, restaurants, transportation spots, and even vehicles, such socio-technical systems could gradually become an integral part of these environments, providing a seamless and natural channel for businesses to engage with their customers. These channels could play a significant role in advancing customer relationships on the one hand, while increasing the amount of relevant feedback for organizations on the other, because they enable immediate interaction at the place where customers acquire new experiences about a certain service or product.

Acknowledgements. The authors would like to thank Payam Hossaini, Pasi Karppinen, Sitwat Langrial, Tuomas Lehto, Seppo Pahnila, Anssi Öörni, and collaboration partners Andris Blaka, Uldis Dzenis, Mārcis Ešmits, and Virpi Roto, who helped with this research. This is part of OASIS research group of Martti Ahtisaari Institute, University of Oulu. The study was partly supported by the Foundation of Nokia Corporation, as well as by the Someletti research project on Social Media in Public Space (grant 1362/31) and the SalWe Research Program for Mind and Body (grant 1104/10), both provided by Tekes, the Finnish Funding Agency for Technology and Innovation.

References

1. Ajzen, I.: The Theory of Planned Behavior. Organizational Behavior and Human Decision Processes 50(2), 179–211 (1991)
2. Alt, F., Shirazi, A.S., Kubitza, T., Schmidt, A.: Interaction Techniques for Creating and Exchanging Content with Public Displays. In: Proceedings of the SIGCHI Conference on Human Factors in Computing Systems, pp. 1709–1718. ACM (April 2013)
3. Bandura, A.: Social Foundations of Thought and Action: A Social Cognitive Theory. Prentice Hall, Englewood Cliffs (1986)

4. Chatterjee, S., Price, A.: Healthy Living with Persuasive Technologies: Framework, Issues, and Challenges. Journal of the American Medical Informatics Association 16(2), 171–178 (2009)
5. Cialdini, R.B., Kallgren, C.A., Reno, R.R.: A Focus Theory of Normative Conduct: A theoretical Refinement and Reevaluation of the Role of Norms in Human Behavior. Advances in Experimental Social Psychology 24(20), 1–243 (1991)
6. Crano, W.D., Prislin, R.: Attitudes and Persuasion. Annu. Rev. Psychol. 57, 345–374 (2006)
7. Deutsch, M., Gerard, H.B.: A Study of Normative and Informational Social Influences upon Individual Judgment. The Journal of Abnormal and Social Psychology 51(3), 629 (1955)
8. Fehr, E., Fischbacher, U.: Social Norms and Human Cooperation. Trends in Cognitive Sciences 8(4), 185–190 (2004)
9. Festinger, L.: A Theory of Social Comparison Processes. Human Relations 7(2), 117–140 (1954)
10. Fogg, B.J.: Persuasive Technology: Using Computers to Change What We Think and Do. Morgan Kaufmann, San Francisco (2003)
11. Hair, J.F., Ringle, C.M., Sarstedt, M.: PLS-SEM: Indeed a Silver Bullet. The Journal of Marketing Theory and Practice 19(2), 139–152 (2011)
12. Huang, E.M., Koster, A., Borchers, J.: Overcoming Assumptions and Uncovering Practices: When Does the Public Really Look at Public Displays? In: Indulska, J., Patterson, D.J., Rodden, T., Ott, M. (eds.) PERVASIVE 2008. LNCS, vol. 5013, pp. 228–243. Springer, Heidelberg (2008)
13. Kock, N.: WarpPLS 4.0 User Manual. ScriptWarp Systems, Laredo, TX (2013)
14. Langrial, S., Lehto, T., Oinas-Kukkonen, H., Harjumaa, M., Karppinen, P.: Native Mobile Applications for Personal Well-being: A Persuasive Systems Design Evaluation. In: Pacific Asia Conference on Information Systems (PACIS), p. 93 (2012)
15. Lehto, T., Oinas-Kukkonen, H., Drozd, F.: Factors Affecting Perceived Persuasiveness of a Behavior Change Support System. In: ICIS Proceedings, Orlando, Florida (2012)
16. Malone, T.W., Lepper, M.: Making Learning Fun: A Taxonomy of Intrinsic Motivations for Learning. In: Snow, R.E., Farr, M.J. (eds.) Aptitude, Learning and Instruction: III. Conative and Affective Process Analyses, pp. 223–253. Erlbaum, Hillsdale (1987)
17. Mangold, W.G., Faulds, D.J.: Social Media: The New Hybrid Element of the Promotion Mix. Business Horizons 52(4), 357–365 (2009)
18. Mathew, A.P.: Using the Environment as an Interactive Interface to Motivate Positive Behavior Change in a Subway Station. In: CHI 2005 Extended Abstracts on Human Factors in Computing Systems, pp. 1637–1640. ACM (April 2005)
19. May, M.A., Doob, L.W.: Cooperation and Competition. Social Science Research Council Bulletin 125 (1937)
20. Mead, M.: Cooperation and Competition among Primitive Peoples. McGraw-Hill, New York (1937)
21. Müller, J., Alt, F., Michelis, D., Schmidt, A.: Requirements and Design Space for Interactive Public Displays. In: Proceedings of the International Conference on Multimedia, pp. 1285–1294. ACM (2010)
22. Oinas-Kukkonen, H., Harjumaa, M.: Persuasive Systems Design: Key issues, Process Model, and System Features. Communications of the Association for Information Systems 24(1), 28 (2009)
23. Oinas-Kukkonen, H., Oinas-Kukkonen, H.: Humanizing the Web: Change and Social Innovation. Palgrave Macmillan, Basingstoke (2013)
24. Payne, A.F., Storbacka, K., Frow, P.: Managing the Co-creation of Value. Journal of the Academy of Marketing Science 36(1), 83–96 (2008)

25. Rafaeli, S., Ariel, Y.: Online Motivational Factors: Incentives for Participation and Contribution in Wikipedia (2008)
26. Rashotte, L.: Social Influence. The Blackwell Encyclopedia of Social Psychology 9, 562–563 (2007)
27. Rottiers, S.: The Sociology of Social Recognition: Competition in Social Recognition Games (No. 1004) (2010)
28. Schoenau-Fog, H.: Teaching Serious Issues through Player Engagement in an Interactive Experiential Learning Scenario. Eludamos. Journal for Computer Game Culture 6(1), 53–70 (2012)
29. Stibe, A., Oinas-Kukkonen, H., Bērziņa, I., Pahnila, S.: Incremental Persuasion Through Microblogging: A Survey of Twitter Users in Latvia. In: Proceedings of the 6th International Conference on Persuasive Technology: Persuasive Technology and Design: Enhancing Sustainability and Health, p. 8. ACM (2011)
30. Stibe, A., Oinas-Kukkonen, H., Lehto, T.: Exploring Social Influence on Customer Engagement: A Pilot Study on the Effects of Social Learning, Social Comparison, and Normative Influence. In: 46th Hawaii International Conference on System Sciences (HICSS), pp. 2735–2744. IEEE Press, New York (2013)
31. Vassileva, J.: Motivating Participation in Social Computing Applications: A User Modeling Perspective. User Modeling and User-Adapted Interaction 22(1-2), 177–201 (2012)
32. Wilson, S.R., Benner, L.A.: The Effects of Self-Esteem and Situation upon Comparison Choices During Ability Evaluation. Sociometry, 381–397 (1971)
33. Wood, J.V.: What is Social Comparison and How Should We Study It? Personality and Social Psychology Bulletin 22(5), 520–537 (1996)
34. Zajonc, R.B.: Social Facilitation. Science 149, 269–274 (1965)

Appendix A: Measurement Items and Combined Loadings

Constructs	Indicators	Load
Social Learning	The system helped me learn from others.	.810
	Observing tweets by others in the system helped me to learn from them.	.808
	I was able to learn from tweets sent by others.	.789
Social Comparison	I was able to compare others' performances in the system.	.869
	In the system, I noticed users with similar behaviors.	.720
	In the system, I was able to compare others based on their activity.	.798
Normative Influence	The system informed me about how most people behave.	.846
	The system displayed common patterns that people generally follow.	.844
	The system explained how people generally respond.	.879
Social Facilitation	I noticed others who were using the system.	.833
	In the system, I was able to observe others participating.	.739
	In the system, I could notice the number of others participants.	.806
Cooperation	The system allowed the users to cooperate.	.850
	The system showed me the results of cooperative efforts among users.	.748
	I noticed that the system enabled cooperation among users.	.834
Competition	The system allowed competition between the users.	.854
	The system stimulated its users to compete.	.859
	I noticed the results of competition among users in the system.	.776
Recognition	Users of the system were publicly recognized for their participation.	.894
	The system recognized its active participants publically.	.701
	I noticed public recognition of active users of the system.	.875
Perceived Persuasiveness	I felt motivated to engage with the system.	.806
	The system motivated me to participate.	.916
	The system influenced my thoughts while I was using/observing it.	.737
Behavioral Intention	I would be willing to try such a system in the future.	.967
	I would like to use the system in the future.	.942
	I would consider using the system in the future.	.932

Analyzing Non-Textual Arguments with Toulmin

Kristian Torning

Danish School of Media and Journalism,
Emdrupvej 72, DK-2400 Copenhagen
krt@dmjx.dk

Abstract. This paper seeks to advance existing research on persuasive design, opening up new research opportunities by addressing the notion of technology embedded arguments. The prevailing literature does not offer models for analyzing technology embedded arguments, and thus in order to explore some basic ideas on the analysis of arguments in technology, Toulmin's traditional argument pattern is used on two simple persuasive design examples. The main findings are: 1) it is difficult to analyze non-textual persuasive designs with Toulmin's pattern due to the less explicit nature of technology embedded arguments and 2) there are ethical implications if users cannot systematically assess the validity of technology embedded arguments.

Keywords: Persuasive design, technology embedded arguments, technology arguments, Toulmin's argument pattern, argument model.

1   Introduction

The goal of this paper is to take a first small step in theorizing about the contours of an argument model for persuasive designs, which is done by exploring the notion of non-textual technology embedded arguments as opposed to text based arguments. Currently we do not have models for analyzing non-textual technology embedded arguments. In this paper, as an explorative experiment, two persuasive design artifacts are examined using Stephen Toulmins' argument model [19], which is commonly used for analyzing textual communication. The paper is structured in three sections. First some background information is offered, secondly two designs are analyzed and lastly findings are discussed.

2   Background

Traditionally, when we speak of 'persuasion' the 'readers' (including 'listeners' and 'viewers') are persuaded by a deliberate message comprised of words containing an appeal in some form. Traditional arguments are thus textual. They are put forth in speech or writing using words. The most classical taxonomy of means of textual persuasion is comprised by rhetorical appeal, as defined by Aristoteles (/455 b.c.) [2]: logos (reason), pathos (abrupt emotion) or ethos (~credibility). Still to this day, it seems that these are the primary ways in which we influence humans. We may speak

A. Spagnolli et al. (Eds.): PERSUASIVE 2014, LNCS 8462, pp. 236–246, 2014.
© Springer International Publishing Switzerland 2014

to their minds offering reason, their hearts offering compassion or justice, or we can ask them to accept our claims with reference to some form of authority.

Seen from the textual perspective, the process of uttering persuasive communication may begin with crafting such appeals into 'symbols': "Coercion takes the form of guns or economic sanctions, while persuasion relies on the power of *verbal and nonverbal symbols*" [14] (emphasis added). Here, persuasion is anchored in a voluntary change of behavior or attitude. Viewed from this perspective, we can observe the 'speaker' as a person shaping and communicating textual 'symbols' with a clear intention and outcome in mind, and the 'listener' may then accept or reject his proposal. For thousands of years, we have been able to embed such symbols in speech and writing, employing context aware strategies for doing so (Aristotle, Cicero and Quintilian [10]).

Researchers and philosophers have created models for analyzing such symbolic transactions in order to assess the validity of, i.e., 'logos' appeals [19], [20]. When addressing an informed audience with speech or writing, listeners thus have the ability to evaluate the soundness of the reasoning, employing either common sense or the aforementioned models. For instance, when faced with a claim supported by logos, the audience might ask: "Based on what?" Requesting clarification for the backing of the claim, the listeners might assess whether the speaker's claim is indeed probable (logos) or they could question the authority (ethos) used to bolster the claim. In a similar manner, listeners might reject a pathos appeal if they do not find it moving. From this perspective, textual persuasion can be regarded as an inter-human symbolic transaction, where symbols are shaped by a 'speaker' who might (or might not) persuade listeners to change their behavior or attitude towards something. This is the essence of any rhetorical act.

Persuasive design has surfaced as an approach towards designing behavior changing technologies [4], [7], [8]. Persuasive design is marked by the explicit intention of the designers to change users' behaviors or attitudes in a deliberate fashion. The explicit aim is behavior transformation achieved by constructing either physical objects or software that, on behalf of the designer, persuade the user of a predetermined target behavior. Persuasive design is also a rhetorical act that takes the form of intentional symbolic transactions. Designers thus engage in a rhetorical act, as they craft designs with a predetermined outcome in mind. The effort is grounded in the designer's wish for causing a transformation in users − their act of design is intentional. The designer thus delegates the rhetorical act of persuasion to non-human entities. The most obvious difference between arguments embedded in text and arguments embedded in technologies is that the latter to a large degree seem *user experience based* rather than textual. Persuasive designs persuade users by offering them a persuasive experience with the design. To avoid any confusion (i.e., anthropomorphizing [3]), persuasive designs are not persuasive as such. Interactive- or analogue technologies do not pose their own intentions; they merely act as a medium for the designer's intention − a vehicle for persuasion [18]. However, it is not always clear what kind of 'persuasion' we are dealing with.

Notably, some multimedia based persuasive designs employ a mix of textual and non-textual argumentation. For instance, applications may persuade users both by compelling interaction design and by video, where textual arguments are presented, but often times designs do not explicitly pose arguments composed of words. In crafting persuasive designs, designers can somehow embed both non-textual and textual arguments into interactive and analogue technologies. It seems thus that for many applications and designs, the influence actually sits in the crux of the designer's intentions, the user and the experienced usage of the designed object. Users are thus influenced or moved towards a certain behavior or attitude change, but not necessarily via cogent arguments.

Persuasive design is not the first discipline to encounter this issue. In their description of visual arguments, Birdsell and Groarke [6] note that most scholars who study argumentation theory are preoccupied with verbal elements, i.e., words. They explore the notion that photos, art, pictures etc., might pose a different type of argument, speculating if textual arguments are, in fact, just a subset of influencing. The same strand of thought seems applicable to persuasive designs and the arguments embedded in them.

As we begin to explore the notion that arguments may somehow be presented in material form [17], we add a confusing complexity to our previous understanding of 'persuasion.' From a hermeneutical perspective, it can be argued that readers are indeed interacting with the text they read. In interactive systems this becomes more accentuated, as interactions are more explicit and clearly marked by the designers' intention; interactions are explicitly modeled, carefully crafting each possible outcome. However, the more explicit 'interaction' of many computer systems does not advance our understanding of 'persuasion' in such artifacts. In moving from 'speakers' (or 'writers') to 'designers,' things soon become blurry. For instance, persuasive design methods [9], [12], [13], [15] seemingly advocate the view that persuasion resides in the right mix of strategies; however, one obvious problem is that none of the suggested tactics suggested in the models individually appears to be persuasive. To what degree can 'tunneling' and 'reduction', for example, be specific persuasive design tactics? Can persuasive design models be reduced to a process for deploying collages of tactics adopted from various other fields of research? A Pandoras box with a whole plethora of large questions opens as we begin to observe persuasive design as the rhetorical act of embedding symbols into technologies. Thus the experiment below of analyzing non-textual arguments with a textual model for arguments is only a smaller part of a far larger picture.

3   Analyzing Technology Embedded Arguments with Toulmin

There is a need to develop models for analyzing non-textual arguments that are embedded in technologies where they offer user experience based persuasion. While researchers and philosophers have developed models for analyzing traditional textual arguments and appeals (e.g., enthymeme, syllogism and rhetorical appeals), it is unclear how 'users' are persuaded with technology embedded arguments. To form basic ideas on the analysis of technology embedded arguments, Stephen Toulmin's argument pattern [19] has been applied to two persuasive designs in order to explore its utility in regards to analyzing technology embedded arguments. Toulmin's pattern - selected as an acclaimed modern model for enthymemic argumentation - is a form of argumentation that has previously also been used in the field of information systems [21]. The pattern has been very influential in modern rhetoric, as it deals with the inadequacies of formal logic when addressing everyday disputes in a very convincing and decisive manner by favoring the 'probability' of claims made rather than their formal 'truth.'

Toulmin's pattern (as seen in Figure 1) is centered on the analysis of verbal statements in speech or writing, and can be employed for analyzing arguments in writing and speech by making the internal dynamics of arguments explicit.

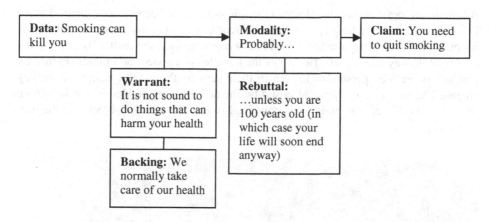

Fig. 1. Toulmin's argument pattern applied to an anti-smoking argument

The general concept of Toulmin's model based on an argument pattern is that the 'claim' is the conclusion put forth by the speaker. When persuading, we pose our 'claim' and then support it by adding a 'warrant' that would allow the listener to actually agree with us, based on the 'data' we present – in essence resulting in persuasion. The 'data' is typically something that the audience finds easier to accept than the claim itself. 'Modality,' 'rebuttal' and 'backing' are elements that are often times omitted. The 'modality' concerns the level of certainty that we put behind our claim; the 'rebuttal' signifies exceptional conditions that may defeat or rebut the conclusion; and the 'backing' indicates why the 'warrant' is applicable in this particular case. Notably, when we apply Toulmin's pattern on arguments, we will often find that elements are missing; for instance, we may say: "You need to quit smoking; it causes cancer" without any explicit 'modality', 'rebuttal' or even a 'warrant' or 'backing.' Thus, a difficult aspect of the pattern is that such elements can be implicit. To complicate things further, each element can be regarded as its own claim.

For instance, consider the 'data' in the example above: "Smoking can kill you." This statement can in itself be considered a claim. If someone were to question this, we would have to provide (another set of) data and a warrant that would justify this data/claim in order to persuade that this was actually the case. Thus, we are often faced with deep hierarchies of arguments – entangled arguments. Claims in one argument may be used as data in another, reflecting how arguments are formed in everyday argumentation. In analyzing the persuasive designs (below) with the pattern, the approach was simple. The only viable option seemed to be to determine the target behavior, the behavior that the design is clearly attempting to invoke and regard this behavior as the 'claim' made by designers via the design.

3.1   A Key Chain That Persuades

A simple analogue persuasive design example is the hotelkeeper's key chain. Latour [5], [11] describes a hotelkeeper who feels great distress that his guests do not turn in room keys when leaving the hotel. The hotelkeeper resolves the matter by altering the *design* of the key chain itself. He makes the key chains heavier and bulkier (Figure 2), and guests are then persuaded to turn in their keys by the altered design of the key chains. The non-textual argument posed by the artifact is embedded in the key chain itself. The hotelkeeper's intention is conveyed in the usage of the object – in the user experience

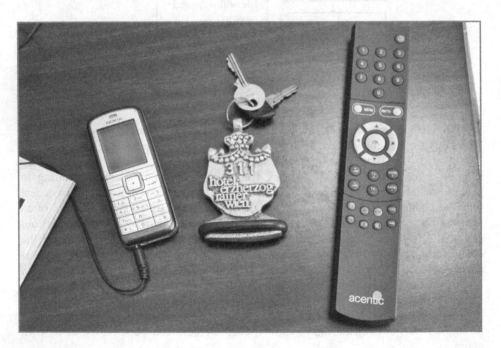

Fig. 2. Bulky hotel key chain example

What happens then if we try to force the persuasive design example into Toulmin's argument pattern? The claim seems to be the only easy element to fill in (Figure 3):

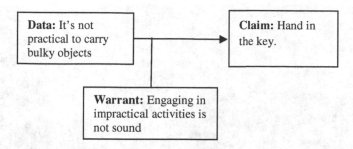

Fig. 3. Toulmin's basic argument pattern applied to the hotelkeepers key chain design

The reasoning is anchored in the user's experience of the key: It will be more troublesome for *the user* to carry a bulky key chain, although one could freely choose to do so. To some degree, the argument posed by the key chain is implicit or even covert. Users are not explicitly alerted to the intention or motives of the hotelkeeper. Notably, the key chain poses only one primary argument, which we can only truly grasp when using it or in the example above (Figure 3), where both data and warrant are objects of interpretation or even *speculation*. Others might have rivaling theories as to why the guests should hand in the key. We could easily invent other data supporting the claim, e.g., "There is a fine for losing a key."

3.2   Speed Feedback Sign

Another example for analysis is found in public space. Public space offers us many examples of technology made to afford a behavioral change. In traffic, a common behavioral issue is to get motorists to lower their speed. A digital sign designed to address this issue employs a persuasive approach (Figure 4). The sign is hard to overlook. It flashes lights and will claim the attention of drivers exceeding the legal travelling speed. The drivers are then left with the option of slowing down or ignoring it. The motorists already have their own speedometer, but the external sign initially offers a form of reduction, making it easier to read the traveling speed, since drivers do not have to look down at their own speedometer to read their current traveling speed.

This is an example of 'kairos' [1], [16], addressing the user at the most opportune moment. Signs are placed where drivers predictably tend to ignore their own speed, that is, they are not paying attention to their own dashboard. A common behavioral reaction is that drivers look down and check if their own speedometer does indeed indicate the same speed as the sign does. Thus, the persuasive design results in the very behavior that the drivers should be exhibiting. As in the previous example, the design artifact is centered on one primary argument: the user should obey the speed limit. Regardless, many of the elements in Toulmin's argument pattern are open for speculation:

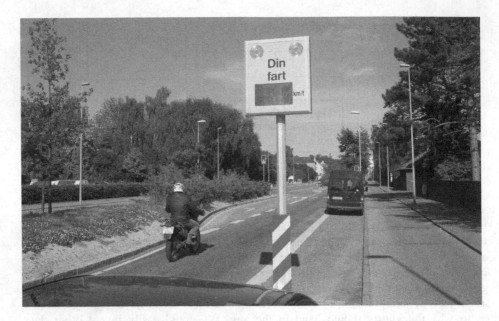

Fig. 4. The external speedometer sign shows the speed (50 km/h) of passing motorists

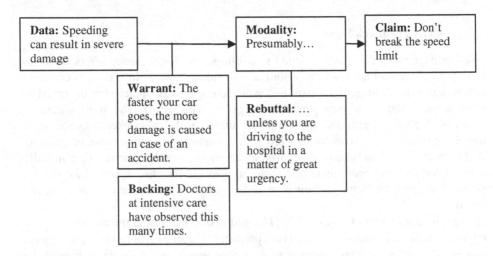

Fig. 5. Toulmin's full argument pattern applied to the external speedometer sign

In the extended model applied in Figure 5, the problem is that other interpreters might extrapolate the argument in a different manner. For instance, you could argue that the claim is: "lower your speed"; "speeding is dangerous"; "you should obey the law"; "it's unethical to put other motorist in danger"; "speeding is not worth the risk," etc. Thus, it seems that if we regard this design artifact as posing a textual argument, there are multiple possible interpretations at play.

4   Discussion and Ethical Implications

In stretching Toulmin's argument pattern to encompass design, the model is being pushed towards the boundary of what can be justified. The pattern does shed some light as an exploration of the unique properties of designs crafted with the intention of persuading users; however, it is less clear how a synthesis between textual and non-textual could occur using this model. When working with the model, many questions surfaces.

A clear problem, methodology wise, is that the elements in Toulmin's model are even less explicit in persuasive designs than they are in oral or written communication. In the two examples analyzed here, the internal dynamics of the user experienced based technology embedded arguments are largely invisible; in the analysis the target behavior was diagnosed as being the 'claim' made by designers. The rest of the elements in the model, even in these very simple designs analyzed, are very much a matter of interpretation, to a degree where one can argue that subjectivism is lurking. For instance, the data and the warrants in the two examples emerged from a common sense stance, from *speculating* how such arguments might be posed in text employing a common sense approach. They cannot explicitly and directly be extracted from the designs; in essence, the designer's reasoning is invisible. The same is the case for both modality and rebuttal. It is unclear which force claims are being put forth in the designs analyzed.

From the perspective of Toulmin's pattern, the designs can be regarded as presenting postulates. They are in essence suggesting a behavior change based on the assumed existence of facts or truth supporting the designer's covert reasoning. From a research perspective, the lack of clearer parameters to analyze arguments posed in design is frustrating. There is little doubt that the two design artifacts presented here are arguing a point, each clearly putting forth suggestions for behavior transformation. The designs have been made for a reason. They are intentional, not accidental; however, it is questionable how the embedded arguments work. How can we tell if a technology artifact is convincing if we cannot determine whether or not it is posing a cogent argument? What kind of pattern would capture all the issues at play here?

The application of Toulmin's pattern indirectly sheds some light on a potentially strong ethical implication. If the non-textual user experience based technology embedded arguments are not identical or interchangeable with verbal arguments, are they real 'arguments'? If users in reality have no means of evaluating the quality or the internal dynamics of technology embedded arguments or the force with which they are being put forth via a 'persuasive' user experience, are we then in reality talking about 'persuasion' or perhaps some form of manipulation or even propaganda? One could argue that it is unethical to influence users towards a change in their behavior or attitudes, without any hint as to why such recommendations might be right. Also, in influencing users, without revealing our motives or reasoning, we are implicitly passing judgment on their current behavior, hinting that the users' current behavior or attitude is somehow wrong.

There seems to be a foundational ethical issue in regards to symmetry between designers and users. If persuasive designs often times are an asymmetrical form of communication, the receivers of the communication do not have a fair chance of evaluating the behavior or attitude change being suggested via the designs.

Practically, if users, for instance, are faced with two mobile health technologies, each designed to invoke the same behavior change as well as addressing the same audience of users, which one is then posing the better 'argument'?

Facing similar challenges in defense of visual arguments, Birdsell and Groarke [6] argue that visual arguments are simply a different type of argument. They claim that textual arguments and visual arguments are at the same level, while 'influencing' is a level above both. Perhaps user experience based arguments are to be regarded in the same manner. While visual and user experience based arguments might have different qualities than textual explicit argumentation, they are perhaps still arguments, albeit of a different kind. In all fairness, we should not be too surprised that very compelling user experiences can influence users in a manner that cannot be translated directly into textual arguments, for we cannot fully translate *experience* into language; this is the case for many experiences ranging from love to riding a bicycle. We should also remember that explicit textual arguments are objects of interpretation, but such interpretations have the advantage that they are a matter of interpretation of the explicit texts. If one were to discuss rivaling interpretations, they would be anchored in the text. User experience based arguments embedded in technology are elusive; who is to tell if an 'experience' of the designed object is perceived uniformly between different users? How do we point to the central argument posed? How do we share a feeling of truth invoked by a design?

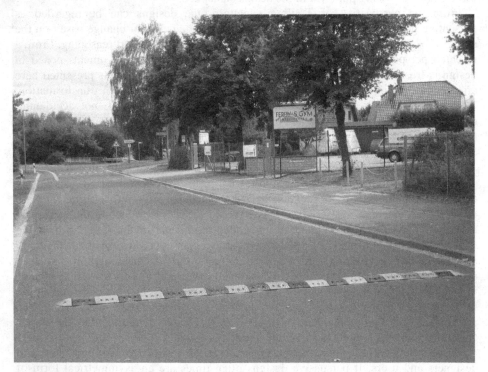

Fig. 6. Speed bump forcing drives to slow down or feel discomfort (Photo by Marco: http://flic.kr/p/5iqxpN)

Regardless of the above-mentioned difficulties, Toulmin's model does offer a clearer perspective on coercion, also in technology design. As with arguments posed in speech, if the intention of the data or warrant or backing in an argument in essence is to invoke *discomfort*, coercion is taking place. In the traffic sign example given above, motorists are offered a free choice. They can still choose to speed if they so choose. However, as speeding is a common behavioral issue, other solutions have also been designed to address the same problem, such as "speed bumps" (see Figure 6 below). Speed bumps are deliberately crafted to make driving bumpy, and - from a persuasive design perspective - if the driver does not slow down, the speed bumps can be considered to be coercive. Motorists are not left a real choice in whether or not they want to speed; thus, there is no persuasion. Notably, the claim might be the same: "Don't break the speed limit," but the data would be, e.g., "*Or else* we will make your driving uncomfortable," making it a clear cut example of physical coercion. It is easy to determine coercion in physical designs. Determine the claim and ask "Or else what?" If the answer is anything other than "nothing," coercion is at play.

In conclusion, since a prevailing pattern for analyzing arguments relatively fails at addressing the complexity posed of two simple persuasive designs, there seems to be support for Redstrøm's claim, that is, we are indeed faced with a new form of "arguments in material form" [17]. User experience based non-textual arguments are seemingly a new form of arguments. In this researcher's mind, there is no doubt that we are in many cases dealing with 'persuasion'; however, unless we can invent new models or patterns for systematic evaluation of designs, it is difficult for users (and researchers) to decode the arguments embedded in technologies. Admittedly, there is a wider context than the application itself for many designs. For instance, a good manual to a product or instruction might provide many of the arguments that the designed object by itself does not. Another circumstance might be one that could opt for a solution where the persuasive design employs a mix of user experience based persuasion as well as traditional persuasion in the form of text or audio visual feedback, i.e., speech and writing. Such elements are quite easy to embed in interactive technologies, and might alleviate some of the ethical issues in regards to symmetry between senders and receivers. Thus, some ethical considerations might be practically solved by ensuring that textual arguments are presented in the applications.

As persuasive design becomes an increasingly common design approach, users should at least have the guarantee that researchers and practitioners are aware of this issue. Toulmin's pattern is not fitting for analyzing persuasive designs, but the pattern can help us in understanding arguments and thus it may serve as a starting point; however, if we are to push further, we need the ability to reach consensus about arguments posed in designs. Otherwise, it might be difficult for us (and others) to determine if we are actually researching the same phenomena. We are still in need of an argument model or pattern for technology embedded arguments.

Acknowledgments. I would like to thank my reviewers for offering exceptionally valuable and thought provoking feedback.

References

1. Andrew, A., Borriello, G., Fogarty, J.: Toward a Systematic Understanding of Suggestion Tactics in Persuasive Technologies. In: de Kort, Y.A.W., IJsselsteijn, W.A., Midden, C., Eggen, B., Fogg, B.J. (eds.) PERSUASIVE 2007. LNCS, vol. 4744, pp. 259–270. Springer, Heidelberg (2007)
2. Aristotle: Rhetoric (2010), http://classics.mit.edu/Aristotle/rhetoric.html
3. Atkinson, B.M.C.: Captology: A Critical Review. In: IJsselsteijn, W.A., de Kort, Y.A.W., Midden, C., Eggen, B., van den Hoven, E. (eds.) PERSUASIVE 2006. LNCS, vol. 3962, pp. 171–182. Springer, Heidelberg (2006)
4. Berdichevsky, D., Neunschwander, E.: Toward an Ethics of Persuasive Technology. Commun. ACM 42, 51 (1999)
5. Bijker, W.E., Law, J.: Shaping technology/building society: Studies in sociotechnical change, 2nd edn. MIT Press (1994)
6. Birdsell, D.S., Groarke, L.: Toward a Theory of Visual Argument. Argumentation and Advocacy 33, 1 (1996)
7. Fogg, B.J.: Persuasive Technologies. Commun. ACM 42, 26–29 (1999)
8. Fogg, B.J.: Persuasive Computers: Perspectives and Research Directions. In: CHI 1998 Los Angeles USA, April 18-23, p. 225 (1998)
9. Fogg, B.J., Hreha, J.: Behavior wizard: A method for matching target behaviors with solutions. In: Ploug, T., Hasle, P., Oinas-Kukkonen, H. (eds.) PERSUASIVE 2010. LNCS, vol. 6137, pp. 117–131. Springer, Heidelberg (2010)
10. Kjær Christensen, A.-K., Hasle, P.: Classical Rhetoric and a Limit to Persuasion. In: de Kort, Y.A.W., IJsselsteijn, W.A., Midden, C., Eggen, B., Fogg, B.J. (eds.) PERSUASIVE 2007. LNCS, vol. 4744, pp. 307–310. Springer, Heidelberg (2007)
11. Law, J.: A Sociology of Monsters - Essays on power, technology and domination. The Sociological Review, Great Britain (1991)
12. Lockton, D.: Design with Intent Toolkit Wiki (2013), http://www.danlockton.com/dwi/Main_Page
13. Lockton, D., Harrison, D., Stanton, N.A.: The Design with Intent Method: A Design Tool for Influencing User Behaviour. Appl. Ergon. 41, 382–392 (2010)
14. Miller, G.: R.: On Being Persuaded: Some Basic Distinctions. In: Dillard, J.P., Pfau, M.W. (eds.) The Persuasion Handbook: Developments in Theory and Practice, Sage Publications, Inc., Thousands Oaks (2002)
15. Oinas-Kukkonen, H., Harjumaa, M.: Persuasive Systems Design: Key Issues, Process Model, and System Features. Communications of the Association for Information Systems 24, 28 (2009)
16. Räisänen, T., Oinas-Kukkonen, H., Pahnila, S.: Finding kairos in quitting smoking: Smokers' perceptions of warning pictures. In: Oinas-Kukkonen, H., Hasle, P., Harjumaa, M., Segerståhl, K., Øhrstrøm, P. (eds.) PERSUASIVE 2008. LNCS, vol. 5033, pp. 254–257. Springer, Heidelberg (2008)
17. Redström, J.: Persuasive Design: Fringes and Foundations. In: IJsselsteijn, W.A., de Kort, Y.A.W., Midden, C., Eggen, B., van den Hoven, E. (eds.) PERSUASIVE 2006. LNCS, vol. 3962, pp. 112–122. Springer, Heidelberg (2006)
18. Torning, K., Oinas-Kukkonen, H.: Persuasive System Design: State of the Art and Future Directions, pp. 1–8 (2009)
19. Toulmin, S.E.: The uses of argument, updated edn. Cambridge University Press, New York (2003)
20. Walton, D., Reed, C., Macagno, F.: Argumentation schemes. Cambridge University Press, New York (2008)
21. Yetim, F.: A Framework for Organizing Justifications for Strategic use in Adaptive Interaction Contexts (2008)

Embodied Persuasion

Visual-Spatial Dimensions of Meaning Portrayal in Visual and Interactive Media

Thomas J.L. Van Rompay

University of Twente, Faculty of Engineering Technology,
Department of Product Design, De Horst, Drienerlolaan 5, 7522NB, Enschede
t.j.l.vanrompay@utwente.nl

Abstract. Research on embodied cognition indicates that abstract meaning attributions are to a large extent grounded in our own (and at the same time shared) bodily interactions in and with the environment. One particularly interesting finding relates to visual-spatial aspects inherent in these interactions that bring about specific experiential qualities. In this paper we will show how such visual-spatial dimensions may be applied across visual and interactive media in order to induce specific beliefs, feelings and behaviors. In addition, future directions are discussed, amongst others addressing the feasibility of applying the insights presented in interface and interactive product design.

Keywords: Persuasive visualization, embodiment, interactive products, sensory experience, consumer decision making.

1 Introduction

Starting within the field of cognitive linguistics, and later emerging as one of the most studied topics in social psychology, embodiment is now widely considered one of the key pillars involved in human decision-making, affect, and behavior (Johnson, 1987; Lakoff & Johnson, 1999). But although embodiment has been studied extensively in relation to language and cognition, it has hardly been studied in relation to visual and interactive media. In this latter context, recent developments have paved the way for embodied types of user input (e.g., gesture and multi-touch input). As these trends require active participation of users 'through' their bodies, insights into how bodily actions carry meanings are called for. The goal of this article is therefore to show how different types of meaning portrayal can be traced to visual-spatial patterns originating in our bodily interactions. Four such embodied structures will be discussed. Focus in the first part of this paper will be on graphic design and research from our own lab[1]. In the second part, the insights and implications issuing forth from these studies will be discussed in the context of interactive products, backed up by research in human computer interaction and social psychology.

---

[1] All participants in our experiments were informed of the purpose of our research and signed an informed consent form.

A. Spagnolli et al. (Eds.): PERSUASIVE 2014, LNCS 8462, pp. 247–252, 2014.
© Springer International Publishing Switzerland 2014

2   Visual-Spatial Dynamics in the Consumer Context

Image schemas (Johnson, 1987) capture structural visual-spatial aspects of our daily interactions in and with the environment. Examples are the schemas for containment, verticality, angularity, and expansion. Consider, for instance, the containment schema. Containment in everyday life (e.g., being inside a closed space such as one's house or car, or a baby in his mother's arms) is generally correlated with experiencing security and safety. The embodied basis for such associations can be traced to the experiential given that containment involves the notion of a protective frame which shields one off from forces acting on the outside (e.g., feeling safe and warm inside one's living room when it is cold and wet outside). At the same time, however, containers limit freedom of movement and may therefore also trigger associations with restraint and limitation.

In line with these notions, Van Rompay, Hekkert, Saakes, and Russo (2005) showed that everyday containers providing increasing degrees of closure to their contents (i.e., a closed versus an open pitcher or vase) are perceived as more secure, but at the same time as more restricting. As for graphic design, consider the following example of an advertisement for a baby lotion (see Figure 1) featuring either a depiction of a baby without a clearly articulated visual border (low containment) or a solid, visually salient, protective frame (high containment; Strien, 2008). Although in no way indicative of product benefits or functioning, participants (assigned to one of these two conditions) rated the solid-border variant higher on skin protection (and related qualities such as hydrating).

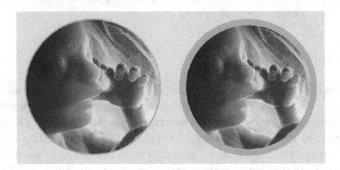

Fig. 1. Advertising imagery and containment (from: Strien, 2008)

Another pervasive schema is the verticality schema. Verticality in daily language is often used to convey a sense of power, success or exclusivity as indicated by figurative phrases such as 'looking up to someone', 'we made it to the top', and a 'high-end fashion store'. The relationship between verticality and power-related concepts is embodied in so far we ourselves experience that it takes bodily effort to overcome gravitational forces, but that doing so also inspires a sense of success or achievement, and that being high grants us a sense of (visual) control over those below. Because of these couplings, we intuitively associate verticality with power-related concepts such as success and luxury.

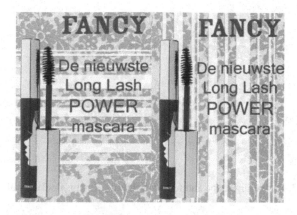

Fig. 2. Advertising background imagery and containment (from: Van Rompay et al., 2012)

In a recent study, we argued that visual representations of this schema (Figure 2) might boost (economic power-related) perceptions of exclusivity and value (Van Rompay, De Vries, Bontekoe, & Tanja-Dijkstra, 2012). Specifically, orientation of background imagery was manipulated such that a target product was either pitted against a vertically oriented or a horizontally oriented background. In line with embodied reasoning, exclusivity and price perceptions (reflecting value) were higher in the vertical background condition, showing that the 'verticality-power' relationship is not a mere linguistic curiosity but actually structures the way we think and perceive. Hence, because in our embodied interactions, the vertical dimension is associated with power-related qualities, we attribute such qualities to displays articulating verticality or a 'rising upward'.

3   Shaping Expectations and Transforming Sensory Experiences

In order to further explore the persuasiveness of embodied meaning portrayals, in a follow-up study (Becker, Van Rompay, Schifferstein, & Galetzka, 2011) we sought to demonstrate its influence on actual consumer experience (rather than mere consumer perceptions of product or brand). Specifically, we assessed the impact of packaging shape on taste experience. The manipulation (shape angularity versus roundedness; Figure 3) was based on the embodied given that in our daily interactions with objects, angular form features are experienced as conflicting or imposing as they present conflict between stimulus and surroundings (Zhang, Feick, & Price, 2006). For instance, a sharp angle of a saloon table is rather imposing in interaction with one's forehead, whereas rounded form features are 'easy' on their surroundings (and our bodies). Hence, this embodied given explains why we entertain 'common' associations between rounded form features and harmoniousness on the one hand, and angular form features and forcefulness on the other.

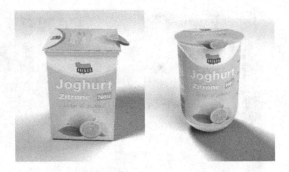

Fig. 3. Packaging shape and form articulation (from: Becker et al., 2011)

In order to test whether such associations triggered by product appearance would transpire in subsequent sensory experiences, we had participants taste a sample (identical across the conditions) of neutral-tasting yoghurt, after which they evaluated taste intensity. Results showed that the angular (as opposed to the rounded) package inspired a more intense taste experience. Hence, embodied expectations triggered by visual perception of packaging shape are not trivial or negligible but can actually steer evaluations of cross-sensorial input, further underlining their persuasive impact.

4   Embodiment in the Online Context and in Interaction Design

Recently, several studies have attested to the applicability of embodied representations in online and dynamic media. For instance, Landau, Vess, Arndt, Rothschild, Sullivan, & Atchley (2011) reasoned that people perceive their inner 'self' as an entity that may either expand or contract. That is, in our daily interactions we implicitly associate expansiveness of bodily posture with qualities such as self-confidence, whereas a contracted posture is readily associated with shyness or weakness. Interested in whether exposure to expanding or contracting stimuli might activate these self-related constructs, participants were primed with dynamic representations of a series of expanding (growing in size) or contracting (decreasing in size) squares. Results showed, amongst others, that participants primed with entity expansion perceived themselves as more self-actualized, showing that (dynamic) visualizations of image schemas may also induce affective states. Similarly interested in expansiveness and its embodied basis, Carney, Cuddy, and Yap (2010) directly manipulated bodily contraction/expansiveness through seating posture. Participants taking in an expansive posture not only felt more confident, they were also more assertive in a subsequent negotiation task.

This latter finding is of particular relevance in light of recent trends in interactive product development making use of gesture input. For instance, gaming consoles such as Wii and PlayStation Move can sense movement in space, paving the way for interactive games such as yoga, pilates, and dance where bodily postures and movements take center stage. Furthermore, ever more e-learning applications (e.g., social networking, management training, healthy lifestyle coaching) solicit feedback from users revolving around abstract concepts such as liking, importance, conflict, status, and emotional impact. It is especially with respect to such abstract concepts that bodily-based image schemas may prove a particularly fruitful starting point.

For instance, Hurtienne et al. (2010) showed that participants (holding a handheld device) intuitively understand the connection between positive abstract concepts such as familiarity and liking on the one hand and gestures 'towards' (as opposed to 'away from') the body on the other. Furthermore, as these relationships are embodied (from childhood on, positive stimuli are associated with bodily approach and nearness), these do not require cognitive processes to be learned and understood. Hence, relationships between abstract concepts and gestures are intuitively understood, even by target groups with little or no experience with interactive products (Hurtienne et al., 2010).

5   Discussion

Concluding, visual-spatial elements can induce meaning perceptions, desirable states of mind, and related behaviors. Furthermore, the different studies discussed suggest that such effects can be brought about in different ways. First of all, they may be 'primed' as suggested by Landau et al. (2011). For instance, in the context of a management training application, animations of expanding shapes may be used in order to boost self-confidence, subsequently 'put to the test' in role-playing scenarios. But as interactive applications allow for active user participation, users may also be prompted to, for instance, track shapes using handheld motion controllers. In our example, shapes with angular, straight features may (in line with Becker et al., 2011) be used to instill a sense of empowerment. Additionally, the discussed relationship (Van Rompay et al., 2012) between verticality and power may be exploited by using vertically oriented shapes that solicit rising arm movements. Such bodily actions could likewise prime dominance or power, transpiring in more efficient decision-making, for example. Finally, full body movements may be solicited (e.g., by having users simulate full-body movements presented on screen).

Further demonstrating that such bodily enactments may be particularly suited to get a grip on abstract content, we recently explored the bodily basis of envisioned product expressions in the design context. To this end, design students acted out episodes in which they felt dominant or involved with respect to another person or object interacted with, paying particular attention to bodily posture. Analyses showed that dominance-related postures involved stretching trunk movements (making oneself tall) and bodily balance (taking in a balanced, stable position), whereas 'involved' postures involved the creation of a protective container. Through these bodily enactments, participants could re-experience the abstract quality (i.e., product expression) designed for. These (albeit preliminary) findings further demonstrate the potential of gesture input in soliciting desired states of mind in serious gaming or e-learning applications.

Finally, with new media such as tablets providing increasing opportunities for small-scale bodily actions (e.g., dragging or swiping objects on an iPad), future research could explore to what extent parameters such as direction of movement and expansiveness of finger-hand movements can likewise induce meanings and affective states. In sum, the insights presented not only allow one to explain (seemingly) obvious relationships between visual-spatial features and meaning portrayal encountered in design, they may also open up avenues for creating new types of human-product interaction.

References

1. Becker, L., Van Rompay, T.J.L., Schifferstein, H.N.J., Galetzka, M.: Tough package, strong taste: The influence of packaging design on taste impressions and product evaluations. Food Quality and Preference 22(1), 17–23 (2011)
2. Carney, D., Cuddy, A.J.C., Yap, A.: Power posing: Brief nonverbal displays affect neuro-endocrine levels and risk tolerance. Psychological Science 21(10), 1363–1368 (2010)
3. Hurtienne, J., Stößel, C., Sturm, C., Maus, A., Rötting, M., Langdon, P., Clarkson, J.: Physical gestures for abstract concepts: Inclusive design with primary metaphors. Interacting with Computers 22(6), 475–484 (2010)
4. Johnson, M.: The body in the mind. The University of Chicago Press, Chicago (1987)
5. Lakoff, G., Johnson, M.: Philosophy in the flesh. Basic Books, New York (1999)
6. Landau, M.J., Vess, M., Arndt, J., Rothschild, Z.K., Sullivan, D., Atchley, R.A.: Embodied metaphor and the "true" self: Priming entity expansion and protection influences intrinsic self-expressions in self-perceptions and interpersonal behavior. Journal of Experimental Social Psychology 47(1), 79–87 (2011)
7. Strien, M.L.: Visuele oriëntatiemetaforen in advertenties (Master's thesis). University of Twente (2008)
8. Van Rompay, T.J.L., De Vries, P.W., Bontekoe, F., Tanja-Dijkstra, K.: Embodied product perception: Effects of verticality cues in advertising and packaging design on consumer impressions and price expectations. Psychology & Marketing 29(12), 919–928 (2012)
9. Van Rompay, T.J.L., Hekkert, P., Saakes, D., Russo, B.: Grounding abstract object characteristics in embodied interactions. Acta Psychologica 119(3), 315–351 (2005)
10. Zhang, Y., Feick, L., Price, L.J.: The impact of self-construal on aesthetic preference for angular versus rounded shapes. Personality and Social Psychology Bulletin 32(6), 794–805 (2006)

Embedded Disruption: Facilitating Responsible Gambling with Persuasive Systems Design

Kristen Warren, Avi Parush, Michael Wohl, and Hyoun S. Kim

Department of Psychology, Carleton University, Ottawa, ON, Canada
{kristen.mitchell,avi.parush,michael.wohl,
hyoun.kim}@carleton.ca

Abstract. Principles of Persuasive Systems Design (PSD) have been implemented in various applications designed to promote attitude or behaviour change. In order to facilitate responsible gambling, current practices call for gamblers to preset monetary limits and adhere to them. In this study, PSD principles were combined with a "just-in-time" embedded disruption in order to facilitate adherence to preset monetary limits in online gambling. A user-centred design process, including focus groups and a heuristic evaluation, was employed to define needs and requirements, and evaluate the tool. A lab study with a virtual casino showed that the embedded disruption tool was associated with more players quitting when they reached their preset monetary limit compared with the current monetary limit tool, demonstrating the principle of embedded disruption is effective.

Keywords: Persuasive Systems Design, Embedded Disruption, Heuristic Evaluation, Validation Study, User-Centred Design.

1 Introduction

1.1 Background

The principles of Persuasive Systems Design (PSD) have been applied to various domains where behaviour change is desired, such as obesity [1][2], Borderline Personality Disorder [3], smoking cessation [4], alcohol consumption management [5][6], and weight loss/exercise [7][8]. In the existing examples of applications intended to aid users in reducing a harmful behaviour or attitude, it is of note that the mechanism intended to prevent the adverse behaviour is dissociated from the behaviour itself. For example, in some quit-smoking and alcohol management applications, users are required to fill out a daily log after the negative behaviour targeted for change has already occurred. While shown to have some effectiveness, these applications are limited in their reach due to their inability to intervene at precise times in which the user would benefit from motivational or persuasive messages.

Embedding persuasion so the user is reminded of their target behaviour at specified points such as the user's decision point to engage in the negative behaviour or just

A. Spagnolli et al. (Eds.): PERSUASIVE 2014, LNCS 8462, pp. 253–265, 2014.

before, has had very little attention when combined with PSD principles. The four principles of "just-in-time" persuasion (i.e. Present an easy to understand message, at just the right time, at just the right place, in a non-annoying way; [9]) can potentially facilitate the necessary disruption to a user's negative behavior, and increase the persuasive efficacy of a tool designed to promote behaviour or attitude change [10]. We tested this approach in a tool aimed at facilitating responsible gambling.

1.2 Gambling and Responsible Gambling

Online gambling is becoming increasingly popular, especially among young adults [11][12]. This form of gambling is particularly problematic as it allows 24/7 access to virtually any gambling game, including electronic gambling machines (EGMs) – the most addictive form [11]. Research shows that individuals who partake in online gambling are far more likely to become disordered gamblers compared with offline gamblers [13][14]. As such, it is becoming increasingly important to give attention to means of facilitating responsible online gambling, particularly as online gambling becomes more ubiquitous.

Gambling research shows that one of the most popular and effective means of promoting responsible gambling is through the use of pre-commitment tools. The aim of such tools is to help users set a time or spending limit for their gambling session prior to beginning play - when they are in a cool affective state and their reasoning is unhindered [15]. The rationale, as illustrated in Figure 1, is that the pre-commitment tool will be persuasive enough for the user to shift from the current behaviour, i.e. possibly gambling beyond their limits, to the desired behaviour: quitting once the pre-set limit is reached.

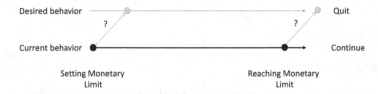

Fig. 1. Current approach to facilitate RG using preset limits and limit reached points

The most common way to help facilitate pre-commitment is by communicating its responsible gambling (RG) utility through pop-up messages displayed during game-play (see [16]). Once engaged, users find pre-commitment messaging via pop-ups helpful in terms of monitoring time or money spent [17]. Additionally, research has found that using pop-up messaging successfully reduces the user's flow state [18][19], which increases limit adherence [18, 20]. The procedure is as follows: each user is shown a pop-up message before they begin play asking them to set a limit for their gambling session (Figure 2a). Then, each user receives a second pop-up message when their pre-set limit has been reached (Figure 2b).

Although the aforementioned research is promising, another research study showed that 80% of gamblers spent more money than their pre-set monetary limit even though they were using an RG tool similar to the standard tool shown below [21]. This clearly demonstrates the need for further research focused on methods of increasing effectiveness, engagement and appeal of pre-commitment tools such as the pop-up message.

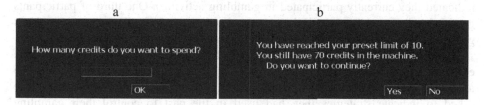

Fig. 2. Standard monetary limit pop-up window (a), and the monetary limit reached pop-up window (b)

1.3   The "Just-In-Time" Principle and Embedded Disruption

A flow state is characterized by user dissociation from their surroundings, and promotes continuous play and enjoyment [22]. Although a flow state is beneficial in that flow is correlated with pleasure, it has been shown that computer interfaces that entice users into a state of flow have greater addictive power than those that do not [23]. The progression and maintenance of disordered gambling behaviour is correlated with the ease with which a user enters, and remains in, a flow state [24]. Therefore, in order for an RG tool to be effective, a user's flow state necessarily has to be disrupted to shift their attention to the RG messages that aim to motivate the target behaviour of gambling responsibly whilst maintaining the user's enjoyment of the game [18]. By incorporating "just-in-time" motivational principles [9], it is hypothesized that the user's flow can be disrupted, enjoyment maintained, and adherence to the preset limit facilitated.

1.4   Objectives of the Study

The objective of the current research is to examine whether the inclusion of PSD and "just-in-time" motivation principles as embedded disruption during gambling game-play can increase user engagement and efficacy with the RG tools.

One of the most important objectives of a persuasive RG tool is to carefully embed disruptive elements so users can maintain the fun and exciting aspects of gambling, but are simultaneously reminded of their desired behaviour (i.e. adhering to their pre-set limit) at key moments with the intent of facilitating responsible gambling.

2   Needs Assessment

Focus groups served as the primary needs assessment, and included several objectives: 1. To obtain insight as to how and why individuals gamble; 2. To explore what RG strategies gamblers have used in the past; and 3. To determine aspects of RG tools which are appealing and effective.

Participants included 17 undergraduate students (9 female; mean age = 19.7) who indicated they currently participated in gambling activities. One third of participants gambled online, and 4 indicated they gambled online regularly. There were two focus groups each lasting 1.5 hours, and both were moderated by a professional facilitator.

A key finding of the focus group was that a monetary limit tool would be more effective than a time limit tool. Participants also indicated that the tool cannot be annoying or "kill the fun", otherwise it will not be engaging. When participants were asked to indicate strategies they had used in the past to control their gambling expenditure, several participants spontaneously indicated that having time to "cool down" after a gambling session (5-30 minutes) was effective and significantly decreased their craving to gamble. These findings translated into several design requirements for the creation of a persuasive, embedded disruption RG tool.

3   Embedded Disruption and PSD Principles

In order to design an embedded disruption RG tool, "Just-in-time" motivation was adopted from Intille's 2004 research [9], and PSD principles were adopted from Oinas-Kukkonen and Harjumaa's research on Persuasive Systems Design [25]. The intent of the embedded disruption tool is to facilitate responsible gambling: Specifically, quitting the gambling session once a user's preset limit is reached. The principles of interest to the embedded disruption RG tool are:

1. Embedded disruption
2. Self-monitoring
3. Reminders/Suggestion
4. Tailoring
5. Liking

3.1   Embedded Disruption

In contrast to the current approach, the rationale of the proposed embedded disruption (Figure 3) is to disrupt the flow of the user's gambling session through modification of the existing pop-up windows to include persuasive elements, and introducing an additional persuasion opportunity with the intent of facilitating responsible gambling through motivating the user to quit when they reach their pre-set limit. This was implemented by adding a popup window warning users that they are approaching their pre-set limit (See Figure 7).

"Just-in-time" motivational principles [9] informed the number of pop-up messages (one reminder before reaching the limit and one notification at the decision point immediately when the user has reached their limit), the type of messages used (informative opposed to punitive), and when the persuasive messages were delivered (at the point of decision and a reminder shortly before). The three popup windows corresponding to each of these three points in the flow are presented in figures 6, 7, and 8, respectively

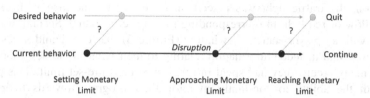

Fig. 3. Proposed approach to facilitate RG using the initial preset limit point, the embedded disruption limit approaching point, and concluding limit reached points

As per the focus group findings, careful attention was paid to ensuring the pop-up windows were not presented too frequently (based on duration of play) or presented in a way that would annoy users. This resulted in selecting one pop-up message to set the limit before beginning play, and two pop-up messages during play: the first presented when the user reaches the last 10% of their pre-set credit limit (which reminds the user that they originally wanted to quit soon), and the last when the user reaches their pre-set limit. Although limited research was available to aid in deciding what percent users should view the "approach limit" message, it was hypothesized that 10% would be effective in maximizing the amount of time users could spend enjoying their gambling experience in a flow state (i.e. approx. 90% of their gambling session), while giving the user enough time to psychologically prepare for their approaching limit (i.e. approx. the last 10% of play).

Several elements were designed into the embedded disruption RG tool to interrupt flow. When users view a pop-up message, the rest of the screen fades to a dark grey hiding the colours underneath, breaking the visual flow of the game. Also, the user is required to wait a set duration before either returning to the game or quitting play, i.e. 10 seconds upon approaching their limit and 5 minutes upon reaching their limit. This was hypothesized to act as a mechanism to shift the user's attention from the game to something else for a short duration. Based on the findings of the focus group, such a time delay could serve as a "cool down" period, which gambling theorists and research often put forth as a key RG strategy [26]. Finally, the user is required to make a choice, by pressing the relevant button, whether to continue playing or quit the game.

3.2   Self-monitoring

Several features were designed to engage the principle of self-monitoring [27] in users. First, a traffic light metaphor was placed statically on the screen at all times

(Figure 4). Due to the different traffic light states (green, yellow or red), status information can be conveyed through the graphical icon without text, meaning very little cognitive load is required in order for the user to determine how many credits remain in relation to their pre-set limit. This use of a metaphor not only helps the user remain aware of their current credit status, but also makes the conveyance of status information unobtrusive and easily interpreted both when the icon is attended to (conscious awareness) and when the icon is not attended to (subconscious awareness).

To solidify the association between the traffic light metaphor and status information, the traffic light was placed on each pop-up message with either the green, yellow or red light lit (corresponding to the user's status). Second, users were provided with a "player statistics" window (Figure 5) that they could access at any point in time, and included information relating to their wins and losses, time played, and how many credits they had spent in relation to their pre-set limit. This provides users with the ability to constantly monitor their progress towards their pre-set monetary limit, which aids the user in feeling in control of their gambling session. Additionally, the process of self-monitoring increases the chance that the user will be in a cool affective state when they do reach their limit, facilitating responsible gambling behaviour.

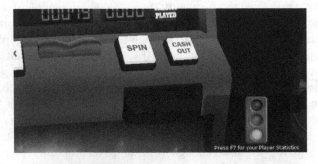

Fig. 4. Traffic light metaphor to facilitate self-monitoring

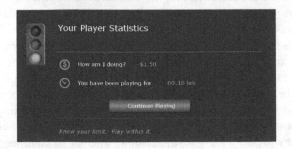

Fig. 5. Player's statistics panel to facilitate self-monitoring

3.3   Reminders/Suggestion

The PSD principle of Reminders/Suggestion [27] was employed by placing an informative message at the bottom of each pop-up window (Figures 6, 7 & 8) in a distinct colour and font to attract attention. Examples of such informative messages include: *Know Your Limit, Play Within It*; *Gambling within your limit will allow you to play again and have more fun*; and, *Think about it – How much can you afford to lose?*. Additionally, the "approach limit" pop-up message also serves as a clear reminder to the user (Figure 7).

3.4 Other Design Aspects

3.4.1 Tailoring

Implementation of the Tailoring [27] PSD principle can be seen in the careful choice of wording within the pop-up messages. First, on the pop-up window that allows users to choose a monetary limit, the text reads, "Please select how many credits you are willing to lose. . ." (Figure 6), which focuses the user's attention on the high probability that they will be losing the money they are about to spend. Similarly, on the final pop-up message, the text reads, "You have reached your credit limit" (Figure 8), both priming the user with a reference to reaching a limit on a credit card (which has a negative affective association), as well as focusing their attention on the fact that they have lost all of the credits they had originally intended to spend.

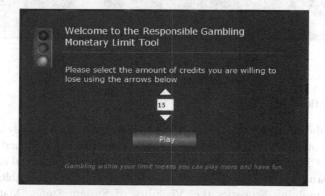

Fig. 6. Initial monetary limit setup window

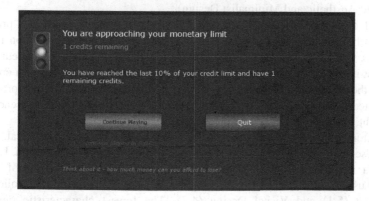

Fig. 7. The embedded disruption window: Approaching the preset monetary limit

3.4.2 Liking

To ensure the principle of Liking [28] was adequately considered, after initial prototypes were developed a professional graphic designer was hired to create the visual design of the embedded disruption RG tool. Attention was paid to various visual design principles such as colour theory, alignment, font selection, focus, and depth. It was hypothesized that this attention to visual design would increase the appeal of the tool and subsequent engagement with the tool, which would in turn positively impact limit adherence.

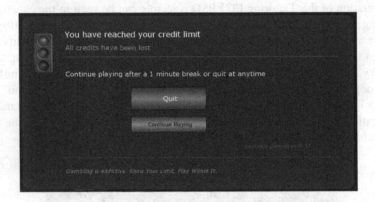

Fig. 8. Limit reached popup window

3.5   Evaluation of the Design

The basic usability of the embedded disruption tool was qualitatively assessed via heuristic evaluation [29]. Evaluators were a mix of usability experts and non-experts (n = 6, and n = 5, respectively; mean age = 26; 6 male), and were asked to analyze the embedded disruption RG tool individually, with 5 principles applicable taken from Nielsen's 10 usability heuristics (i.e. Visibility of System Status, Match Between System and the Real World, Consistency and Standards, Recognition rather than Recall, and Aesthetic and Minimalist Design).

Several evaluators indicated that the traffic light metaphor was not prominent enough to be effective, and several also thought the 5-minute delay upon reaching one's limit was excessive. One common issue identified was that the monetary value of a credit is not clear. Although casinos intentionally guise the value of a credit and therefore the association between a credit and its monetary value was not practical to incorporate, the other findings were implemented by increasing the prominence of the traffic light, and reducing the 5 minute mandatory delay to 1 minute.

Evaluators were asked to rate the tool on five usability characteristics: Satisfaction, Ease of Use, Enjoyableness, Likely to use in the Future, and Visual Design. Each was rated on a 1-7 Likert scale, and each was analyzed by frequency. Ease of Use and Likely to use in the Future were rated highest (6 and 5.8, respectively), followed by Satisfaction (5.1) and Visual Design (4.7). The lowest characteristic rating was

Enjoyableness (4). These results show promise, as Likeliness to use in the Future and Visual Design were thought to directly impact fundamental requirements of the embedded disruption RG tool: engagement and overall appeal.

4   Testing the Embedded Disruption

Since both RG tools involve users setting a monetary limit and receiving a notification when their limit is reached, the main goal of the study was to compare whether participants in each condition quit or continued playing upon reaching their pre-set limit. Additional metrics were incorporated to aid in the explication of why participants quit or continued playing, such as determining the engagement and satisfaction users felt while gambling and appeal of the tool itself, as well as posing additional questions to users in the embedded disruption RG tool condition regarding their perception of tool aspects unique to the persuasive tool.

4.1   Method and Procedure

Fifty-six undergraduate students (19 male) who reported that they currently engage in gambling activities (e.g., slots, casino, poker, etc.) were recruited to participate. The age of participants ranged from 18 to 39 years ($M = 20.38$, $SD = 4.27$).

Participants were recruited for a one-hour gambling session and were asked to gamble using a simulated online casino slot machine, as well as fill out an HCI questionnaire after they had finished their gambling session. Participants were randomly assigned to one of two conditions: 1. Gambling with the standard RG tool ($n = 27$; Figure 2a & 2b); or 2. Gambling with the RG tool with embedded disruption ($n = 29$; Figures 4, 5, 6, 7, 8). Participants were given a total of $20 (80 credits) with which to gamble in the simulated online casino. To make the session as realistic as possible, participants were informed that the odds of winning were identical to those in local casinos. Each participant was informed that they could stop gambling at any time and would be able to keep any remaining money. Participants gave their informed consent and were fully debriefed after their gambling session.

4.2   Findings

A chi-square analysis was performed to determine whether there was a significant difference in the number of participants who quit or continued gambling when they reached their pre-set limit as a function of which RG tool was used. The results showed a significant difference ($\chi^2_{1, n = 48} = 5.21$, p = .033), with more participants in the embedded disruption tool condition quitting when they reached their limit ($n = 23$) than those in the standard RG tool condition ($n = 15$) (Figure 9).

Participants were asked to rate on a 1-7 Likert scale (1 = strongly disagree; 7 = strongly agree) their level of agreement with several statements, which were then analyzed using one-way ANOVA to reveal any differences between conditions. In response to the statement, "I found the monetary limit tool to be engaging", results showed a significant difference ($F_{1, 52}$ = 5.22, p = .03) with the embedded disruption tool rated as more engaging (M = 5.1, SE = .22) than the standard RG tool (M = 4.3, SE = .28). In response to the statement, "During play, I was aware of how many credits I had spent in relation to the limit I set", results showed no significant differences between groups ($F_{1, 53}$ = .01, p = .93).

Since there were motivational elements in the embedded disruption tool, several additional questions were posed to participants in this condition that were not relevant to those in the standard RG tool condition. In response to the statement, "I found the traffic light helpful in keeping track of where I was in relation to my limit", results showed that 59% of participants chose 1 (strongly disagree), and 30% of participants chose either 2 or 3 (M = 1.9, SD = 1.5). Participants were also asked to comment after giving their 1-7 rating, which were analyzed qualitatively. Nine users indicated that they did not notice the traffic light, and 9 noticed it but did not know what it was for. The remaining participants did not comment.

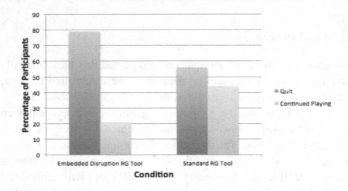

Fig. 9. Proportion of participants quitting vs. continuing to play as a function of the RG tool

Participants were also asked to select from a "Yes", "No", or "Not Sure" response set to the following question: "Did you notice the player statistics window?". For those participants who did notice the player statistics window, they were then asked to rate on a 1-7 Likert scale (1 = strongly disagree; 7 = strongly agree) their level of agreement with the statement, "I found that the player statistics were helpful in monitoring my expenditure". Only 7 participants (12.5%) indicated they noticed the player statistics window. Of those 7, most (5) indicated they disagreed that the player statistics window was helpful in monitoring expenditure (M = 2.67, SD = 2.18). However, of those participants who viewed their player statistics while gambling, 2 out of 4 decided to quit immediately after viewing them, and before they had reached their pre-set limit.

5   Conclusions and Implications

The most important indicator of preset limit adherence - whether participants quit or continued playing - was significant, and therefore it can be concluded that the embedded disruption tool is more effective at motivating gamblers to adhere to their pre-set limit than the standard RG tool. This finding shows the viability of PSD principles and "just-in-time" motivation in creating guidelines for designing effective and persuasive RG tools to facilitate responsible gambling. Moreover, participants indicated that the embedded disruption tool was more engaging than the standard RG tool. This is an interesting and promising result, as it indicates that the embedded disruption tool was effective in its disruption while allowing participants to be engaged during their gambling session, addressing one of the most important needs of gamblers. This effect can potentially be explained by the percent at which the approach limit message was presented: Since participants did not see the approach limit until the last 10% of their credits remained, they were able to enjoy 90% of their gambling experience without disruption.

The traffic light metaphor was not effective as a status indicator, as 89% of participants indicated they either strongly disagreed or disagreed with the statement that the traffic light was helpful in keeping track of where they were in relation to their limit. Also, the qualitative comments showed that participants did not notice the traffic light, and the majority of those that did, failed to realize its purpose. It is hypothesized that this pattern can be explained by the phenomenon of inattentional blindness: a common occurrence where an individual does not notice features in a scene when other attention-demanding tasks are performed simultaneously [30][31]. Participants may have been consumed by the task of playing the slot machine, and therefore became oblivious to items elsewhere.

The player statistics were also not readily noticed, however the few that did notice them were appreciative of the information contained. Given the location of the player statistics was immediately below the traffic light, it is hypothesized that participants did not notice this for the same reason as they did not notice the traffic light – attention is paid to the constantly changing foreground items and background or external items become less salient. Therefore, increasing the salience of the traffic light may also increase the salience of the player statistics through association.

References

1. Toscos, T., Faber, A., An, S., Gandhi, M.: Chick clique: persuasive technology to motivate teenage girls to exercise. In: CHI 2006 Ext. Abstr. .... (2006)
2. Tsai, C.C., Lee, G., Raab, F., Norman, G.J., Sohn, T., Griswold, W.G., Patrick, K.: Usability and Feasibility of PmEB: A Mobile Phone Application for Monitoring Real Time Caloric Balance. Mob. Networks Appl. 12, 173–184 (2007)
3. Carroll, D., Rizvi, S.L., Dimeff, L.A., Linehan, M.M., Skutch, J.: A Pilot Study of the DBT Coach: An Interactive Mobile Phone Application for Individuals With Borderline Personality Disorder and Substance Use Disorder (2011)
4. Lehto, T., Oinas-Kukkonen, H.: Persuasive features in six weight loss websites: A qualitative evaluation. In: Ploug, T., Hasle, P., Oinas-Kukkonen, H. (eds.) PERSUASIVE 2010. LNCS, vol. 6137, pp. 162–173. Springer, Heidelberg (2010)
5. Cohn, A.M., Hunter-Reel, D., Hagman, B.T., Mitchell, J.: Promoting behavior change from alcohol use through mobile technology: the future of ecological momentary assessment. Alcohol. Clin. Exp. Res. 35, 2209–2215 (2011)

6. Yap, M., Jorm, A., Bazley, R., Kelly, C., Ryan, S., Lubman, D.: Web-based parenting program to prevent adolescent alcohol misuse: rationale and development. Australas. Psychiatry 19, 339–344 (2011)
7. Purpura, S., Schwanda, V., Williams, K., Stubler, W., Sengers, P.: Fit4Life: The Design of a Persuasive Technology Promoting Healthy Behavior and Ideal Weight. Comput. Eng., 423–432 (2011)
8. Lehto, T., Oinas-Kukkonen, H.: Persuasive features in six weight loss websites: A qualitative evaluation. In: Ploug, T., Hasle, P., Oinas-Kukkonen, H. (eds.) PERSUASIVE 2010. LNCS, vol. 6137, pp. 162–173. Springer, Heidelberg (2010)
9. Intille, S.S.: Ubiquitous computing technology for just-in-time motivation of behavior change. Stud. Health Technol. Inform. 107, 1434–1437 (2004)
10. Brownell, K.D., Stunkard, A.J., Albaum, J.M.: Evaluation and modification of exercise patterns in the natural environment. Am. J. Psychiatry 137, 1540–1545 (1980)
11. Griffiths, M., Wardle, H., Oxford, J., Sproston, K., Erens, B.: Internet Gambling, Health, Smoking and Alcohol Use: Findings from the 2007 British Gambling Prevalence Survey. Int. J. Ment. Health Addict. 9, 1–11 (2011)
12. McBride, J., Derevensky, J.: Internet Gambling Behavior in a Sample of Online Gamblers. Int. J. Ment. Health Addict. 7, 149–167 (2008)
13. Griffiths, M., Barnes, A.: Internet Gambling: An Online Empirical Study Among Student Gamblers (2008)
14. Ladd, G.T., Petry, N.M.: Disordered gambling among university-based medical and dental patients: A focus on Int. gambling. Psychol. Addict. Behav. 16, 76–79 (2002)
15. Ladouceur, R., Blaszczynski, A., Lalande, D.R.: Pre-commitment in gambling: a review of the empirical evidence. Int. Gambl. Stud. 12 (2012)
16. Monaghan, S.: Review of Pop-Up Messages on Electronic Gaming Machines as a Proposed Responsible Gambling Strategy (2008)
17. Blaszczynski, A., Gainsbury, S., Karlov, L.: Blue Gum gaming machine: An evaluation of responsible gambling features. J. Gambl. Stud., 1–16 (2013)
18. Stewart, M.J., Wohl, M.J.A.: Pop-Up Messages, Dissociation, and Craving: How Monetary Limit Reminders Facilitate Adherence in a Session of Slot Machine Gambling (2012)
19. Nelson, S.E., LaPlante, D.A., Peller, A.J., Schumann, A., LaBrie, R.A., Shaffer, H.J.: Real limits in the virtual world: self-limiting behavior of Internet gamblers. J. Gambl. Stud. 24, 463–477 (2008)
20. Wohl, M.J.A., Stewart, M.J., Gainsbury, S., Sztainert, T.: Facilitating Responsible Gambling: The Relative Effectiveness of Education-Based Animation and Monetary Limit Setting Pop-up Messages Among Electronic Gaming Machine Players (2012)
21. Broda, A., LaPlante, D.A., Nelson, S.E., LaBrie, R.A., Bosworth, L.B., Shaffer, H.J.: Virtual harm reduction efforts for Internet gambling: effects of deposit limits on actual Internet sports gambling behavior. Harm Reduct. J. 5, 27 (2008)
22. Davis, M.S., Csikszentmihalyi, M.: Beyond Boredom and Anxiety: The Experience of Play in Work and Games (1977)
23. Chou, T.-J., Ting, C.-C.: The role of flow experience in cyber-game addiction (2003)
24. Jacobs, D.F.: Evidence for a common dissociative-like reaction among addicts (1988)
25. Oinas-kukkonen, H., Harjumaa, M.: Persuasive Systems Design: Key Issues, Process Model, and System Features. Communications of the Association for Information Systems 24 (2009)

26. Wohl, M.J.A., Christie, K.-L., Matheson, K., Anisman, H.: Animation-based education as a gambling prevention tool: correcting erroneous cognitions and reducing the frequency of exceeding limits among slots players. J. Gambl. Stud. 26, 469–486 (2010)
27. Fogg, B.: Persuasive Technology: Using Computers to Change what we Think and Do. Morgan Kaufmann (2002)
28. Cialdini, R.: Influence. Morrow, New York (1984)
29. Nielsen, J., Blatt, L.A., Bradford, J., Brooks, P.: Usability Inspection. Methods, 413–414 (1994)
30. Mack, A., Rock, I.: Inattentional Blindness. MIT Press, Cambridge (1998)
31. Most, S.B., Scholl, B.J., Clifford, E.R., Simons, D.J.: What you see is what you set: sustained inattentional blindness and the capture of awareness. Psychol. Rev. 112, 217–242 (2005)

(Re)Defining Gamification: A Process Approach

Kevin Werbach

The Wharton School, University of Pennsylvania, Philadelphia, PA
werbach@wharton.upenn.edu

Abstract. Gamification is a growing phenomenon of interest to both practitioners and researchers. There remains, however, uncertainty about the contours of the field. Defining gamification as "the process of making activities more game-like" focuses on the crucial space between the components that make up games and the holistic experience of gamefulness. It better fits real-world examples and connects gamification with the literature on persuasive design.

Keywords: Gamification, games, persuasive design, persuasive technology.

1   Gamification as a Process

There is a long history of organizations leveraging games, play, and competitions in the workplace, school, and elsewhere. Around 2008, a variety of examples combining game-derived concepts and digital platforms for motivation suggested that a new field was emerging. Practitioners settled on the term "gamification" to describe it [11]. The term has stuck, despite criticisms of both the word and the phenomenon [12]. Over the intervening years, gamification has enjoyed significant growth in both adoption and academic interest.[1] Yet questions remain regarding what is unique and valuable about gamification. Some critics even argue that gamification is inherently exploitative [3].

If gamification is to mature as a field, its boundaries must be better understood. Gamification is should be understood as a process. Specifically, it is *the process of making activities more game-like*. Conceiving of gamification as a process creates a better fit between academic and practitioner perspectives. Even more important, it focuses attention on the creation of game-like experiences, pushing against shallow approaches that can easily become manipulative. A final benefit of this approach is that it connects gamification to persuasive design.

Of course, defining gamification in certain ways will not necessarily alter practices. The "correct" understanding of gamification is ultimately what exists in the world. The goals of the exercise here are two-fold. First, in a new and contentious field, designers, users, and commentators sometimes do look to prevailing definitions to understand what is considered mainstream or a best practice. Second, investigating

---

[1] As of February 27, 2014, Google Scholar returned 6,120 results for the term, "gamification."

A. Spagnolli et al. (Eds.): PERSUASIVE 2014, LNCS 8462, pp. 266–272, 2014.

definitions can reveal aspects of gamification that are not obvious from examples themselves.

In the tradition of ordinary language philosophy, this paper takes the view that a gamification definition should be evaluated based on the common usage of terms. Specialized language may enhance precision within discourse communities, but when a phenomenon cuts across many such communities, it can obfuscate more than it clarifies.

In the existing literature, the most widely-used formal definition of gamification is "the use of game design elements in non-game contexts," as proffered by Sebastian Deterding and three co-authors in 2011 [5]. Others, including myself, offered similar definitions around the same time [17]. Because the distinguishing feature of this approach is the emphasis on game design elements, I label it the *elemental* definition.

This definition is valuable in many ways, but the concepts of "game design elements" and "non-game contexts" are both contestable. As Deterding et al concede, there is no universal list of game elements. This inherent uncertainty is problematic. For example, if, according to Koster, narrative is not a game mechanic [9], but it is to other game design theorists, does applying narrative to business processes constitute gamification? In fact, some definitions of game mechanics expressly exclude the points and reward structures that are typical features of gamification.

A related problem concerns the relationship of elements to experiences. Clearly not everything that includes a game element constitutes gamification. Examinations in schools, for example, give out points and are non-game contexts. If virtually every test were an example of gamification, the term would lose all meaning. Worse, by singling out atomic elements, the definition reinforces the notion that they are the most important aspects of games. Critics of gamification have effectively attacked this perspective [12].

By defining gamification as a process, we can talk about activities being more or less game-like, without needing to define a point where the designed system crosses over into gamification. This framing encourages designers to think about how to enhance and deepen the game-like aspects of their designs, rather than thinking their job is done once they drop in points or badges. Moreover, a key aspect of games is that they are voluntary [4][14]. If gamification designers view their task as pushing towards experiences that players engage with voluntarily, it may help to combat the possibility for manipulation or exploitation highlighted by Bogost and others [3].

Moreover, with this approach there is no need to limit the definition of gamification artificially. Deterding et al separate gamification (involving parts of games) from serious games (involving whole games). However, the dividing line is often difficult to see. Systems such as Foldit (for crowdsourced protein folding research) and Duolingo (for language learning) are game-like but not immersive simulations like the typical serious game. With the process approach, these can be seen as gamification examples, without struggling over whether they involve "non-game contexts."

Similarly, there is no need to insist that games cannot be gamified. Microsoft's XBox Live online service, for example, incorporates an additional experience of gameful achievements on top of an existing game environment. It operates exactly like many other gamification systems, yet Deterding et al state they would exclude it, in order to separate the enterprises of game design and gamification [5]. This is unnecessary: Someone can be engaged in game design and also engaged in gamification, without conflating the two. One activity seeks to create games; the other seeks to make *games or non-games* more game-like.

The deeper reason to reconceptualize gamification as a process is to focus attention on the types of experiences it seeks to create, and the mechanisms to do so. To be sure, the question of what constitutes a game has long bedeviled game designers, theorists, and even philosophers [4][14]. There is even a view, most prominently expressed by Ludwig Wittgenstein, that a game cannot be formally specified at all [18]. A useful definition of gamification need not resolve this debate. "Game-like" implies a constellation of attributes (Wittgenstein's term is "family resemblances") associated with certain kinds of experiences, without necessarily giving primacy to any of them.

As Huotari and Hamari note, the experiences games create may involve hedonic pleasure, suspense, or feelings of mastery [8]. A successful game is engaging; players commit to playing it voluntarily. As a practical matter, gamification operates as an applied practice in business (conceived broadly), which seeks to tap into that engagement to serve goals associated with some underlying activity. Those might involve signing up new customers, encouraging students to complete assignments more conscientiously, or any number of behavioral objectives.

What exactly does it mean to make something more game-like? Mollick and Rothbard capture this well when they say, in distinguishing gamification at work from simple sales contests, "[a] game is designed when it is purposefully created with reinforcing contexts, interactions, and mechanisms that create a more immersive feeling of play" [10]. Game elements are one means to the end of gamification, but what matters is how those elements are selected, deployed, implemented, and integrated. Experts recognize that, to use Schell's term, many "lenses" can be employed in game design [13].

Gamification is the process of making activities more game-like. In other words, it covers coordinated practices that objectively manifest the intent to produce more of the kinds of experiences that typify games. The designer's subjective mental state is relevant, but ultimately gamification is a process in the world manifesting that intent. Similarly, the player's subjective experience is an aspect of the gamification process, but not a necessary condition.

For example, the designer of the Stack Exchange developer question-and-answer site modeled it on the game Counter-Strike, in which "working *together* [is] the most effective way to win" [1]. The resulting design incorporated game elements such as badges, but what made it successful was this deeper effort to create a collaborative experience around an activity that would normally be highly individualized.

Another means of making activities more game-like is to try to make them more fun. Fun is a contestable term, but on some level it captures the ineffable qualities that distinguish games. Volkswagen's The Fun Theory contest illustrates how a process of incorporating fun into activities can produce valuable results. Volkswagen asked for entries that illustrated the concept that "fun can change people's behavior for the better."

One of the winning entries was "the deepest trashcan in the world" [7]. It enticed people to avoid littering by simulating the sound of a deep cavern when trash was thrown into an ordinary receptacle. Under the process definition, this would be understood as gamifying the activity of throwing out the trash, even though it does not involve any specific game design elements. The design of the physical trashcan is a concrete manifestation of the gamified activity.

There is an existing definition of gamification that uses the language of process, but it goes in a different direction. Drawing on concepts from the theory of service marketing, Huotari and Hamari define gamification as "a process of enhancing a service with affordances for gameful experiences in order to support user's overall value creation" [8]. In this way, they avoid the over-focusing on specific attributes and static nature of the elemental definition. In doing so, however, they resort to specialized language, which may not be accessible to researchers in other fields or to practitioners.

A bigger consideration is where the service marketing analogy leads. First, to Huotari and Hamari, drawing on the service marketing literature, the "value of a game service, be it 'pleasure', 'suspense', 'mastery' or 'gamefulness', is always determined by the player's individual perception." The trouble with this conception is that it implies that a bad game is somehow not a game at all. If I happen to feel that *Call of Duty* lacks challenge, suspense, and hedonic qualities, it does not call into question whether the developer is engaged in game design. Huotari and Hamari acknowledge that attempts at gamification may be more or less successful in creating the requisite player experience However, their player-centric perspective goes too far in disregarding the designer's intent. The subjective gamefulness of a system is an important factor in assessing gamification, but not the only one.

A further difference in the service marketing definition is its conception of gamification as an enhancing service that supports a core service. This leads Huotari and Hamari to claim that the social location app Foursquare is "not a gamified service in itself [8]," but a gamified enhancement to restaurants and bars. This seems unnecessarily constrained. Foursquare users who enjoy checking in are experiencing gamification, regardless of what they are checking in to. Many of the badges on Foursquare (such as the swarm badge for checking in with many other people) do not directly involve an underlying business. If what matters is the experience, why isn't that enough?

2   Definitional "Fit"

From an ordinary language perspective, a good definition should cover the systems that are generally understood to involve gamification, and exclude those that aren't. The important question isn't whether a definition is "right" in an abstract sense, but whether the distinctions and boundaries it creates are useful. Three examples illustrate how the process approach meets this test.

Virgin Healthmiles is a program that employers deploy in order to encourage health and wellness among their employees [16]. The program uses challenges, competitions, and virtual points redeemable for real-money rewards to encourage healthy behaviors. It is widely recognized as a gamified service [2], and all the leading definitions properly classify it as such. For the elemental definition, the key is that Virgin Healthmiles uses game design elements such as points and challenges. For the service marketing definition, the key is how the system's interface uses feedback to promote outcomes the user values. For the process definition, the key is that the program takes otherwise dull healthful behaviors and makes them more fun, rewarding, or attractive as competitive challenges.

The process definition therefore works as well as the other definitions for the classic PBL ("points, badges, leaderboards") systems [17] that are the most familiar examples of gamification. Where it shines is for examples closer to the periphery.

The Face Game is embedded in the intranet log-in process at online retailer Zappos [19], as a way to promote community and cross-organizational collaboration. When a worker signs in, they see a randomly chosen photo of another employee, with several options for their name. If the employee selects the wrong one, they see a page about their colleague from the company directory, and an invitation to connect with that co-worker to get to know them better.

The Face Game uses no common game design elements, unless that concept is expanded to include things as basic as guessing an answer from a list of choices. If that satisfied the elemental definition, gamification would be so broad as to lose any distinctiveness. Under the service marketing definition, the Face Game would not be an enhancement to a core service, because the goal is to promote camaraderie, not to improve the log-in process. Yet it is usefully identified as a gamified system. The Face Game is an effort to make an activity (logging in) and a business objective (fostering collaboration) more game-like, if only a little. The Face Game is not really a game at all, because the interaction is so lightweight. It is gamification because it involves leveraging curiosity or fun to serve business goals. Only the process definition covers it.

If the Face Game illustrates the insufficient coverage of existing definitions, the opposite scenario is where they are overbroad. LinkedIn's use of a progress bar to encourage users to add details to their online profiles has been cited as an example of a gamified activity [17]. And indeed, it meets the test of the elemental definition, because progress bars are used in game design.

If this is the only condition, however, the definition is radically over-expansive. Microsoft uses progress bars for Windows software installation. A strict reading of the elemental definition would call this gamification, yet that seems implausible. The process definition properly excludes the Windows progress bars, because they involve no gameful intent. LinkedIn uses progress bars to create an experience; Microsoft doesn't. The service marketing definition would get hung up on whether LinkedIn's online profile and the Windows installer are core services, which is not the real issue.

3   Gamification as a Form of Persuasive Design

Because gamification seeks to influence behavior, the literature on persuasive design can be brought to bear. Fogg's behavior model for persuasive design, for example, situates systems within a continuous space defined by motivation on one axis and ability on the other [6]. The desired action is triggered at a certain point, but designing the appropriate trigger involves an understanding of where the user sits within the graph. Game-like experiences can promote both motivation (by making activities feel more engaging) and ability (by promoting learning, achievement, and feelings of confidence).

Viewed as a process, therefore, gamification can function as a specialized tool to enhance the behavior change interventions that Fogg and others describe. And indeed, when a system such as the Zamzee fitness tracking and motivation platform for underprivileged youth utilizes game structures like rewards, levels, and challenges, it does so in service of persuasive design [20]. The process definition makes this clear and thus focuses attention on how the game-like attributes contribute. The elemental definition would founder on the artificial games/gamification distinction (Zamzee's tagline is "The Game That Gets Kids Moving") and de-emphasize the persuasive aspects relative to the design elements. The service marketing definition would search – perhaps with difficulty – for a "core service," and de-emphasize the persuasion in favor of co-creation and user value propositions.

Viewed through the lens of the process definition, gamification and persuasive design mesh well. A game is an inherently persuasive artifact, because it is by nature voluntary and goal-directed [14]. Games push toward objectives, but they do so in a non-coercive way, as do persuasive technologies [6]. Tromp, Hekkert, and Verbeek define a matrix of four ways that design can influence behavior: coercive, persuasive, seductive, or decisive [15]. Gamification techniques can be deployed in each quadrant. When offered voluntarily to users, as a marketing inducement or behavior change opportunity, gamification is likely to fit into the persuasive or seductive categories. When mandated in a workplace, it could be decisive or coercive.

It is these later applications, especially coercion, that raise the greatest concerns about manipulating or exploitation. A coercive experience may use game design elements, but arguably it would be *less* game-like due to its departure from voluntariness. To reiterate, the process definition will not itself prevent gamification designers from exploiting participants. However, to the extent that a definition helps to clarify norms and focus conversations around player-respecting attributes, it could make a positive contribution.

Gamification is still a young field. How scholars and practitioners define it will affect the coherence of their efforts, and shape the critical debate over its legitimacy. A definition of gamification as "the process of making activities more game-like" best captures the essential aspects of the practice. It fits what gamification is today, and provides valuable direction for the future.

References

1. Attwood, J.: The Gamification, Coding Horror (October 12, 2011),
   http://blog.codinghorror.com/the-gamification/
2. Boese, S.: Scoring Serious Results Through Gamification. HREOnline.com (May 13, 2013), http://www.hreonline.com/HRE/print.jhtml?id=534355401
3. Bogost, I.: Persuasive Games: Exploitationware. Gamasutra (May 3, 2011),
   http://www.gamasutra.com/view/feature/6366/
   persuasive_games_exploitationware.php
4. Carse, J.: Finite and Infinite Games. Ballantine, New York (1986)
5. Deterding, S., Dixon, D., Khaled, R., Nacke, L.: From Game Design Elements to Gamefulness: Defining "Gamification". In: MindTrek 2011, pp. 9–15. ACM Press, New York (2011)
6. Fogg, B.: A Behavior Model for Persuasive Design. In: Persuasive 209: 4th International Conference on Persuasive Technology, April 26-29 (2009)
7. Fun Theory, The: The World's Deepest Bin (September 21, 2009),
   http://www.thefuntheory.com/worlds-deepest-bin
8. Huotari, K., Hamari, J.: Defining Gamification: a Service Marketing Perspective. In: MindTrek 2012, pp. 17–22. ACM Press, New York (2012)
9. Koster, R.: Narrative is Not a Game Element. RaphKoster.com (January 20, 2012),
   http://www.raphkoster.com/2012/01/20/
   narrative-is-not-a-game-mechanic/
10. Mollick, E., Rothbard, N.: Mandatory Fun: Gamification and the Impact of Games at Work (June 10, 2013), http://ssrn.com/abstract=2059841
11. Paharia, R.: Loyalty 3.0: How Big Data and Gamification are Revolutionizing Customer and Employee Engagement. McGraw-Hill (2013)
12. Robertson, M.: Can't Play, Won't Play. Hide & Seek (October 6, 2010),
    http://hideandseek.net/2010/10/06/cant-play-wont-play/
13. Schell, J.: The Art of Game Design: A Book of Lenses. Morgan Kaufmann, San Francisco (2008)
14. Suits, B.: The Grasshopper: Games, Life and Utopia. Broadview Press (2005)
15. Tromp, N., Hekkert, P., Verbeek, P.-P.: Design for Socially Responsible Behavior: a Classification of Influence Based on Intended User Experience. Design Issues 27(3), 3–19 (2011)
16. Virgin Healthmiles: Employees "Got Game?" Press Release (August 23, 2011),
    http://us.virginhealthmiles.com/news/Pages/
    PR_110823_Gamification.aspx
17. Werbach, K., Hunter, D.: For the Win: How Game Thinking Can Revolutionize Your Business. Wharton Digital Press, Philadelphia (2012)
18. Wittgenstein, L.: Philosophical Investigations. Wiley-Blackwell (2010)
19. Zappos: You've Been Faced, http://zappified.com/face
20. Zamzee, https://www.zamzee.com/

Persuasion in the Car: Probing Potentials

David Wilfinger, Magdalena Gärtner,
Alexander Meschtscherjakov, and Manfred Tscheligi

Christian Doppler Laboratory for "Contextual Interfaces",
HCI & Usability Unit, ICT&S Center, University of Salzburg
{david.wilfinger,magdalena.gaertner,
alexander.meschtscherjakov,manfred.tscheligi}@sbg.ac.at

Abstract. The automotive domain has recently investigated interfaces
to persuade drivers to drive safer or in a more sustainable way. So far,
these systems are rather technology driven and mostly do not follow a
user centered design process. Our aim is to widen the scope of automotive persuasive interfaces and bring the user into the loop. We present
a probing study aiming at the identification of persuasion potentials in
the car. We describe findings related to inappropriate behavior, past behavior changes, and persuasion for passengers. Our study is a qualitative
approach to inform the design of innovative persuasive interfaces in the
automotive domain. We present the setup and results of the probing
study including a discussion of its potentials and limitations.

Keywords: automotive interfaces, car, cultural probing, persuasion.

1 Introduction and Related Work

Car traffic is known to be the cause of several problems affecting individuals,
as well as society. In general, driving in a car can be very stressful and frustrating. On a more dramatic level, environmental pollution and accidents due to
distraction or speeding cause injuries and may even kill people. Some of these
problems can be solved by laws or by means of technology, but the behavior of
each individual traffic participant also has a significant impact.

Persuasive technology has already been researched to change driver behavior
focusing mainly on eco-friendliness (e.g., [1]), as well as safe driving (e.g., [4]).
So far, research is missing the extent to which drivers and passengers want
to be supported in their behavior change and what areas hold potential for
persuasive efforts. We assume that drivers and passengers are often aware of a
potential disadvantageous behavior by themselves but have no support to initiate
or foster the actual behavior change. To close that gap from the perspective of
user centered design, this paper presents the results of a probing study aiming at
the identification of persuasion potentials in the car. We understand the study
as a preliminary approach, which holds the potential to help orientate the design
of persuasive interfaces and play an important role in the future of driving.

In the last years, automakers and researchers have included a range of persuasive interfaces in vehicles either to reduce fuel consumption or to improve

A. Spagnolli et al. (Eds.): PERSUASIVE 2014, LNCS 8462, pp. 273–278, 2014.

driver safety. Nissan, for example, introduced the Eco Pedal, which pushes back when the driver is accelerating too fast[1]. Honda presented their Eco Assist[2] system which let the speedometer background glow in different colors according to the driver's behavior, while Ford's Smart Gauge[3] tries to persuade drivers by visualizing green leaves when the driver behaves eco-friendly.

From the researcher's side, Ecker et.al. [1] developed "EcoChallenge", a community- and location-based in-car persuasive game with the goal to motivate and support behavioral change towards a fuel-reducing driving style. Tulusan et.al. [6] proved that a smartphone application can improve fuel efficiency by 3.23% even when the drivers do not pay for the fuel because they use, for example, a corporate car. Miranda et. al. [4], to the contrary, focused on "texting while driving"-behavior in their research. They proved the efficacy of combining a persuasive video documentary with text message reminders to decrease "texting while driving". Shepherd et. al. [5] influenced college students with the help of peers posing as passengers to drive risky (or not) in a driving simulation. The peers used verbal persuasion to affect the driving behavior of the students in one direction or the other. Their findings highlight the substantial influence of peers as passengers in a risk-related situation. This non-exhaustive list proves that both, industry and academia, are putting effort into the design, improvement, and implementation of persuasive in-car technologies.

2   The Probing Study

Media reports about the consequences of negative behavior are omnipresent and traffic participants learn about appropriate behavior in driving schools. Nevertheless, drivers do not always act accordingly. The motivation for our study is to identify persuasive potentials to overcome this hurdle by initiating a process of self reflections in the drivers, utilizing the probing methodology.

With the presented study, we aim at identifying aspects of driving where drivers are aware that their (or others) behavior is inappropriate and, thus, unsafe with regard to the current traffic situation. We want to receive information on past behavior changes and use the reasons for these changes for future designs to assist drivers who have not changed their behavior yet. We also aim at identifying potentials for passenger interfaces in the car that help the passengers to alter their behavior, in order to improve the situation for everyone (e.g., drivers, other traffic participants).

2.1   Study Method and Setup

We used probing as our research method. Thereby, participants received a "probing package" consisting of items that foster creativity and are returned to researchers for analysis [2]. Probes can help the users to express their feelings and

---

[1] www.nissan-global.com/EN/TECHNOLOGY/OVERVIEW/eco_pedal.html

[2] world.honda.com/INSIGHT/eco/index.html

[3] smartdesignworldwide.com/work/ford-smart-gauge/

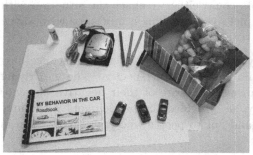 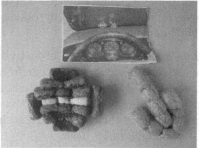

Fig. 1. Left: Probing package including road book, digital camera, colored markers, play corn, glue, two DIN A3 paper posters, three toy cars. Right: Probe 6 "My little helper" illustrating a system, which supports the driver during passing maneuvers

provide information on what caused the experience and how to address these experiences with interactive technology.

In order to conduct the probing study, we designed probing packages given to participants at the beginning of the study along with a short introduction and the signing of an informed consent. The central study instrument was a road book. In it, double pages were attributed to each probe, including instructions, graphical elements to cut out, and removable postcards. In addition to the road book, it consisted of a digital camera, colored markers, a bag full of play corn, glue, two DIN A3 paper posters, and three toy cars (see Figure 1). The study was centered on different topics related to behavior change in the car. The basic concept was to introduce participants to these topics (e.g., "The younger me") and then propose an activity (e.g., "draw a storyboard") to probe experiences made regarding that topic. In the following, these study topics and activities are introduced.

Probe 1 When I act in a way that is not safe: The first activity aimed at unveiling traffic situations in which drivers are aware that their behavior is unsafe and should be altered. Therefore, the participants were asked to create a collage to illustrate these situations with the help of comic-style pictures they had to glue on a sheet of paper. Missing elements they had to draw themselves.

Probe 2 The younger me: The goal of this probe was to gather information about what made drivers change their behavior in the past and potentially deduce how persuasive interfaces could support a behavior change using the same approach. Participants were encouraged to draw some sort of a storyboard. On the left side they sketched their behavior from earlier days, on the right side they sketched their current behavior.

Probe 3 Idiots on the road: This probe made use of the fact that it is often easier to report on other drivers' negative behaviors than on ones own misbehavior. The goal was, on the one hand, to collect traffic episodes, while on the other hand, to understand what other drivers would have needed in order to refrain from behaving that way. Participants could either re-enact the situation with toy-cars and document it by taking pictures or making a movie, or write down what happened.

Probe 4 Dear driver, ... : This activity aimed at gathering information concerning the driver's behavior in the car from a passenger's perspective. The underlying concept is that drivers might not always be aware of their negative behavior but passengers are. For this activity, we provided the participants with three postcards that they were asked to hand out to people who travel with them in the car on a regular basis.

Probe 5 Crime scene passenger seat: For this probe, participants were asked to probe situations where they had passengers in the car, who behaved in a bad way. They received graphical elements illustrating a crime scene (e.g., crime scene tape, a car, a subject) to cut out and glue on a sheet of paper. To summarize the crime scene, participants were encouraged to write up a small newspaper article to describe what exactly happened (e.g., who committed the crime and why).

Probe 6 My little helper: This activity asked participants to build a mock-up of a behavior changing systems they would like to have. The underlying concept is that rather than getting final design ideas, researchers get information on participants' requirements and desires that are integrated in the mockup. To build the mock-up the participants were provided with play corn, a craft material made of maize that sticks together when dampened.

Overall, 16 participants (6f, 10m) were recruited based on a recruitment profile (car driver, holding a driving license for at least 5 years, a yearly mileage travelled by car of at least 5,000 kilometers, driving with passengers regularly) through different mailing lists of our department. They were aged between 21 and 69 years and experienced drivers holding their driving license between 5 years and 51 years. The yearly mileage travelled by car varied between 7,000 up to 35,000 kilometers. All participants received 20 Euros for participating.

2.2   Analysis

When the participants returned the probing package after a three weeks period, they went through each probe (see, Figure 1) together with a researcher.

For the analysis of the probes, two workshops were conducted with three and four researchers respectively. Within the workshops, we made use of the essentials of the affinity diagram technique by Holtzblatt [3] to organize the information we deduced from the probes. Each probe was looked at by one researcher, who then presented it to the others. This presentation was followed by a discussion on the meaning of the probe in relation to the research goal. Each identified core content of the probe was written on paper cards and pinned to a wall. Further cards containing corresponding themes, ideas, and thoughts were placed next to each other. When the information of the probe had been exploited, the process was repeated with the next probe. Finally, the paper cards on the wall were grouped across probes, according to the identified themes.

3   Results

In the following, we present the main findings from the study. They include reflection-in-action, time perception, persuasion for passengers, as well as behavior change over time aspects.

Reflection-in-action: We identified a range of situations in which drivers were actually aware that their behavior was not appropriate but deliberately did not change it until they had to face the consequences. Utilizing the metaphor of a mirror, we envision a persuasive system which allows self reflection about one's negative actions and provide experience of what consequences the behavior (potentially) has. Above that, providing not only information on possible consequences but having users experience them without actually getting harmed is a major challenge and innovation potential. Persuasive strategies are also potentially more successful when drivers or passengers are told how their behavior might affect others in a negative way.

Time perception: The perception of time and stress was another relevant reason for inappropriate behavior. One reason for that is the unpredictability of time, when traveling by car. The time for commuting, for example, can vary considerably from day to day. Thus, it is possible that a trip that should not take more than 10 minutes takes an hour or more. Persuasive interfaces in this context can reduce frustration by showing how little time is won through stressful behavior (e.g., tailgating), by allowing a realistic estimation of travel times and by providing means of positive distraction when a journey takes longer than expected. This can include accurate feedback about the expected delay, information about the deviation from the average trip duration and the invitation to conduct alternative activities such as proposing a new audio book.

Persuasion for passengers: Passengers also play an important role when it comes to inappropriate behavior in traffic. We definitely identified front-seat passengers who do not behave appropriately and pose a risk to the driver and others (e.g., in reaching for the steering wheel) as targets for persuasion. In the probes, drivers complained specifically about passenger's missing understanding for their situations. Accordingly, persuasion for passengers includes making visible which effects certain behaviors have on the driver. Supporting the passengers in giving appropriate feedback and being a real help is a challenge for the future.

Behavior change over time: The probes revealed several reasons for behavior changes, including key experiences (e.g., accidents and traffic fines), the change of available vehicle technology (e.g., automatic transmission), and learning processes over time (e.g., the awareness that driving fast, and braking hard does not pay of in terms of a cost-benefit calculation). Interestingly, changes towards a more negative behavior were also probed. The experience one gains over the years results in a loss of attention on the road. And while the cars got safer over time, other emerging technologies such as mobile services lead to novel, unsafe driving behaviors. We conclude that both, momentary experiences and unconscious but continuos changes, may inform the design of future persuasive interfaces.

4 Conclusions

Our findings reveal various potentials and challenges that may be addressed when developing persuasive technology for the car. Thereby, we have experienced that probing is a meaningful method to get initial insights into persuasive potentials within the car, especially when empirical research data are absent. We also found the user's subjective reactions, impressions, and experiences to be useful for researchers and designers, although we faced some methodological challenges by applying the probing method in this context. First, we are aware that our results can not be generalized. They are subjective experiences from individuals, which have an unknown validity. Second, we often probed typical episodical experiences, which might not always include a novelty factor. Third, behavior changes often seemed to occur unconscious or at least not well reflected due to the fact that driving is habitual in nature. Nevertheless, at least some of these changes were hidden implicitly in the probes and could be made explicit in the analysis process.

We have found that past behavior changes of drivers can serve as a fruitful source of information. In a next step, our findings have to be transformed into persuasive designs. Making these concepts actually work in a vehicle in a safe and technologically sound way is part of our future work in automotive persuasion.

Acknowledgments. The financial support by the Federal Ministry of Economy, Family and Youth, the National Foundation for Research, Technology and Development and AUDIO MOBIL Elektronik GmbH is gratefully acknowledged (Christian Doppler Laboratory for "Contextual Interfaces").

References

1. Ecker, R., Holzer, P., Broy, V., Butz, A.: Ecochallenge: a race for efficiency. In: Proc. MobileHCI 2011, pp. 91–94. ACM, New York (2011)
2. Gaver, B., Dunne, T., Pacenti, E.: Design: Cultural probes. Interactions 6(1), 21–29 (1999)
3. Holtzblatt, K., Wendell, J., Wood, S.: Rapid contextual design: a how-to guide to key techniques for user-centered design. Morgan Kaufmann Publishers, San Francisco (2005)
4. Miranda, B., Jere, C., Alharbi, O., Lakshmi, S., Khouja, Y., Chatterjee, S.: Examining the efficacy of a persuasive technology package in reducing texting and driving behavior. In: Berkovsky, S., Freyne, J. (eds.) PERSUASIVE 2013. LNCS, vol. 7822, pp. 137–148. Springer, Heidelberg (2013)
5. Shepherd, J.L., Lane, D.J., Tapscott, R.L., Gentile, D.A.: Susceptible to social influence: Risky "driving" in response to peer pressure. Journal of Applied Social Psychology 41(4), 773–797 (2011)
6. Tulusan, J., Staake, T., Fleisch, E.: Providing eco-driving feedback to corporate car drivers: what impact does a smartphone application have on their fuel efficiency? In: Proc. UbiComp 2012, pp. 212–215. ACM, New York (2012)

SubRosa: Supporting a Proper Learning Atmosphere through Subtle Cues with Immediate Feedback

Paweł Woźniak[1,2], Bartosz Koczorowicz[2],
Morten Fjeld[1], and Andrzej Romanowski[2]

[1] t2i Interaction Lab, Department of Applied IT
Chalmers University of Technology, Gothenburg, Sweden
pawelw@chalmers.se
[2] Institute of Applied Computer Science
Lodz University of Technology, Lodz, Poland

Abstract. *SubRosa* is a persuasive ambient display system designed to reduce sound levels in areas used for quiet study. We have constructed a high-fidelity prototype that visualises ambient noise levels, in this case as a rotting tomato. *SubRosa* is different from similar systems in that it uses immediate feedback and targets a dynamic user group with a high member turnover. An experience study we conducted in two different locations showed positive influence on ambient noise conditions. Based on the study results, we discuss insights into the design of persuasive ambient displays, the effectiveness of our approach, and types of ambient feedback that could be used in similar systems. By comparing the experience study results, we show how immediate feedback for ambient displays is suitable for environments with dynamic user groups.

Keywords: persuasive technology, ambient display, behavioural change, ubiquitous computing.

1 Introduction

Research by Kjellberg et al. shows that high noise levels negatively affect learning ability [1]. To mitigate this, university buildings often have study rooms or spaces meant for students to work in silence. Students often forget to maintain a low volume when using them, defeating the purpose of these spaces. This can be caused by several activities, such as students talking to each other or the distracting one-sided conversation of mobile phone use. The learning process is also affected by the navigation of personal privacy in these shared spaces [2] i.e. privacy in study spaces is a complex issue *per se*. However, in our busy modern world many events often disturb this precious silence. As a consequence, we need extra means to keep the quiet study room truly quiet and to move noise-generating activities outside.

SubRosa is an ambient display system that aims to counter this problem by providing students with ambient feedback that will affect their everyday behaviour and improve learning conditions. One of the original purposes of ambient

A. Spagnolli et al. (Eds.): PERSUASIVE 2014, LNCS 8462, pp. 279–290, 2014.

displays—a core concept in ubiquitous computing since its creation (as reported by Weiser and Brown [3])was to provide information about the environment. More recent research has shifted to the field of ambient influence, where ambient displays are used to affect behaviour and habits. *SubRosa* (Figure 1) is a new effort in this field, investigating the feasibility of implementing ambient influence in a public setting. By prototyping and evaluating the system, we hope to learn how ambient displays can affect the behaviour of dynamic user groups.

In the remainder of this paper, we discuss related science projects, describe the design and implementation of the *SubRosa* system, and report on a field study conducted in two separate locations. This work contributes: (1) a novel idea for an ambient display-based persuasive system (i.e. a system that uses computer technology for behavioural change) aimed at noise reduction in spaces where intellectual work takes place, and (2) an implementation and field study of the aforementioned system in a real-life campus environment.

2   Related Work

In our research we aimed to build on the results of previous systems. The power-aware cord by Gustafsson and Gyllenswärd visualised energy consumption by varying light levels [4]. Nakajima et al. showed a virtual aquarium in which the objective was to promote proper tooth brushing habits. A key element of the project was for the user to develop an emotional attachment to the system [5]. While that study showed significant effects, it is hardly scalable to public spaces and multiple users. Consequently, our system does not attempt to stimulate emotions. Coralog by Kim et al. proposes embedding ambient displays in the user's everyday computational environment [6], and Nakajima and Lehdonvirta suggest personalised art installations as a means of influencing behavioural change [7]. Fortmann et al. [8] show how work environments can be augmented to motivate users to exercise during the day. These systems have informed the design of *SubRosa* by showing how ambient persuasion can be embedded in everyday environments.

One notices that while all these systems are focused on a specific user, influencing group behaviours through ambient displays is an unexplored area. In contrast, *SubRosa* provides collective feedback to a group of users who spend their time in a given place and at a specific moment. This strategy is shared with The Clouds [9], which is *SubRosa*'s main inspiration. Rogers *et al.* built a persuasive system that convinced users to use the stairs in a building, rather than the elevator, via an interactive installation—a wall-sized display accompanied by light-emitting diodes embedded in the floor. The Clouds was targeted at regular users of a particular building, who could be treated as similar people because they worked at the same institution. Another ambient display system that was designed for group use was Nimio [10], which created a social information channel with a set of translucent silicone toys. With *SubRosa* we aim to learn more about how dynamic groups of users who use a shared space—groups with a high member turnover—can be influenced by ambient displays.

Where The Clouds used accumulated feedback (*i.e.* showed status based on historical statistics), *SubRosa* explores how immediate responses can factor in influencing behaviour effectively. In order to achieve this, we had to choose a proper form of representation. As previous successful systems have used both approaches (i.e. immediate and accumulative feedback) and incorporated representational strategies (water ripples in ambientROOM [11]) or abstract strategies (lighting levels in [12]), with *SubRosa* we investigated how these choices of representation are motivated, and which are appropriate for use as immediate feedback. Indeed, immediate feedback has been used to stimulate behaviours. Ham et al. used immediate light colour feedback to motivate thermostat adjustments [13] and Froehlich presented an array of technologies promoting green behaviours, some of which utilised immediate feedback.

Our system is heavily inspired by recent works in the area of pervasive displays. Like Schmidt et al. [14], we believe displays will soon pervade everyday environments, and we aim to capitalise on their potential to promote positive behaviour. A study by Memarovic et al. [15] revealed that public displays are likely to engage strangers and are often treated as a community resource. This fact makes an impact on the design of our system, as social engagement is required if we would like users to actively maintain the proper conditions for their own learning. Claes and Vande Moere [16] show that displays in public spaces may create intrigue. Reveal-It! [17] illustrates how users may be prompted to reflect on their actions in the wild. These systems influenced the design of our own and suggested that a public display was the right medium for *SubRosa*.

3   Design

SubRosa was designed in two major stages. First, we identified the target space and conducted a preliminary study. Secondly, we designed and evaluated the final prototype.

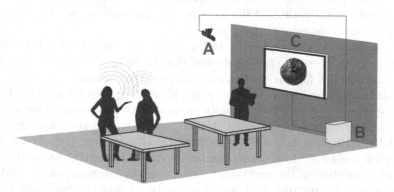

Fig. 1. The basic components of *SubRosa* : A. Noise level measurement, B. Hidden computer, C. Display

3.1   Initial Phase

We chose a quiet study room of the International Faculty of Engineering (IFE) of the Lodz University of Technology building as the setting for our study. The building is primarily a teaching facility for approximately 1200 students. It also provides a large open space with a bistro and two adjacent spaces for individual study: a computer lab and the study room under investigation. From informal interviews with both students (13) and academic personnel (3), we inferred that noise in the shared study rooms was a well-known issue. While many were looking forward to fill their breaks between classes with additional course work, this was often rendered impossible by the lack of suitable space.

Our first core activity was conducting semi-structured interviews with 9 students randomly chosen from the occupants of the study room at different times. We used a script in which we asked if the person was a regular user of the room and how the atmosphere could be improved. 8 out of the 9 participants listed reducing noise levels as a desired improvement. To further understand the problem, we spent two days a week for three weeks inside the room and monitored the sound levels. We determined that perceived noise levels varied significantly, and the noise was generated by several sources, such as conversations, phone calls, chairs scraping against the floor, or doors slamming.

The next step was to establish a rule that would enable us to determine when the noise levels had a negative impact on the environment. We recruited five volunteers to sit in the study room for one day, one at a time. The sound levels were constantly recorded. The volunteers used a simple dedicated application (nicknamed *the woodpecker*) to record their subjective opinion of the noise level in the room. Users were asked to press a button when the noise level was excessive. By comparing the obtained timestamps with noise levels, we could estimate the annoyance threshold for each of the participants. We used a mean of those thresholds to establish a reference noise level. All participants stated that while a low level of steady noise is easily tolerable, there existed a clear threshold above which work performance was affected. The exact level of that threshold may be subject to change. The participants also mentioned that sudden outbursts of noise greatly affected the learning environment, so we endeavoured to incorporate this requirement into *SubRosa*.

The remaining challenge was to find a proper visualisation for the different noise levels. Our literature review showed that there is no standard design procedure that applies for our particular situation. Past research has shown that immediate understanding by the user is not always required for a successful persuasive system [9]. The Clouds clearly showed that a persuasive system does not need to be obvious and explicit. Consequently, we explored ambiguity as a potential contributing factor. As suggested by Gaver et al. [18], we employed information ambiguity to generate user interest. We explored imagery that had no direct connection to the problem of excess noise in common spaces. Additionally, we looked for pictures that would easily blend into the background when the noise levels were as desired, but may become noticeable in case of excess noise.

We chose to compare images varying in their levels of dynamism and abstractness by projecting them onto a canvas mounted inside the study room and inviting users (a total of 11 students) to individually provide feedback in closed sessions (so as not to spread the news of the system too soon). We used three alternatives. The tomato (Figure 2a) rots when noise levels increase, the sun (Figure 2b) hides behind the horizon and the pipe man (Figure 2c) decreases in size. The tomato is representational and dynamic, the sun representational and subtle and the pipe man has an abstract connection to the sound. We asked our participants to order the three visualisations according to subjective preference by asking: "Which of these you would most gladly see in the study room?" This way, we aimed for our display to provide a pleasant aesthetic addition to the room when in low-noise condition. Our preliminary study showed that the tomato was the most suitable choice (first choice for 7 out of 11 participants). Because user feedback indicated the tomato was the most desirable choice, we decided to use it in our long-term study. An illustration of a man's head was perceived as boring (*"This guy doesn't impress me much. The tomato was cool."*). Users found it difficult to relate to the video of a setting sun (*"The time is not right for a sunset."*).

3.2   Designing the Final Prototype

Having agreed that the tomato was to be our visualisation medium, we had to address the issue of how it would relate to the state of the learning environment. A challenge faced by *SubRosa* was the need to influence the users of the room as quickly as possible. Unlike The Clouds, which was mainly targeted at repeat users of a certain space, our system was required to appeal and be acceptable to everyone whether they were a first-time user of the room or a seasoned IFE veteran. As the targeting of a dynamic group whose behaviour determines the state of the display has not been previously explored, we had to use new means to convey the message. Due to the context of the room, the users desire for a high noise level to reduce immediately .Consequently, we decided not to use accumulated feedback (for example, average noise levels for the day) as the basis for the visualisation, but to make the tomato respond to the noise level almost immediately. In our design we embraced Weiser and Brown's notion of the periphery [3]. We tried to make *SubRosa* an ambient display in its low-noise

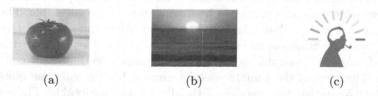

(a)   (b)   (c)

Fig. 2. The three visualisations used in the pilot study. The tomato (a), sunset (b), and the pipe man (c). Our preliminary study showed that the tomato was the most suitable choice. All images were sourced from royalty-free repositories.

state and have it "step out of the periphery" when noise levels needed to be reduced, prompting users to take action. We also revisited and adapted guidelines presented by Claes and Vande Moere [16] and applied them to *SubRosa*'s design. In fact, we introduced a twist to those guidelines in order to adapt them from urban space display to our particular environment. While our display may be affective, as it has a direct relationship to the environment (in line with the guidelines), we decided that it should only be immediately noticeable in the undesired condition if it is out of context with the visual nature of the location. While there are contexts where a picture of a rotten tomato may be expected (e.g. an art museum), it is surely surprising in a study room. This is contrary to the guidelines. However, we have still embraced the need for a metaphor that can be understood by everyone, regardless of skill and social position. A tomato is an everyday object, to which users can easily relate. Finally, just as Claes and Vande Moere suggest, we took utmost care so that the display always presented correct, up-to-date information, as precision is strictly required to create the potential for positive effect.

4   Implementation

A high-fidelity prototype of *SubRosa* was constructed to conduct our experience study. A microphone connected to a personal computer was mounted and hidden in the ceiling to gather noise levels. The computer was connected to a screen displaying the rotting tomato. See Figure 3 for technical details of the implementation. The display was strategically located within the room so that it was noticeable from all directions, and the seating and table arrangement were modified to increase the screen's visibility. As we sought to provide full anonymity to all participants in the study, sound from the room was never recorded. For the purposes of data collection, noise levels were measured, cached, averaged in 3 second windows, and then saved to a file. The system was only active during regular work days and during working hours. We used a single omnidirectional microphone mounted centrally in the ceiling of the room. The microphone was placed in the middle of the room and belowe ceiling-level to avoid unwanted amplification. This provided us with an overview of the global noise levels. As the source of the noise is not important for our users—as long as there is excess noise, learning conditions will be affected—we saw no need for determining and localising the source of noises. The rotting tomato was a collection of images, frames from a short video clip. The frame numbers were mapped to noise levels so that excessive noise was presented by a poor state of the vegetable. This way, the display was always dynamic, providing a pleasing ambiance to the room when the learning atmosphere—noise level—was acceptable. We added a small amount of constant sinusoidal movement to the tomato so that it seemed not to be static. The state of the tomato was determined by the real-time noise level delayed by $0.5s$ so that the reaction of the display was noticeable. The software was implemented with Processing (graphics) and Minim (audio). The noise level values we used were root-mean-square amplitudes obtained in real time from Minim's audio buffers.

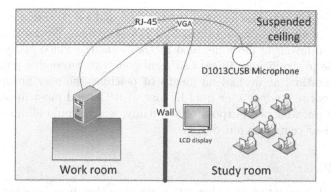

Fig. 3. The technical setup used to deploy *SubRosa* in a quiet study room

5   Field Study

SubRosa was evaluated in a field study at two distinct sites. The study respected applicable professional code of conduct and it did not qualify as coercion or deceit. The first location was the study room where we conducted our pilot study—an open space for students with a variety of users having different backgrounds. The other site, Chalmers University of Technology, was a space with a limited set of users who were academic and administrative personnel. Student access to this location was limited. Chalmers served as our control location—our research hypothesis was that *SubRosa* is more effective in the case of a dynamic user group and, therefore, we expect little effect in the case of Chalmers. It is worth noting that while the group at Chalmers has a low member turnover, the nature of their work is rather dynamic and noise is also an issue. There are dedicated discussion spaces, but loud conversations and answering telephone calls is a reported problem. This assessment was obtained from an independent, external employee survey. An important feature of both environments was the fact that we could limit our privacy considerations when deploying *SubRosa*. Both countries where the system was deployed do not have laws preventing recording in public spaces and CCTV systems are commonplace. Both universities have CCTV systems in operation and the room at IFE was already monitored by security 24/7.

5.1   Study Design

Studies in both locations lasted for approximately twelve weeks and data was collected simultaneously. Our deployment was performed outside of office hours in order to avoid being noticed. Initially, the visualisation module was disabled and measurements (root mean square (RMS) noise intensity values) were saved. Afterwards, *SubRosa* was activated during a weekend (the system allows for predefining activation times and remote management). The time of the study was correlated with the academic calendar in both locations, thus eliminating the possibility of a place being less frequented during a particular period, generating false-positive lower noise levels. The collected data consists of a qualitative component—the RMS noise levels in the rooms—and a qualitative component—a set of time stamped notes obtained by the researchers. We took the decision to use notes in favour of more detailed methods such as video analysis or voice recording due to significant ethical and legal concerns. Surveying users was also out of the question, as we had no means of reaching the user group using the system (the entire student user pool in case of IFE), and most importantly we feared communicating the purpose of the study, which would eliminate the ambiguous element central to our design.

5.2   Results

The measured noise intensity values are specific to the given location as the system was calibrated each time, so the absolute values cannot be easily compared between locations. Mean differences, however, are relevant. Table 1 presents a summary of pre- and post-study RMS noise values at the two locations. We have discarded low ambient noise levels since the pilot study found that these do not cause a significant disturbance. Figure 4 presents the results obtained at IFE and Chalmers as a plot of noise level over time. In order to relate to previous studies and identify practical consequences of our results, we replicated the statistical methodology used by Rogers et al. [9]. In the IFE case, a decrease in mean noise level of $\mu_{pre} - \mu_{post} = 0.0134$ (a 9% decease) was observed. While this value is small in absolute terms, it is statistically significant as we obtained $t(1258) = 6.0182$ and $p < 0.001$. We calculated the Pearson product-moment coefficient in order to determine whether the effect was not related to time and we found no correlation between the time after the installation and the noise level with $r = 0.059$ with $p > 0.05$. On the other hand, we observed a slight, but non-significant increase in noise level for Chalmers ($\mu_{pre} - \mu_{post} = -0.0041$, $t(1265) = -3.3279$ and $p < 0.05$). As a result, we can conclude that *SubRosa* produced a significant reduction in the noise levels in the case of a dynamic user group, but failed to produce a significant result in the stable group. User reactions to the system were varied. Generally, the system piqued the curiosity of those in the rooms. We observed that the constantly changing users at IFE noticed the display at different stages of their stay in the room. Some would notice the display immediately, while others were prompted by fellow users. We noted several cases of the users performing actions to try and determine the cause of the tomato's changes. Having discovered that the display responded to sounds, several users proceeded to generate noise in order to cause a reaction (*"Is that thing on?"* was by far the most common comment). This intrigue, however,

Table 1. Mean (μ) and standard deviation (σ) for measurements before and after the installation of *SubRosa* in the two locations

Location	μ_{pre}	σ_{pre}	μ_{post}	σ_{post}
IFE	0.1454	0.0463	0.1320	0.0306
Chalmers	0.1345	0.0314	0.1386	0.0276

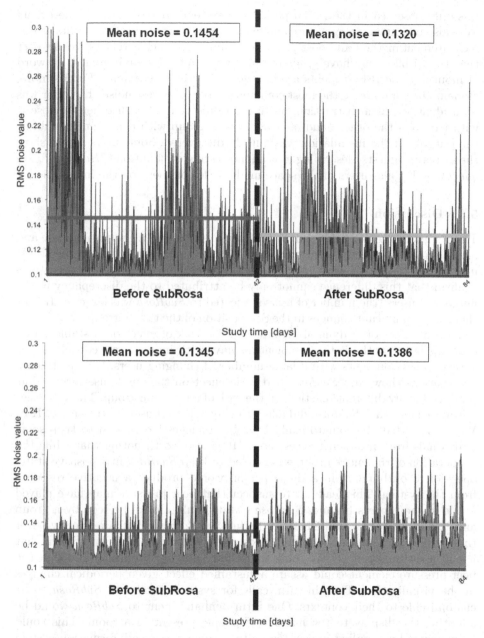

Fig. 4. RMS noise levels in the study period at IFE (a) and Chalmers (b). Note that IFE is a place with a constantly changing user group and *SubRosa* was used by a fixed group at Chalmers. Noise values below a threshold established with a pilot study were discarded. In the case of IFE, two weeks immediately preceding the installation of the system were discarded to factor out the novelty effect. The values shown represent deviations above the established noise level threshold and are derivatives of microphone- and environment-specific values—values between sites are not comparable.

was only observed in the initial period the system's deployment. These events were also of a momentary nature and cannot affect our qualitative results as our measurement method and post-processing eliminated such artefacts. We suspect that the display may have gradually integrated into the environment by word of mouth as the IFE students are a large and active community. Furthermore, students began noticing the most common sources of excess noise. The door was soon identified as a distraction and users would remind each other to close it with care. On the other hand, at Chalmers, a group with consistent members, the purpose of the installation was quickly discovered. Some users would show the display to guests, describing it as an interesting contraption (*"Here's a funny gadget."*). Regular users of the space made little comment on the installation.

5.3   Discussion

The key finding of our field study is that *SubRosa* elicited a greater response and intrigue in the dynamic user group of the study room rather than in the stable user group, the group with low member turnover. The qualitative observations confirm that this difference cannot only be attributed to the discrepancy in the number of users (the number of users subjected to *SubRosa* was larger at IFE as there were significant changes in the composition of the target group). *SubRosa*'s significant effect on a dynamic group, and the lack of effect on a stable group confirms our hypothesis that ambient displays with immediate feedback are effective in environments with a large number of changing users. Our qualitative observations show that *SubRosa* had little effect on the stable user group, but produced many different reactions in the case of a dynamic group. There is a significant chance that *SubRosa* did affect the behaviour of users in the case of IFE. We suspect that the tomato could have been suggestive enough to keep some individuals from producing excess noise. It is also worth noting that while the cooperation of the entire group was needed to keep *SubRosa* in a positive state, one violent outburst from a single person would produce a negative response from the system. This leads us to suspect that peer pressure may have played a role in the process because *SubRosa*'s state could always be seen by a group and it did not target individuals. Whether *SubRosa* will remain effective over time is uncertain, even though our six-week evaluation period has shown that it had a sustained effect. We think that the results are promising and that the peer-pressure element could assure a sustained effect given periodical changes in the visualisation. This, in turn, calls for systems similar to *SubRosa* to be customisable to their contexts. One future enhancement to *SubRosa* would be adapting the display to the number of people present in a room. This could be achieved by coupling our system with a room presence information system similar to the one presented in [19].

SubRosa's ambiguity was an interesting aspect of the study. Unlike The Clouds, our system featured no elements that would suggest a desired behaviour. A deteriorated tomato was the only representation of an undesirable state for the environment. We have created an ambient display to which users can easily relate, which is in line with the findings of Nakajima and Lehdonvirta [7].

However, the way each user relates to the display is different. We used imagery that may produce negative feelings. *SubRosa* shows that there are potential benefits from using a less abstract metaphor for ambient displays. Through our study, we hope to inspire more exploration by further design of similar systems. Rogers et al. [9] explored accumulated feedback for a stable group and we investigated immediate feedback for stable and dynamic groups. That leaves one more alternative to be explored and we need more research to understand the interplay between these parameters.

6   Conclusions and Future Work

This paper described the design, implementation and in situ study of *SubRosa*, an ambient display system offering immediate feedback, targeting the problem of excessive noise in study environments. Our study has confirmed the persuasive potential of ambient displays, as suggested by past research. *SubRosa* targets a highly dynamic group and the results of the study indicate that immediate feedback is appropriate for influencing the behaviour of users of public spaces in dynamic groups. Intrigue was a significant element in the interactions with the system. We replicated the methodology, study length, and statistical apparatus from previous similar studies, and determined that our system was significantly effective in case of a group with a high member turnover. We hope to inspire new interventions and new systems that positively affect larger groups, and use different metaphors to achieve that goal. Furthermore, we would like to see approaches similar to *SubRosa* applied to other public spaces where noise is an issue.

Acknowledgements. The research leading to these results has received funding from the People Programme (Marie Curie Actions) of the European Union's Seventh Framework Programme FP7/2007-2013/ under REA grant agreement no. 290227. Thank you to Barrie Sutcliffe for his editorial work. Paweł Woźniak is an Early Stage Researcher in the DIVA Marie Skłodowska-Curie ITN. The authors thank the International Faculty of Engineering for help in conducting the studies.

References

1. Kjellberg, A., Landström, U., Tesarz, M., Söderberg, L., Akerlund, E.: The effects of nonphysical noise characteristics, ongoing task and noise sensitivity on annoyance and distraction due to noise at work. J. Environ. Psychol. 16, 123–136 (1996)
2. Stone, N.J.: Designing effective study environments. Journal of Environmental Psychology 21, 179–190 (2001)
3. Weiser, M., Brown, J.S.: Beyond calculation, pp. 75–85. Copernicus (1997)
4. Gustafsson, A., Gyllenswärd, M.: The power-aware cord: energy awareness through ambient information display. In: CHI EA 2005, pp. 1423–1426. ACM (2005)

5. Nakajima, T., Lehdonvirta, V., Tokunaga, E., Kimura, H.: Reflecting human behavior to motivate desirable lifestyle. In: Proc. DIS 2008, pp. 405–414. ACM (2008)
6. Kim, T., Hong, H., Magerko, B.: Design requirements for ambient display that supports sustainable lifestyle. In: Proc. DIS 2010, pp. 103–112. ACM (2010)
7. Nakajima, T., Lehdonvirta, V.: Designing motivation using persuasive ambient mirrors. Pers. Ubiquit. Comput. 17, 107–126 (2013)
8. Fortmann, J., Stratmann, T.C., Boll, S., Poppinga, B., Heuten, W.: Make me move at work! an ambient light display to increase physical activity. In: Proceedings of PervasiveHealth 2013, Brussels, Belgium, pp. 274–277. ICST (2013)
9. Rogers, Y., Hazlewood, W.R., Marshall, P., Dalton, N., Hertrich, S.: Ambient influence: can twinkly lights lure and abstract representations trigger behavioral change? In: Proc. Ubicomp 2010, pp. 261–270. ACM (2010)
10. Brewer, J., Williams, A., Dourish, P.: A handle on what's going on: Combining tangible interfaces and ambient displays for collaborative groups. In: Proceedings of TEI 2007, pp. 3–10. ACM, New York (2007)
11. Wisneski, C., Ishii, H., Dahley, A., Gorbet, M., Brave, S., Ullmer, B., Yarin, P.: Ambient displays: Turning architectural space into an interface between people and digital information. In: Yuan, F., Konomi, S., Burkhardt, H.-J. (eds.) CoBuild 1998. LNCS, vol. 1370, pp. 22–32. Springer, Heidelberg (1998)
12. Occhialini, V., van Essen, H., Eggen, B.: Design and evaluation of an ambient display to support time management during meetings. In: Campos, P., Graham, N., Jorge, J., Nunes, N., Palanque, P., Winckler, M. (eds.) INTERACT 2011, Part II. LNCS, vol. 6947, pp. 263–280. Springer, Heidelberg (2011)
13. Ham, J., Midden, C., Maan, S., Merkus, B.: Persuasive lighting: the influence of feedback through lighting on energy conservation behavior. In: Proceedings of Experiencing Light 2009 International Conference on the Effects of Light on Wellbeing, Eindhoven, the Netherlands, October 26-27, pp. 122–128. Eindhoven University of Technology, Eindhoven (2009)
14. Schmidt, A., Pfleging, B., Alt, F., Sahami, A., Fitzpatrick, G.: Interacting with 21st-century computers. IEEE Pervasive Computing 11, 22–31 (2012)
15. Memarovic, N., Langheinrich, M., Alt, F., Elhart, I., Hosio, S., Rubegni, E.: Using public displays to stimulate passive engagement, active engagement, and discovery in public spaces. In: Proceedings of MAB 2012, pp. 55–64. ACM, New York (2012)
16. Claes, S., Vande Moere, A.: Street infographics: raising awareness of local issues through a situated urban visualization. In: Proceedings of PerDis 2013, pp. 133–138. ACM, New York (2013)
17. Valkanova, N., Jorda, S., Tomitsch, M., Vande Moere, A.: Reveal-it!: the impact of a social visualization projection on public awareness and discourse. In: Proceedings of CHI 2013, pp. 3461–3470. ACM, New York (2013)
18. Gaver, W.W., Beaver, J., Benford, S.: Ambiguity as a resource for design. In: Proceedings of CHI 2003, pp. 233–240. ACM (2003)
19. Woźniak, P., Romanowski, A.: Everyday problems vs. ubicomp: a case study. In: Proceedings of WIMS 2012, pp. 57:1–57:4. ACM (2012)

Systematic Review of Behavioral Obesity Interventions and Their Persuasive Qualities

Anna Xu[1,*], Taridzo Chomutare[2], and Sriram Iyengar[1]

[1] University of Texas, Health Science Center at Houston, Houston, TX
[2] University of Tromsø, Tromsø, Norway
anna.xu@uth.tmc.edu

Abstract. In this systematic review of weight loss interventions, we reviewed interventions aimed at maintaining weight loss, and identify persuasive elements that drive weight maintenance.

Methods: We searched the Medline database for long-term obesity interventions, and targeted randomized control trials that aimed to reduce weight among adults for over 12 months, and extracted outcomes related to body weight change.

Results: Seventeen publications were in the final review. Tailoring, or group counseling led by a health care professional, was shown to have a significant effect on long-term weight loss. Positive effects were also obtained by personalization (one-on-one counseling), competition (competing against other people trying to lose weight), and reminders.

Conclusion: Maintaining weight loss long-term as so far eluded researchers, but results suggest that that some elements of the interventions are more greatly associated with weight maintenance than others. Future interventions might be more effective if they were based on persuasive technology.

Keywords: Persuasive technology, obesity, systematic review, behavior.

1 Introduction

Obesity is known to be a major problem in the United States and has a major influence on chronic health conditions such as type 2 diabetes, hypertension, and cardiovascular disease [5, 11]. Obesity is also associated with increased healthcare costs [14, 21]. The prevalence of obesity shows that current interventions to reduce obesity have so far been inadequate. There is a need to identify elements of effective intervention strategies to decrease the health and economic costs of obesity. Although many obese individuals intend to change their dietary and exercise habits, only a few succeed. Even though interventions are usually successful in short term weight loss, long-term weight loss intervention effects are often not sustained [2, 3, 9, 23].

Lifestyle factors, such as an excess intake of calories and low levels of physical activity, have been shown to be the main causes of obesity [11, 15]. Promisingly,

---

* Corresponding author.

A. Spagnolli et al. (Eds.): PERSUASIVE 2014, LNCS 8462, pp. 291–301, 2014.

long-lasting weight loss has been shown to occur with long-term diet and physical activity [8, 18, 19]. Behavioral interventions, first introduced in the 1970s, attempt to change diet and exercise habits by modifying the environment such as restricting types of food available, or change behavior, such as receiving rewards for healthy behaviors [7]. Behavioral modification interventions therefore may help overweight people lose weight, especially if they target lifestyle changes such as reducing caloric intake and increasing physical activity.

However, most behavioral approaches to date have been quite complex, featuring multiple design elements in any one intervention. Previous reviews have typically classified obesity interventions into diet, physical activity and behavior counselling [4] – and these classes are not necessarily mutually exclusive. A serious drawback with this kind of classification is that it is simplistic in nature and therefore does not capture the persuasive essence of many of the interventions. There are many meta-analyses of obesity interventions, but there have been much fewer studies of how the design of health interventions affects outcomes [1, 10, 12, 13]. Consequently, there is limited evidence of the efficacy of the persuasive qualities in weight loss maintenance. However, the methods used to study design elements have been used previously [10, 12, 13] and in more limited ways in standard meta-analyses [1].

An existing framework, Persuasive Systems Design (PSD), has identified a number of design features that can influence and change a user's behavior. First discussed by Oinas-Kukkonen [16], the PSD model provides a classification method that can be used to analyze behavioral weight loss interventions. The model allows us to abstract the important concepts in complex interventions by providing a uniform platform for comparison, without the diversity of every case. In this paper, we map persuasive qualities of the interventions to the PSD model and aim to discover the most effective elements that "drive" long-term weight loss.

1.1   Aims

In this paper, we aim to use the PSD model to extract and analyze persuasive system features in interventions to find the most effective elements that "drive" long-term weight loss. Persuasive technology, as defined by BJ Fogg, is a term for software designed to provoke change in human behavior in a prescribed way [6]. We have used a derivative of Fogg's model, Oinas-Kukkonen's Persuasive Systems Design (PSD) model, as a framework to explain our approach. PSD also has been successful in changing user's behaviors other systems, such as Fit4Life, which used an earpiece that guided a user through explicit verbal suggestions, such as when specific foods should be eaten or avoided [17].

We aim to answer these two questions:

(1) Are weight loss and weight loss maintenance interventions for adults more effective when there are elements of persuasive systems design theory underlying the intervention?

(2) What specific persuasive elements of interventions work best for sustaining weight loss?

2   Methods

We conducted an electronic literature search for randomized controlled trials (RCTs) relating to weight loss and weight loss maintenance among adults. The relevant literature was found by a search of the°medical database Medline (1977 to present), previous systematic reviews of interventions for the overweight and obese, and citations in reviews and papers. Main keywords were obesity, overweight, weight reduction program, and randomized control trial.

2.1   Inclusion Criteria

The first criterion was that the article should be a randomized control trial (RCTs) that evaluated the effectiveness of interventions for treatment of obesity and weight loss maintenance. We focused on behavioral-based interventions for adults. RCTs that did not include a lifestyle or behavioral based component were not included in this review. For example, a "diet only" intervention, or an intervention that only used diet as a modification without a behavioral component, would not be included. A second criterion is that the study should observe participants for at least 12 months, whether the time was spent on the duration of the intervention itself or by length of follow-up. Interventions are only deemed effective if the weight loss is maintained long term. A third criterion is that the study must have had at least 300 participants at the start of the intervention. Loss due to follow up was not included in this figure. Because the rate of weight loss maintenance is less than 5% [3], a large study population is better equipped to detect those numbers.

2.2   Exclusion Criteria

We excluded interventions that targeted those with several mental illnesses such as bipolar disorder, or included surgical interventions, like gastric balloons. Although we accepted lifestyle interventions with an additional pharmacotherapy aspect, such as Orlistat, exclusive drug-based interventions were not considered.

Intervention details were retrieved from the articles themselves. If the research design was already published in a previous or associated publication, the previous paper was consulted. To be considered, studies must have included a measure of weight change, such as pounds or kilograms of weight lost.

2.3   Mapping and Data Abstraction

Mapping between the PSD model and the persuasive qualities of the reviewed interventions involved two authors going through papers independently, and then meeting for consensus analysis. The two authors (AX, TC) initially agreed on a set of definitions for the PSD model, adapting the definitions to suit the weight loss case where necessary. Instead of considering the inter-rater agreement, the goal of the consensus meeting was to ensure we identified all the persuasive elements as written in the reviewed studies, and that we coded them correctly. Each paper finally selected in the review was carefully read to identify the results reported with regard to weight loss.

Table 1. Definitions of 9 most common persuasive design elements in interventions

Self-monitoring	A system that helps track one's own performance or status supports in achieving goals.	An intervention that allows a participant to track his own health habits, such as a food diary or exercise spreadsheet.
Personalization	A system that offers personalized content or services has a greater capability for persuasion.	One-on-one counseling with a nutritionist or dietician.
Tunneling	Using the system to guide users through a process or experience provides opportunities to persuade along the way.	An intervention that guides participants through a process to lose weight. Examples include two phase interventions, such as a rapid weight loss phase followed by a weight maintenance phase, or exercise interventions that gradually increase physical activity.
Reduction	A system that reduces complex behavior into simple tasks helps users perform the target behavior and it may increase the benefit/cost ratio of a behavior.	A weight-loss intervention that reduces the cognitive load of losing weight. Examples include meal-replacement drinks, tokens that represent caloric values, and point systems.
Reminders	If a system reminds users of their target behavior, the users will more likely achieve their goals.	Reminders in interventions can take the form of mailings to non-responders to encourage participation, or by email to set new weight loss goals.
Similarity	People are more readily persuaded through systems that remind themselves in some meaningful way.	An intervention with similarity will incorporate physical activity behaviors into everyday life. This is after participants reflected on activities they would like to perform 5 days a week and were taught how to cope and adapt with any obstacles they might encounter.
Tailoring	Information provided by the system will be more persuasive if it is tailored to the potential needs, interests, personality, usage context, or other factors relevant to a user group.	Group counseling or education with a nutritionist or dietician. Group tailoring can be also be delivered by group telephone contacts.

Table 1. (*continued*)

Rewards	Systems that reward target may have great persuasive powers.	An intervention that rewards participants with financial incentives for completing goals or sessions.
Competition	A system can motivate users to adopt a target attitude or behavior by leveraging human beings' natural drive to compete.	These include team competitions that allow the teams with the most amount of weight lost to win a prize.

2.4   Statistical Analysis and Tests

Weight loss in the experimental group was deemed statistically significant by self-report of authors, and deemed not statistically significant if authors indicated otherwise (Table 2). Other researchers have used a similar approach to make inferences about the effect of design components on intervention outcome. After they coded papers for persuasive design elements, they compared interventions that had significant differences between intervention and control, non-significant differences, and in some cases, indeterminate differences [10, 12, 13].

After we coded the persuasive design elements of each intervention and judged the weight-loss effectiveness of each experimental-control group, we applied a test of binary proportions. Using this binomial distribution of successful and unsuccessful weight loss interventions, we tested whether the proportion of weight loss is the same in the two groups. Single-tailed P values were calculated.

Table 2. Assessment of effectiveness

Effectiveness of intervention	Definitions
Successful or more effective interventions	Statistically significant weight loss in intervention group compared to control
	Improvement in majority of participants
Unsuccessful or ineffective interventions	Statistically insignificant weight loss in intervention group compared to control
	Intervention no more effective than control group

3   Results

The initial search yielded 1488 articles, as shown in Fig. 1. All papers were reviewed against inclusion and exclusion criteria by the two authors (AX, TC). Any disagreements were resolved by consensus. Based on the title and abstract, this number dropped to 306 after applying the inclusion and exclusion criteria. Of the 306 trials left, 154 were not included due to the trial not lasting longer than 12 months. Another 112 were excluded to do having fewer than 300 participants and another 4 because the researchers used only financial incentives. In the end, we had 17 articles. 4 articles had double experimental groups, leading to 21 interventions total: 13 interventions were unsuccessful, and 8 were successful. The flow chart in Fig. 1 illustrates the study elimination process.

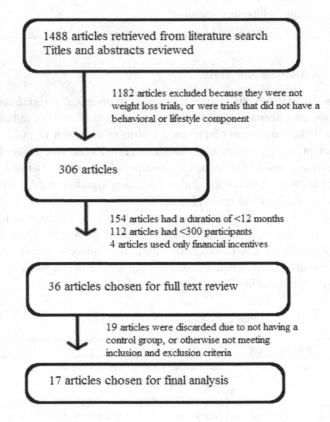

Fig. 1. Flow chart for selection of studies

In figure 2a, we show that there is a difference in weight loss among groups when using author self-report. The average amount of weight lost at 12 months was 1.41 kg for the statistically insignificant or unsuccessful intervention, versus 4.4 kg for the statistically significant or successful intervention.

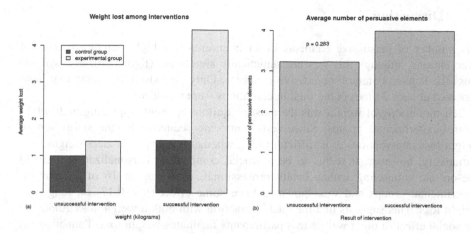

Fig. 2. In figure 2a, successful interventions show a greater amount of weight loss in the experimental group compared to the unsuccessful interventions. In figure 2b, the average number of persuasive elements is higher among successful interventions.

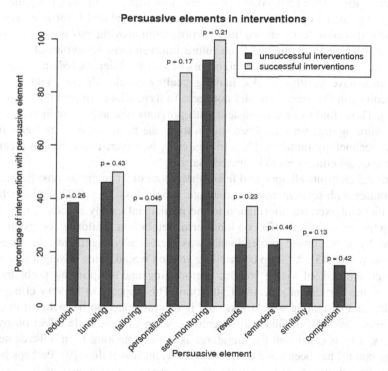

Fig. 3. This figure shows the 9 most common PSD persuasive elements and their frequencies among the successful and unsuccessful interventions

4   Discussion

The number of persuasive elements in an intervention is higher among successful interventions, although this was not statistically significant (figure 2b). We will address the 9 most common persuasive elements. Only persuasive elements that have appeared at least 3 times in the final interventions were included.

Self-monitoring of weight was the most ubiquitous element, appearing in 20 of 21 control-experimental groups. Since self-monitoring seems to be the status-quo of weight loss interventions, it is difficult to tell whether it helps or hinders weight loss. Initiatively, however, it seems to be a crucial component. Personalization, defined one-on-one counseling with a health professional, shows up in 16 of 21 control-experimental groups and was shown to have some effect ($p = 0.17$) on long-term weight loss. This suggests that the dual interaction with both a weight loss guide and the social effect of other weight loss participants facilitates weight loss. Tunneling, an intervention that leads participants through a stepwise program, appears in 10 of 21 interventions, and was not shown to have an effect on weight loss ($p = 0.43$). An example of tunneling is in the 'Keep it Off' group, in which guided participants received the 'Keep It Off' course book, which were worked on with 10 biweekly phone calls with a weight loss coach [20]. Although weight loss was significant among the experimental group, tunneling tends to be somewhat complicated and labor-intensive. It is possible that this complexity serves little purpose in improving and sustaining weight loss, and can be safely eliminated from future interventions. Examples of reduction, changing the environment to make weight loss decisions easier, include making vending machines have healthy snacks, making healthy snacks cheaper, and installing fitness facilities in the workplace, did not seem to have a large impact on weight loss ($p = 0.26$). Those findings are consistent with previous research, as reduction, tunneling, and tailoring together have been shown to be the most common elements in the persuasive technology literature [22]. In this case, however, two common elements, reduction and tunneling seem to be unnecessary.

The other 5 elements all appeared fewer than 6 out of 21 interventions. Reminders, regular contact with participants to encourage weight loss, ($p = 0.23$) and similarity, adapting diet and exercise information to the participant's daily schedule, ($p = 0.46$) both seem to have a limited effect on long-term weight loss. Tailoring, or group counseling led by a healthcare professional, was statistically significant in long-term weight loss ($p = 0.045$). A group counselling session would guide a weight loss attendee through the task of losing weight, customizing and simplifying problems and solutions to the participant's personal situation. This appears to be very effective in maintaining and sustaining weight loss, and is recommended to be included in future interventions. Rewards, or financial incentives, seem to have little effect on overall weight loss. This is consistent the literature, as inadequate long-term rewards needed for weight control has been cited as a cause of weight loss failure [9]. Perhaps people are not motivated by money to lose weight, or the amount of money associated with trials (usually less than \$100, or a return of participant's own money contingent upon losing weight) is not sufficient motivation. Regarding competition, successful interventions had more competitive elements than unsuccessful ones ($p = 0.13$). Although the observed difference between the two was not significant, this finding suggests that competition, in formats similar to 'Biggest Loser' team weight loss challenges, is promising as a weight loss maintenance strategy.

4.1   Limitations

Due to the stringent inclusion criteria of studying long term weight loss in large populations, the number of papers found was not kept high, thus constraining the number of persuasive elements found. Another limitation is that intervention results might be due to concurrent use of multiple persuasive features in the same system.

5   Conclusion

In this study, we reviewed the literature on weight loss among adults that satisfied inclusion and exclusion criteria described above. The aim of this study was to understand weight loss and weight loss maintenance interventions in light of the emerging discipline of persuasive technology (PT). In summary, the 17 publications in the final review show that tailoring, or group counseling led by a health care professional, has a significant effect on long-term weight loss. Positive, but more modest effects, were also obtained by personalization (one-on-one counseling), competition (competing against other people trying to lose weight), and reminders.

Our study indicates that persuasive technology can potentially be a viable framework to analyze the effectiveness of weight loss and weight loss maintenance interventions. PT could also be used to design future interventions, as certain persuasive elements are shown to be more often present in interventions aimed at sustaining weight loss than others. In conclusion, achieving and maintaining long-term weight loss remains a challenge, but results suggest that future interventions may be more effective if they considered elements of persuasive technology in the design.

Acknowledgement. This work was supported by a training fellowship from the Keck Center AHRQ Training Program in Patient Safety and Quality of the Gulf Coast Consortia and in part by the Research Programme for Telemedicine (HST), Helse Nord RHF. We thank the anonymous reviewers whose comments resulted in a greatly improved paper.

References

1. Bacigalupo, R., Cudd, P., Littlewood, C., Bissell, P., Hawley, M.S., Buckley Woods, H.: Interventions employing mobile technology for overweight and obesity: an early systematic review of randomized controlled trials. Obesity Reviews: An Official Journal of the International Association for the Study of Obesity 14(4), 279–291 (2013)
2. Brownell, K.D.: The humbling experience of treating obesity: Should we persist or desist? Behaviour Research and Therapy 48(8), 717–719 (2010)

3. Crawford, D., Jeffery, R.W., French, S.A.: Can anyone successfully control their weight? Findings of a three year community-based study of men and women. International Journal of Obesity and Related Metabolic Disorders: Journal of the International Association for the Study of Obesity 24(9), 1107–1110 (2000)

4. Douketis, J.D., Macie, C., Thabane, L., Williamson, D.F.: Systematic review of long-term weight loss studies in obese adults: clinical significance and applicability to clinical practice. International Journal of Obesity 29(10), 1153–1167 (2005)

5. Flegal, K.M., Carroll, M.D., Ogden, C.L., Curtin, L.: Prevalence and trends in obesity among US adults, 1999-2008. JAMA 303(3), 235–241 (2010)

6. Fogg, B.J.: Persuasive computing: technologies designed to change attitudes and behaviors. Morgan Kaufmann, Elsevier Science, San Francisco, Calif., Oxford (2003)

7. Jeffery, R.W., Wing, R.R., Thorson, C., Burton, L.R., Raether, C., Harvey, J., Mullen, M.: Strengthening behavioral interventions for weight loss: a randomized trial of food provision and monetary incentives. Journal of Consulting and Clinical Psychology 61(6), 1038–1045 (1993)

8. Jeffery, R.W., Drewnowski, A., Epstein, L.H., Stunkard, A.J., Wilson, G.T., Wing, R.R., Hill, D.R.: Long-term maintenance of weight loss: current status. Health Psychology: Official Journal of the Division of Health Psychology, American Psychological Association 19(suppl. 1), 5–16 (2000)

9. Jeffery, R.W., Kelly, K.M., Rothman, A.J., Sherwood, N.E., Boutelle, K.N.: The weight loss experience: a descriptive analysis. Annals of Behavioral Medicine: a Publication of the Society of Behavioral Medicine 27(2), 100–106 (2004)

10. Kelders, S.M., Kok, R.N., Ossebaard, H.C., Van Gemert-Pijnen, J.E.: Persuasive System Design Does Matter: a Systematic Review of Adherence to Web-based Interventions. Journal of Medical Internet Research 14(6), e152 (2012)

11. Kumanyika, S.K., Obarzanek, E., Stettler, N., Bell, R., Field, A.E., Fortmann, S.P.: American Heart Association Council on Epidemiology and Prevention, Interdisciplinary Committee for Prevention. Population-Based Prevention of Obesity: the Need for Comprehensive Promotion of Healthful Eating, Physical Activity, and Energy Balance: a Scientific Statement from American Heart Association Council on Epidemiology and Prevention, Interdisciplinary Committee for Prevention (Formerly the Expert Panel on Population and Prevention Science). Circulation 118(4), 428–464 (2008)

12. Laplante, C., Peng, W.: A systematic review of e-health interventions for physical activity: an analysis of study design, intervention characteristics, and outcomes. Telemedicine Journal and E-Health: The Official Journal of the American Telemedicine Association 17(7), 509–523 (2011)

13. Morrison, L.G., Yardley, L., Powell, J., Michie, S.: What design features are used in effective e-health interventions? A review using techniques from Critical Interpretive Synthesis. Telemedicine Journal and E-Health: The Official Journal of the American Telemedicine Association 18(2), 137–144 (2012)

14. Must, A., Spadano, J., Coakley, E.H., Field, A.E., Colditz, G., Dietz, W.H.: The disease burden associated with overweight and obesity. JAMA: The Journal of the American Medical Association 282(16), 1523–1529 (1999)

15. NHLBI Obesity Education Initiative Expert Panel on the Identification, Evaluation, and Treatment of Obesity in Adults (US). In: Clinical Guidelines on the Identification, Evaluation, and Treatment of Overweight and Obesity in Adults: The Evidence Report, National Heart, Lung, and Blood Institute, Bethesda, MD (September 1998), http://www.ncbi.nlm.nih.gov/books/NBK2003/

16. Oinas-Kukkonen, H., Harjumaa, M.: Persuasive Systems Design: Key Issues, Process Model, and System Features. Communications of the Association for Information Systems 24(1) (2009)
17. Purpura, S., Schwanda, V., Williams, K., Stubler, W., Sengers, P.: Fit4Life: The Design of a Persuasive Technology Promoting Healthy Behavior and Ideal Weight. In: Proceedings of the SIGCHI Conference on Human Factors in Computing Systems, pp. 423–432. ACM, New York (2011)
18. Sarwer, D.B., von Sydow Green, A., Vetter, M.L., Wadden, T.A.: Behavior therapy for obesity: where are we now? Current Opinion in Endocrinology, Diabetes, and Obesity 16(5), 347–352 (2009)
19. Shaw, K., O'Rourke, P., Del Mar, C., Kenardy, J.: Psychological interventions for overweight or obesity. The Cochrane Database of Systematic Reviews (2), CD003818 (2005)
20. Sherwood, N.E., Crain, A.L., Martinson, B.C., Anderson, C.P., Hayes, M.G., Anderson, J.D., Jeffery, R.W.: Enhancing long-term weight loss maintenance: 2 year results from the Keep It Off randomized controlled trial. Preventive Medicine 56(3-4), 171–177 (2013)
21. Sturm, R.: The effects of obesity, smoking, and drinking on medical problems and costs. Health Affairs (Project Hope) 21(2), 245–253 (2002)
22. Torning, K., Oinas-Kukkonen, H.: Persuasive System Design: State of the Art and Future Directions. In: Proceedings of the 4th International Conference on Persuasive Technology, pp. 30:1–30:8. ACM, New York (2009)
23. Wadden, T.A., Foster, G.D.: Behavioral treatment of obesity. The Medical Clinics of North America 84(2), 441–461, vii (2000)

Stop Clicking on "Update Later": Persuading Users They Need Up-to-Date Antivirus Protection

Leah Zhang-Kennedy, Sonia Chiasson, and Robert Biddle

Carleton University, Ottawa, Canada
{leah.zhang,robert_biddle}@carleton.ca, chiasson@scs.carleton.ca

Abstract. Online security advice aims to persuade users to behave securely, but appears to have limited effects at changing behaviour. We propose security advice targeted at end-users should employ visual rhetoric to form an effective, memorable, and persuasive method of communication. We present the design and evaluation of infographics and an online interactive comic developed to persuade users to update their antivirus software. Results show superior learning and behavioural outcomes compared to mainstream text-only security advice.

Keywords: Antivirus, Persuasive Visualization, Usable Security.

1 Introduction

While automated detection systems should be used as the first line of defence against security threats, user education offers a complementary approach to secure computer systems. Online security advice is common and abundant, but typically has little persuasiveness to change behaviour. Persuasive strategies embedded in authentication mechanisms were found to be effective at motivating users to create stronger passwords [11], but little research has investigated whether theories in Persuasive Technology (PT) could be successfully applied to instructional interventions in security.

In this paper, we show that security advice is more persuasive (both perceived and actual) for end-users if it employs visual rhetorical devices that aid in mental model building of secure behaviour. A *mental model* is users' simplified internal concept of how something works in reality [6], and is used in decision making and problem solving. We present the design strategies and prototypes composed of infographics and an online interactive comic that motivate the correct use of antivirus protection. First, we frame the problem in context of computer security and explain how PT strategies in the design can be used to address the challenges. Secondly, we report our user studies that assess the perceived persuasiveness of our prototypes, and the actual persuasiveness at changing users' antivirus management behaviour after one week. Results show that our prototypes provide superior learning outcomes than mainstream text-only security advice. Participants showed high retention, recounted an enjoyable learning experience, and self-reported changes in antivirus management behaviour.

A. Spagnolli et al. (Eds.): PERSUASIVE 2014, LNCS 8462, pp. 302–322, 2014.

2 Challenges of Motivating Antivirus Protection

Fogg's *Functional Triad* identifies *media* as one way that PT can operate to change behaviour [9] — to persuade people by allowing them to explore cause-and-effect relationships, or to provide them with vicarious experiences that motivate or help people to rehearse a behaviour. Work in usable security to address phishing threats (e.g., [14]), privacy policies (e.g., [13]), and data leaks on smartphones (e.g., [2]) has exemplified that media can have positive effects on motivating secure behaviour. Other work successfully applied PT theory in authentication systems to persuade users to create stronger passwords (e.g., [4,11]). The only theoretical exploration of comics in computer security is Security Cartoon [20] that uses short comic strips to explain various security risks. The main theoretical findings suggest that presenting serious topics like computer security as a comic could help users to overcome the "intimidation factor" associated with learning. However, the work does not explore the potential interactive components of web comics, which may help to enhance learning and engagement.

We focus our discussion on the effective use of media to persuade users to maintain an up-to date antivirus software. Antivirus (also known as "AV") prevents, detects, and removes malicious software programs (i.e., malware). *Signature-based* antivirus software scans the contents of the program against a library of known virus signatures, and is effective against existing viruses that are contained in the antivirus database. *Heuristic-based* antivirus software examines programs based on a set of guidelines and rules identifying suspicious behaviour and characteristics. This method of detection is effective against variants of known viruses, and may also detect some *zero-day* viruses[1].

Although PT theory is generalizable in many domains, some unique challenges in computer security require special consideration [11]. We define the main challenges and frame them in terms of antivirus protection:

1) Security is a secondary task [23] that users may choose to bypass if it impedes the completion of a more relevant primary task: Running regular updates and renewing antivirus software subscriptions is a preventative measure that may not directly relate to any specific threat. Most antivirus software checks for updates automatically and sends users reminders, but installing updates, renewing the software, and payment may still require users' attention. Unfortunately, users may ignore prompts and reminders to updates.

2) Security systems are often too complex and abstract for end-users to form proper mental models and use accurately [5]: Most antivirus software automates the virus detection process "behind the scenes" without user interaction. Although automated systems can unburden users from making security decisions, such systems lack vigilant human oversight and therefore cannot handle exceptions and novel patterns. When automation fails, users may be left unprepared to analyze available information, find causality, and take actions to enable system recovery.

---

[1] Unknown malware for which specific antivirus signatures are not yet available.

3   Visual Rhetoric as a Facilitator for Learning

To address the challenges, we aim to use PT as media to persuade users to maintain an up-to-date antivirus software. Specifically, we employ visual rhetoric [18] in security information to construct arguments. Visual rhetoric can be thought of as the analysis of graphical devices using traditional vocabulary from rhetorical theory, such as pathos, logos, and ethos. The construction of images in advertising to make a point or argument is a example of visual rhetoric in practice.

The use of visual rhetoric could work in three ways: 1) foster good mental models; 2) construct arguments to persuade the need for security; 3) overcome the "intimidation factor" associated with security learning. The first two strategies correspond to the traditional mode of Greek rhetoric, logos, and the third strategy to pathos. Images appeal to the users' emotions and help to give reason to our argument of *why* they should follow the advice.

Fogg's behaviour model (FBM) emphasizes that motivation alone may not get people to perform a behaviour if they do not have the ability [10]. When users are unaware or have incomplete mental models of security threats, they may underestimate the risks involved. Furthermore, if security information appears overly technical, time consuming, or uninteresting, users may have low motivation to learn. The FBM model implies that making a behaviour easy to do may be a viable approach to increase behaviour performance [10].

We argue that learning from infographics and interactive comics are relatively easier than other alternatives due to their graphical nature. Infographics are visual representations of information, data, or knowledge [19]. Comics are a form of "sequential art" [8] that use a series of images and text to tell a story. Webcomics with interactivity are capable of persuading users through visual and *procedural rhetoric* [3] by incorporating interactive elements. The media acts as a "facilitator" [10] to signal users that learning about security is easy. Furthermore, infographics and interactive comics have low production costs, and are quicker to produce than film, animation, or games. These characteristics are important as new materials need to be produced rapidly to meet evolving security threats.

4   Prototype Design

The design of our prototypes was guided by the 5-phase ADDIE (Analyze, Design, Develop, Implement, and Evaluate) instructional design model [12]. The *analysis* phase consists of gathering and consolidating information. The *design* phase identifies a "blueprint" of activities and materials required. In the *development* phase, the content and the design are assembled and iterated. Next, the *implementation* phase ensures all material is fully functional before it is revealed to audience. Since ADDIE is an iterative process, evaluation is involved at every stage and may be formal (e.g., pilot study) or informal (e.g., feedback). A final *evaluation* is involved after the *implementation* phase to monitor learning outcomes after a particular time has passed.

Infographic Design: We created two infographics. In the *analysis* phase of the ADDIE process, we reviewed popular online antivirus protection resources as well as antivirus and risk communication literature in computer security. We chose to provide users with practical actionable advice on how to stay safe — explaining the basics of how antivirus software works, why regular updates are necessary, and common myths surrounding malware protection. We selected two metaphors from well-known concepts in security literature, *Surveillance* and *Medical*, to help users build mental models of antivirus protection. *Surveillance* is inspired by physical security metaphors (e.g., [17]), and *Medical* is inspired by biological models used to predict computer virus outbreaks (e.g., [16]). We iterated the two concepts during the *design* and *development* phase and presented sketches to members of our lab for feedback. Each concept was implemented as a infographic (see Figure 1A and 1B) to test its effectiveness against existing text-only advice with no visuals and metaphors. Evaluating two different infographics help to ensure that our findings are not specific to one design. We provided identical textual information on both infographics, first describing how antivirus software works, followed by a tips and myths section.

Comic Design: We expanded the conceptual models included in the infographic designs and explored Fogg's definition of media as interactive technologies that can use both interactivity and narrative to create persuasive experiences that support rehearsing a behaviour or exploring casual relationships [9]. We designed and developed a 10-page online interactive comic that showcases these characteristics. The full comic is available online at [22].

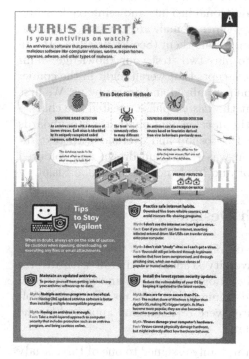
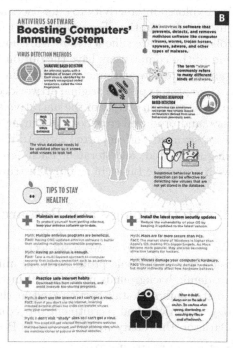

Fig. 1. Infographic prototypes. A) Surveillance. B) Medical.

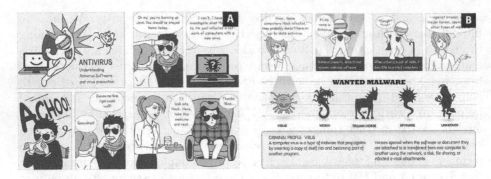

Fig. 2. Individual panels from the comic. A) pg 2 of 10. B) pg 3 of 10.

The characters *Jack* and *Nina* are agents of computer security. They solve computer security crimes and protect users against *Hack*, whose mysterious demeanour is symbolic of all computer security crimes. Jack and Nina take on the role of mentors who teach users about antivirus protection. Conceptually, we extended the medical theme that was found to be successful in the infographic study (discussed in section 6). For example, we subtly allude to the medical theme at the start of the comic, when agent Jack catches a cold, while Hack infects a network of computers with a computer virus (See Figure 2A). The medical concept was used repetitively throughout the comic to strengthen the message. We explored interactivity to offer users additional insights and reinforce learning through exploration. For example, in the "types of malware" section, users can rollover malware silhouettes to learn more about them (See Figure 2B). At the end of the comic, users have the option to play two "test your knowledge" mini games to review and practice important concepts that were taught in the comic.

The prototypes use original artwork conceptualized and drawn by us. We first created written scripts of the narrative at the *design* phase, created the characters, and produced storyboards. During the *development* phase, the storyboards were scanned and imported into Adobe Photoshop and overlaid with text dialogues, tested, and iterated. Each screen was then hand drawn and coloured with a graphic tablet in Adobe Illustrator and implemented in Adobe Flash.

5   Methodology and Research Design

We conducted two between-subject, one-on-one user studies to evaluate the infographic and comic prototypes. 40 university students and staff with diverse academic backgrounds participated in the infographic study, and an additional 16 students and staff participated in the comic study. The research methodology, materials, and recruitment procedures were reviewed and approved by the Carleton University Research Ethics Board.

Infographic Study: Participants were randomly assigned to one of three study conditions: *"Surveillance"* infographic ($n = 15$), *"Medical"* infographic ($n = 15$), and a text-only condition that we will refer to as *"Text"* ($n = 10$). Due to random-ized assignment, the participants' self-reported experiences with antivirus soft-ware were skewed between conditions. Mean self-ratings on a 6 point scale (1 - novice, 6 - expert) were 3.4 for *Surveillance*, 2.7 for *Medical*, and 2 for *Text*. Each infographic was presented on a 20 by 30 inch poster, and the text condition was presented on a letter size printout in 12pt font. We searched for the best writ-ten publicly available online advice, and determined that the most relevant con-tent came from Wikipedia [24], Logical PC Solutions [15] and a security blog [21]. The material was assembled to correspond to the written content of our infograph-ics. We kept all basic text formatting such as headings, indents, and paragraphs to maintain good readability.

Comic Study: After the infographic results were analyzed, we designed a in-teractive comic and conducted a second study. The infographic study provided valuable insights on the types of content and stimulus that should be included in the interactive comic. The purpose of the second study is to investigate whether our comic with a richer interactive user experience helps to further enhance the learning process and effect positive behavioural change. The static infograph-ics were quick to read and provided helpful actionable advice, while the comic uses persuasive technology that incorporates interactivity, a narrative, and mini-games. During the study, participants viewed the comic as a .swf file on a Mac-intosh laptop computer. The average self-rating participants gave on a scale of 1 to 6 (1 - novice, 6 - expert) for prior experience with antivirus software was 2.

Study Instruments: In both studies, participants first completed a *demo-graphic questionnaire*, then a *pretest questionnaire* for evaluating current knowl-edge and behaviour. To elicit more detailed responses, we conducted a interview for the comic study, where we inquired about antivirus management, malware, and how antivirus software works. Next, participants viewed the prototype. Av-erage viewing times were 2 minutes per infographic, 4 minutes for *text*, and between 5 to 8 minutes for the comic. Afterwards, participants were asked to openly comment on their experience and to point out any difficulties they had with the prototype. To elicit further feedback, participants completed a *proto-type evaluation questionnaire* based on Likert scales for measuring the perceived effectiveness and usefulness of the prototypes. In classical models of attitude change, messages are presented, received, processed, and if successful, users' at-titudes shift towards the advocated position [7]. However, the measurement of behavioural intentions is not always a good predictor of behaviour [1]. To mini-mize this intention-behaviour gap, we distributed a *follow-up questionnaire* one week later to assess information retention, and conducted a follow-up interview for the comic study, where participants self-reported the behavioural changes.

We used non-parametric Kruskal-Wallis and Mann-Whitney U significance tests to analyze participants' Likert scale evaluations. McNemar significance tests were used to assess whether knowledge about the antivirus protection significantly changed before and one week after the experiment. In all cases, $p < 0.05$ is considered significant. In the results, all Likert-scale data is pre-sented positively for readability, with 6 = most positive and 1 = least positive.

6   Infographic Study Results

Information Retention: In the *pretest questionnaire*, 40 participants described how antivirus software works to detect malware. The goal was not to test participants' ability to describe technical aspects of detection methods, but to identify their basic mental model of the detection process. We tabulated number of correct responses. Random assignment of participants to conditions led to a varied distribution of correct responses across conditions. 60% (9/15 participants) of correct responses were received for *Surveillance*, 7% (1/15 participants) for *Medical*, and 30% (3/10 participants) for *Text*. The same question was asked verbatim one week later in the *follow-up questionnaire*, where we received 38 completed questionnaires. We tabulated correct responses, then compared these to the *pretest questionnaire*, which was completed prior to viewing the educational materials (Figure 3 summarizes the results). McNemar significance tests were used to analyze the number of correct responses between the two questionnaires. Statistically, there was a significant increase in knowledge for the *Medical* condition ($\chi 2(1) = 1.224, p = 0.031$), but not for *Surveillance* or *Text*.

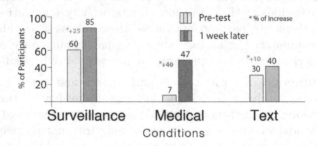

Fig. 3. Participants' ability to describe how antivirus software works before and one week after viewing the infographics and text material

Perceived Effectiveness of the Media: In the *prototype evaluation questionnaire*, participants evaluated the perceived effectiveness of the media based on their experience with the prototype. Our results suggest that communicating security risks through infographics is perceived to be more effective than conveying the information through plain text. *Surveillance* (mean 4.8) and *Medical* (mean 5.3) infographics received higher Likert ratings than the *Text* condition (mean 3.3). Figure 4 (left) shows a Box and Whisker plot[2] that summarize participants' ratings. A Kruskal-Wallis test showed a statistically significant difference between perceived effectiveness of the three conditions ($H(3) = 17.85$ with $p < 0.001$). To determine where the differences lay, Mann-Whitney tests with a Bonferroni corrected p-value of ($p < 0.05/2 = 0.025$) was used. Participants perceived both infographics to be more effective than the *Text*

---

[2] Middle line is the median, whiskers represent the 1*st* and 4*th* quartiles. Outliers are plotted as individual points.

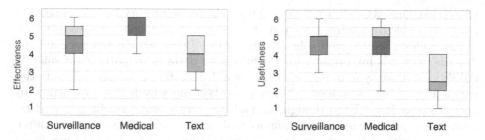

Fig. 4. Likert scale responses assessing the *effectiveness of the prototype at conveying information* (left) and *usefulness of the presented information* (right)

condition: ($U = 18, p = 0.001, r = -0.648$) between *Surveillance* and *Text*, and ($U = 6.5, p < 0.001, r = -0.783$) between *Medical* and *Text*.

There is no statistical difference between *Surveillance* and *Medical* infographics. However, participants' feedback indicate that the medical concept is the most intuitive to understand. One participant noted, "everybody understands how germs and viruses can affect the human body, so they can make meaningful comparisons with how computer viruses work." Another said, "comparing the computer with the human body is vivid and makes it easy to consider the importance of protecting our computer from viruses." Participants said that the bugs in the *Surveillance* infographic are recognizable imagery for viruses, and the surveillance camera is a well understood concept of physical security, but bugs seem "less threatening" than burglars in context of a "home invasion."

Perceived Usefulness of Knowledge Gained: When comparing participants' responses for usefulness of the information (see Figure 4, right), we found a significant difference: $H(3) = 10.394$ with $p < 0.004$. Mann-Whitney tests show a statistical significance between *Surveillance* and *Text* ($U = 27, p = 0.013$, $r = -0.503$), and *Medical* and *Text* ($U = 20, p = 0.001, r = -0.627$), but not between *Surveillance* and *Medical*. This suggests that participants perceived the information shown on both infographics to be more useful than the information shown in the *Text* condition.

Participants' feedback indicates that users would be more likely to remember the main take-away message from the infographics, which is to keep their antivirus up-to-date, even if they could not remember the textual details. A participant said, "graphics would get more attention and draw more people in. It is also easier to commit to memory when there are graphical parallels you can draw upon." Another said, "I definitely think it would be a lot more interesting to read, which would subsequently make the information more memorable. Text can be very daunting to read, so a more visually interesting method of display with pictures and colours would be a lot more useful."

7   Antivirus Comic Results

Information Retention: The *pretest questionnaire* showed that most users do not keep an updated antivirus, and highlighted misconceptions about malware protection. One-week after interacting with the comic prototype, 88% of participants were able to describe how antivirus software works, compared to just 13% in the *pretest* (See Figure 6). In addition, 81% of the participants were able to describe why it is important to perform regular updates. A participant said, "I didn't know that by updating it's actually able to catch more things," and "the comic allowed me to understand how it worked and why is it so important to keep it up to date." Even though the malware terms sound familiar to participants in the *pretest questionnaire*, many could not describe them. One week after interacting with the comic, most participants were able to distinguish various types of malware. 6 participants used scenes from the comic to describe how antivirus software works, such as describing virus signatures as "DNA sequences", and referring to hackers as the "villains." This suggests that visual narratives of Hack helped to emphasize hackers' malicious intentions. Participants found the interactive elements in the comic useful to reinforce concepts learned.

Behavioural Outcomes: In the follow-up interview, participants self-reported positive behavioural changes one week later. Table 1 provides a summary of the results. 31% of participants performed updates during the week. One participant explained, "I updated Avira after our first meeting. I thought I might as well just go and do it, it's not going to be that hard, and I suppose it probably made me more cautious of things that could infect my computer." Another said, "It made me realize that I need to be more aware. You know I went back to my computer and looked at my antivirus software that I had (at work) and went home and looked at my antivirus and made sure that it was up to date."

38% of participants said that learning about malware had made them more cautious when web surfing and/or downloading files. Another 19% said they became more aware of reading the contents of security warnings before performing an action. An encouraging result is that 69% of participants shared the information they learned with family and friends within a week. A participant said "I was explaining it to my parents, especially my dad who has a whole bunch of antivirus on the computer so it made it really slow. So I was trying to explain to him that he doesn't need that many antivirus, he only needs one."

Perceived Effectiveness of the Media: Results from the *prototype evaluation questionnaire* (Figure 5) show that the comic was perceived to be effective. Feedback indicates that the comic was easy to understand, and may be suitable for an audience of all ages. Participants reported a pleasurable user experience, and described the comic as "fun", "cute," and "pleasant". Several participants

Table 1. Antivirus comic: effect of learning on user behaviour

Effects of Learning	# of Participants
Shared knowledge	8 (69%)
More cautious when browsing and downloading	6 (38%)
Updated antivirus within one week	5 (33%)
More conscious of security warnings	3 (19%)
No effect	2 (13%)

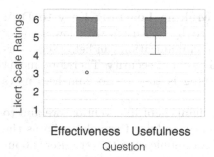

Fig. 5. Likert scale responses for the *effectiveness* and *usefulness* of the comic

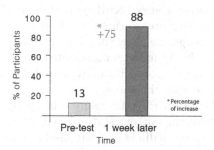

Fig. 6. Participants' ability to describe how antivirus works before and after viewing the comic

wanted to share the information with family and friends. The visual content and interactivity kept users entertained while they learned useful information. A participant said, "If I came across security information and it takes me 30 minutes to read, I probably wouldn't read it. This was quick and easy." Others commented that the characters in the comic made the topic more relatable.

Perceived Usefulness of Knowledge Gained: Results from the *prototype evaluation questionnaire* (see Figure 5) suggest that participants perceived the information taught to them to be highly useful. Feedback indicates that the comic was most useful at clarifying common "myths" surrounding malware and antivirus software. The interactive elements and mini-games were useful to reinforce the information learned.

8   Discussion and Conclusion

In this paper, we show how PT can be used as media to persuade users to update antivirus software. We designed and formally evaluated infographics and a interactive comic that use visual rhetoric to construct arguments. We argue that the strategies proposed in this paper can help to improve computer security understanding, and provide an efficient method for end-user communication of many types of technical information. To summarize, our strategies were:

Use Visual Rhetoric to Construct Arguments: Educating users about how security works may increase motivation to practice secure behaviour because it helps to justify the need. For example, our studies show that learning about antivirus detection methods may motivate users to perform updates because they gained knowledge about *why* regular updates are necessary. Visuals also help to illustrate abstract concepts concretely, thus aid in comprehension.

Build Mental Models of Security Risks: Helping users build mental models of security risks is an important step towards developing long-term motivation and ability. Since not all security threats will occur in the same way each time (e.g., phishing emails), users with a robust mental model would be able to adapt to changing threats and make security conscious decisions.

Increase Users' Ability to Learn (By Making Learning Easy to Do):
Since computer security is often administered by end-users with low security
knowledge, we show that visual methods of communication can help users overcome the intimidation associated with learning about security. Therefore, media
may act as a facilitator to signal that learning is easy to do, and help users
engage with the content.

Although PT offer many other potential channels of intervention, we aim to
address the current state of mainstream security advice through media as the
first step. Media is a widely used channel of communication to warn users about
evolving security threats. We believe a more receptive approach than text-based
security information is to increase the persuasiveness of the message through visual rhetoric, improve users' mental models of security, and to make the learning
process easy to do. The infographics quickly helped users build mental models
of how antivirus software works through metaphors and visually illustrating the
threat of malware. The interactive comic took this one step further to enable
procedural rhetoric through the use of narrative and interactivity to highlight
cause and effect relationships. Results show superior perceived effectiveness and
usefulness of the prototypes over mainstream text-based information, particularly for participants with low security experience. The pretest and follow-up
results confirmed improvements in knowledge and behaviour after one week.

Our future work will address a few limitations, including context, scalabil-
ity, the distribution of participants across conditions, and the control condition.
First, a longitudinal study outside of the lab setting could possibly measure
the prototypes' influences on behaviour over longer time periods and in various learning environments. Second, although we used randomization to assign
participants to a condition to balance the groups, chance distribution of experienced versus inexperienced participants resulted an imbalance between groups
in the infographic study. Third, we carefully adapted mainstream text information from well written online resources as the control condition, but text from
different resources may have varying degrees of effectiveness.

We have successfully extended our proposed strategies to other security topics like password guessing attacks, and are currently working on prototypes for
motivating online privacy. The research resulted in high quality educational materials fully accessible to the general public online [22]. We are actively pursuing
deployment of the material at national and international venues.

Acknowledgements. This project has been funded by the Office of the Privacy Commissioner of Canada (OPC); the views expressed herein are those of
the authors and do not necessarily reflect those of the OPC. S. Chiasson acknowl-
edges funding from NSERC for her Canada Research Chair in Human Oriented
Computer Security.

References

1. Armitage, C.J., Conner, M.: Efficacy of the theory of planned behaviour:
   A meta-analytic review. British Journal of Social Psychology 40(4), 471–499
   (2001)

2. Balebako, R., Jung, J., Lu, W., Cranor, L.F., Nguyen, C.: Little brothers watching you: Raising awareness of data leaks on smartphones. In: Symposium on Usable Privacy and Security (2013)
3. Bogost, I.: Persuasive games: The expressive power of videogames. MIT Press (2007)
4. Chiasson, S., Forget, A., Biddle, R., van Oorschot, P.C.: Influencing users towards better passwords: Persuasive Cued Click-Points. In: British HCI, pp. 121–130. British Computer Society (2008)
5. Chiasson, S., van Oorschot, P.C., Biddle, R.: A usability study and critique of two password managers. In: USENIX Security Symposium (2006)
6. Craik, K., James, W.: The nature of explanation. Cambridge Univ. Press (1967)
7. Crano, W.D., Prislin, R.: Attitudes and persuasion. Annual Review of Psychology 57, 345–374 (2006)
8. Eisner, W.: Comics & Sequential Art. Poorhouse Press, Tamarac (1985)
9. Fogg, B.J.: Persuasive Technology: Using Computers to Change What We Think and Do. Morgan Kaufmann, San Francisco (2003)
10. Fogg, B.J.: A behavior model for persuasive design. In: Persuasive Technology, p. 40. ACM (2009)
11. Forget, A., Chiasson, S., van Oorschot, P.C., Biddle, R.: Persuasion for stronger passwords: Motivation and pilot study. In: Oinas-Kukkonen, H., Hasle, P., Harjumaa, M., Segerståhl, K., Øhrstrøm, P. (eds.) PERSUASIVE 2008. LNCS, vol. 5033, pp. 140–150. Springer, Heidelberg (2008)
12. Gustafson, K.L., Branch, R.M.: What is instructional design? In: Trends and Issues in Instructional Design and Technology, pp. 16–25 (2002)
13. Kelley, P.G., Bresee, J., Cranor, L.F., Reeder, R.W.: A nutrition label for privacy. In: Symposium on Usable Privacy and Security. ACM (2009)
14. Kumaraguru, P., Sheng, S., Acquisti, A., Cranor, L.F., Hong, J.: Teaching Johnny not to fall for phish. ACM Transactions on Internet Technology 10(2), 7 (2010)
15. Logical PC Solutions. 5 Popular Computer Virus Misconceptions, http://www.logicalpcs.com/2012/03/07/5-popular-computer-virus-misconceptions/ (accessed June 2013)
16. Pastor-Satorras, R., Vespignani, A.: Epidemic spreading in scale-free networks. Physical Review Letters 86(14), 3200 (2001)
17. Raja, F., Hawkey, K., Hsu, S., Wang, K.L.C., Beznosov, K.: A brick wall, a locked door, and a bandit: a physical security metaphor for firewall warnings. In: Symposium on Usable Privacy and Security. ACM (2011)
18. Scott, L.M.: Images in advertising: The need for a theory of visual rhetoric. Journal of Consumer Research, 252–273 (1994)
19. Smiciklas, M.: The power of infographics: Using pictures to communicate and connect with your audiences. Que Publishing (2012)
20. Srikwan, S., Jakobsson, M.: Using cartoons to teach internet security. Cryptologia 32(2), 137–154 (2008)
21. Tembhurne, R.: 15 Myths and Misconceptions about Viruses and Security Applications (2013), http://rakesh.tembhurne.com/15-myths-and-misconceptions-about-viruses-and-security-applications/ (accessed June 2013)
22. Versipass. Secure Comics, http://www.versipass.com/edusec
23. Whitten, A., Tygar, J.D.: Why Johnny Can't Encrypt: A Usability Evaluation of PGP 5.0. In: USENIX Security Symposium (1999)
24. Wikipedia. Antivirus Software, https://en.wikipedia.org/wiki/Antivirus_software (accessed June 2013)

Appendix: User Study Materials

Demographic Questionnaire

This information will be held completely confidential. **(Please, do not put your name on this form!)**

Age: _____

Gender: ☐ Male   ☐ Female

At what level are you studying?
☐ Undergraduate   ☐ Masters   ☐ Ph.D.   ☐ Other_____

What year of study are you in? _____

In what academic program are you enrolled?
_____
_____

Have you encountered any educational material about antivirus software before this study? If so, please describe the material.
☐ Yes   ☐ No
_____

Have you ever been in a user study before? If so, please describe the study.
☐ Yes   ☐ No
_____

Pretest Questionnaire

How would you rate your knowledge of how antivirus software works?
Novice   1   2   3   4   5   6   Expert

For each of the computers you use, please indicate the operating system
Computer 1 _____
Computer 2 _____
Computer 3 _____
Computer 4 _____
Computer 5 _____

For each computer listed above, which antivirus is currently installed in your computer?
      Norton
      TrendMicro
      Panda
      Nod32
      Avast!
      OneCare
      McAfee
      Bitdefender
      AVG
      Kaspersky
      F-secure
      Avira
      Other _____
      I don't know
      I don't have an antivirus

Are you currently paying for your antivirus?
      Yes
      No
      I have both paid and free antivirus
      I don't know
      I don't have an antivirus

When was the last time you renewed an antivirus software license/subscription?
      I just renewed
      Last year
      Two years ago
      Three years ago
      Never
      I don't know
      I don't have an antivirus

How often do you update your current antivirus software?
      Daily
      Weekly
      Bi-weekly
      Monthly
      Every six months
      Once a year
      My antivirus automatically updates
      Never
      I don't have an antivirus

How concerned are you with regards to the security of your computer?
☐ Not at all concerned

☐ Not very concerned
☐ Somewhat concerned
☐ Very concerned

I feel antivirus software is too complicated to use
☐ Not at all complicated
☐ Not very complicated
☐ Somewhat complicated
☐ Very complicated

Please rank each operating system based on how secure you think they are. Place "1" beside the OS that you think is the most secure, 2 for the less secure, and 3 for the least secure.
__Macs
__Windows
__Linux

True or false:

Viruses can damage your computer's hardware.
T
F

Running multiple Anti-virus programs on the same computer is beneficial.
T
F

Having an Anti-virus is enough to be secure.
T
F

I can't get a virus if I'm not connected to the Internet.
T
F

I can't get a virus if I don't download anything.
T
F

I can't get a virus if I don't visit "shady" sites, such as porn, gambling, or file sharing websites.
T
F

Macs are far more secure than Windows.
T
F

Do you consider yourself a visual learner?
☐ Yes   ☐ No

In your own words, describe what the following terms mean. Even if you are unsure, write down your best guesses.

What is a computer "virus"? _____

What is a "trojan"? _____

What is a computer "worm"? _____

What is "spyware"? _____

What is "adware"? _____

Please list and describe the ways people can get viruses?

_____

Can you describe how antivirus works to protect your computer? Such as the ways an antivirus can detect viruses?

_____

Prototype Evaluation Questionnaire

Please answer the following questions for the visualization you have examined:

Based on your experience, teaching about antivirus and virus prevention visually is an effective method to communicate about this topic.
Teaching visually is **not effective**   1   2   3   4   5   6   Teaching visually is **very effective**

Presenting the topic in a graphical way has made the information more pleasurable to read.
Not pleasant   1   2   3   4   5   6   Very pleasant

I have gained useful knowledge about <u>antivirus software</u>.
Gained no useful knowledge   1   2   3   4   5   6   Gained a lot of useful knowledge

I have gained useful knowledge about <u>virus prevention</u>.
Gained no useful knowledge   1   2   3   4   5   6   Gained a lot of useful knowledge

The visualization has improved my understanding of how antivirus works.
Did not improve my understanding   1   2   3   4   5   6   Strongly improved my understanding

The information was <u>difficult</u> to understand.
Not at all difficult   1   2   3   4   5   6   Very difficult

The graphics used to portray the topic was <u>confusing</u>.
Not at all confusing   1   2   3   4   5   6   Very confusing

I prefer to learn information from a plain text document instead.
Strongly dislike learning from plain text   1   2   3   4   5   6   Strongly prefer learning from plain text

I will most likely remember what I have learned weeks later.
I won't remember   1   2   3   4   5   6   I will most likely remember

The visualization has convinced me to maintain an up-to-date antivirus.
Not at all convincing   1   2   3   4   5   6   Very convincing

The visualization has taught me useful tips on how to stay safe.
Not at all useful   1   2   3   4   5   6   Very useful

After learning about the topic, I believe I'm already doing all that I can with regards to computer security.
I'm not doing enough   1   2   3   4   5   6   I'm doing everything I can

I would spend time reading this visualization if I came across it elsewhere.
I wouldn't read it at all   1   2   3   4   5   6   I would read all of the visualization

I would recommend this visualization to other people.
Would not recommend   1   2   3   4   5   6   Strongly recommend

I would share the information I learned with other people.
Would not share it   1   2   3   4   5   6   Definitely share it

Did the metaphor help you to understand how computer viruses and antivirus work?
Not at all helpful   1   2   3   4   5   6   Very helpful

Please provide your feedback regarding the information provided (i.e. Was the information useful? Is there other additional information you would like to see?)
_____

Please provide your feedback regarding the graphics provided (i.e., Is it appealing? Is it appropriate for the topic? Did it help to enhance your understanding of the topic?)
_____

How would you interact with this information in a public setting, such as on a wall in a hallway, or perhaps at a bus or train station? (i.e., Would you read it? How long would you spend reading it?)
_____

Follow-up Questionnaire

The following questions give you hypothetical scenarios. Describe what you would do in response to each situation. Please be as specific as possible:

Scenario A: You received an email from your bank in your primary email inbox. The subject line states "Your requested document". You opened the email and everything looks legitimate. The email contains your banks' logo and looks professional. The email explained that they are sending you a confidential document that you have requested online. You have recently logged in to your online bank account. The document is attached to the email reads "Customer_102554009.DOC.exe". How would you proceed?

_____

Scenario B: You found a USB key left on a desk in a conference room. You feel you should return it to the owner, but you are unsure whom the USB key belonged to. You decided to take a look at the contents to see if it can give you hint of who the owner is. How would you proceed?

_____

Scenario C: You received an email from a good friend of yours. The subject line says, "A cool video I found". You opened the mail and it reads, "Hey, I found this thought you might like it. ☺" Below the message there is a link to the video. How would you proceed?

_____

Can you describe how antivirus works to protect your computer? Such as the ways an antivirus can detect viruses?

_____

True or false: (Repeated questions from the pre-test questionnaire)

Viruses can damage your computer's hardware.
T
F

Running multiple Anti-virus programs on the same computer is beneficial.
T
F

Having an Anti-virus is enough to be secure.
T
F

I can't get a virus if I'm not connected to the Internet.
T
F

I can't get a virus if I don't download anything.
T
F

I can't get a virus if I don't visit "shady" sites, such as porn, gambling, or file sharing websites.
T
F

Macs are far more secure than Windows.
T
F

Comic Study Pre-test Interview Questions

Current practice

1. What computer operating system do you use?

2. Do you currently have an antivirus installed on your computer?
If Yes...
I. What type of antivirus do you have?
II. Do you have more than one antivirus programs installed? (If yes, why do you have multiple antivirus programs?)
III. How often do you update your antivirus?
If No...
        I.   Can you give me reasons why not?

Current understanding of viruses

1. How would you define the term "virus"?

2. What is your understanding of viruses and malware? How are they similar or different?

3. Where do you think computer viruses' come from? What is their purpose?

4. Based on your understanding, can you describe how computer viruses could harm your computer?

5. Have you had previous experience with educational material regarding antivirus software? (It may include instructional manuals that came with your antivirus software)
        I. Can you describe the contents of the material?
        II. Did it help with your understanding of how your antivirus works?

Experience of getting infected

1. Have your computer ever been infected with viruses or other types of malware?
If Yes...
        I. Can you describe the experience?
        II. How did it make you feel?
        III. Did you have an antivirus installed when this happened?
        If Yes...
                I. What did you think happened?
        If No...
                I. Do you think if you had an antivirus, this could've been prevented?
                II. Did you install an antivirus software afterwards?
If No...
I. How likely do you think your computer will be infected in the future? Why?

Current knowledge of how antivirus works

1. Are you confident in your knowledge of properly configuring and using antivirus software?
If No...
        I. If you are not confident, can you describe what aspect of the software you don't understand?

2. Can you describe how antivirus software detects viruses or other types of malware?

3. What is the difference between "clean", "quarantine", and "delete"? Which option do you use most often? Why?

4. Can you describe in detail the possible ways you could get infected with a virus?

5. In a hypothetical scenario that your computer is infected, what would you do?

Comic Study Follow-up Interview Questions (One-week later)

Ability to describe viruses and antivirus

1. Based on your understanding, can you describe what are viruses and malware?

2. Can you describe in detail the possible ways you could get infected with a virus?

3. Can you describe how antivirus works? Such as the ways an antivirus can detect viruses?

4. Did the lesson alter the way you currently manage the security on your computer? This includes actions such as installing an antivirus, updating your antivirus, or improved internet surfing behaviours?

5. Did the lesson improve your awareness of the need for antivirus?

Questions about the prototype

1. Did you gain new knowledge after viewing the prototype? If so which part?

3. Which part of the information did you find the most useful?

4. Is there any anything you would like to change/add?

Author Index